Herbal Medicine: Modern Applications of Traditional Formulas

Herbal Medicine: Modern Applications of Traditional Formulas

Editor: Melissa Gould

STATES
ACADEMIC PRESS
www.statesacademicpress.com

States Academic Press,
109 South 5th Street,
Brooklyn, NY 11249, USA

Visit us on the World Wide Web at:
www.statesacademicpress.com

ISBN: 978-1-63989-268-6 (Hardback)

Cataloging-in-Publication Data

Herbal medicine : modern applications of traditional formulas / edited by Melissa Gould.
p. cm.
Includes bibliographical references and index.
ISBN 978-1-63989-268-6
1. Herbs--Therapeutic use. 2. Traditional medicine. 3. Traditional medicine--Formulae, receipts, prescriptions.
4. Medicinal plants. 5. Materia medica, Vegetable. I. Gould, Melissa.
RM666.H33 H47 2022
615.321--dc23

Table of Contents

Preface

I am honored to present to you this unique book which encompasses the most up-to-date data in the field. I was extremely pleased to get this opportunity of editing the work of experts from across the globe. I have also written papers in this field and researched the various aspects revolving around the progress of the discipline. I have tried to unify my knowledge along with that of stalwarts from every corner of the world, to produce a text which not only benefits the readers but also facilitates the growth of the field.

The study and use of medicinal plants is known as herbal medicine. Plant-derived compounds are widely used in pharmaceutical drugs. Herbal medicines are prominently used for patients suffering from chronic diseases such as asthma, diabetes, etc. Herbal teas are the most common form in which herbs are consumed. Herbal teas can be classified as infusions and decoctions. The hot water extracts of herbs are referred to as infusions. Examples of herbs used in infusions are chamomile, mint, etc. The cold infusion of high-mucilage plants is called maceration. The long-term boiled extracts of harder substances are called decoctions. Such substances include barks and roots. This book traces the progress of this field and highlights some of its key concepts and applications. While understanding the long-term perspectives of the topics, the book makes an effort in highlighting their impacts as a modern tool for the growth of the discipline. It includes contributions of experts and scientists which will provide innovative insights into this field.

Finally, I would like to thank all the contributing authors for their valuable time and contributions. This book would not have been possible without their efforts. I would also like to thank my friends and family for their constant support.

Editor

1

Formulation and evaluation of orally disintegrating tablet of Rizatriptan using natural superdisintegrant

Majid Tabbakhian[1,*], Mohammad Ali Shahtalebi[1], Ehsan Salehi[1], Mahtab Keshvari[2]

[1]Department of Pharmaceutics, School of Pharmacy and Pharmaceutical Sciences, Isfahan University of Medical Science, Isfahan, Iran
[2]Isfahan Cardiovascular Research Center, Isfahan Cardiovascular Research Institute, Isfahan University of Medical Sciences, Isfahan, Iran

ARTICLE INFO

Keywords:
Direct compression
Factorial design technique
Orally disintegrating tablets
Rizatriptan benzoate
Superdisintegrants

ABSTRACT

Introduction: Rizatriptan benzoate is a potent and selective 5-$HT_{1B/1D}$ receptor agonist and is effective for the treatment of acute migraine. Difficulty in swallowing is common among all age groups, especially elderly and pediatrics. Orally disintegrating tablets may constitute an innovative dosage form that overcome the problem of swallowing and provides a quick onset of action. This study was aimed to formulate and evaluate an Orally Disintegrating Tablet (ODT) containing Rizatriptan while using semi-synthetic and natural superdisintegrants.
Methods: Orodispersible tablets were prepared by direct compression using natural superdisntegrant (Plantago ovata mucilage) and semi-synthetic superdisntegrant (crospovidone). The prepared tablets were evaluated for hardness, friability, thickness, drug content uniformity, water absorption and wetting time. A 3^2 factorial design was used to investigate the effect of independent variables (amount of crospovidone and Plantago ovata mucilage) on dependent variables [disintegration time, wetting time and Q_5 (cumulative amount of drug release after 5 minutes)]. A counter plot was also presented to graphically represent the effect of independent variable on the disintegration time, wetting time and Q_5. The check point batch was also prepared to prove the validity of the evolved mathematical model. The systematic formulation approach helped in understanding the effect of formulation processing variable.
Results: According to the results of optimized batches, the best concentration of superdisintegrant were as follows: 9.4 mg Psyllium mucilage and 8.32 mg crospovidone gave rapid disintegration in 35sec and showed 99% drug release within 5 minutes.
Conclusion: Plantago ovata mucilage, a natural superdisintegrant, gives a rapid disintegration and high release when used with synthetic superdisntegrant in formulation of orally disintegrating tablet of Rizatriptan.

Implication for health policy/practice/research/medical education:
Plantago ovata mucilage is a natural superdisntegrant that has shown a good disintegration time and wetting effect when used with synthetic superdisntegrant in formulation of orally disintegrating tablet of Rizatriptan.

Introduction

Drug delivery through oral route is the most common and preferred route of drug administration both for solid and liquid dosage forms. However, solid dosage forms are popular because of the ease of administration, accurate dosage, self-medication, pain avoidance, and most importantly the patient compliance (1). Tablets and capsules are the most popular solid dosage forms. However, many people face difficulty in swallowing tablets and hard gelatin capsules (2). It has been found that this problem has been encountered in all groups of patient, but especially with pediatric and geriatric populations. Thus, these conventional dosage forms result in high incidence of noncompliance and ineffective therapy with respect to swallowing specially in the case of pediatric, geriatric, or any mentally retarded persons (3).

***Corresponding author**: Majid Tabbakhian, School of Pharmacy and Pharmaceutical Sciences. Isfahan University of Medical Sciences, Hezarjerib Ave. Isfahan. Iran. E-mail: tabakhian@pharm.mui.ac.ir

It offers several advantages with respect to its stability, administration without water, accurate dosing, easy manufacturing, small packaging size, and handling (4). Its ease of administration in the population especially for pediatric, geriatric, or any mentally retarded persons makes it a very popular dosage form. Due to the presence of superdisintegrants, it gets dissolved quickly, resulting in rapid absorption of drug which in turn provides rapid onset of action (5).

Rizatriptan has a high oral bioavailability of 45%. The half-life is 2 to 3 hours and the T_{max} is 1.5 hours for the conventional tablet and slightly longer for the ODT. 10 mg dose of Rizatriptan benzoate is equipotent to a 100 mg of Sumatriptan, the traditional anti migraine drug. The bioavailability of Rizatriptan benzoate is about 45% which is superior to a poor 14-17% of Sumatriptan (6,7).

In market Rizatriptan is available in freeze dried dosage form which gives rapid disintegration. Main disadvantage of this method is very costly method, process is not feasible and product is highly sensitive to moisture. Freeze drying is cumbersome and it yields a fragile and hygroscopic product (8).

In this study natural superdisintegrants were utilized. Natural superdisintegrants are safer, more biodegradable, better compressible, easier to preparation and cheaper and these advantages can boost the production of ODTs (9).

In the present study, the fast disintegrating tablets were prepared by the method of direct compression using various pharmaceutical excipients. The excipients used were avicel pH 102,

crospovidone, Plantago ovata mucilage, mannitol, aspartame, aerosil and magnesium stearate.

Materials and Methods

Rizatriptan benzoate was bought from Farabi Pharmaceutical Company. Aerosil and aspartame was obtained as gift from Isfahan University of Medical Science Lab and other ingredients were bought from market.

Preparation of orally disintegrating tablets

Orally disintegrating tablet of Rizatriptan was prepared by direct compression method. All the ingredients were passed through 60 mesh sieve separately. The Rizatriptan, crospovidone, Psyllium mucilage, avicel PH 102, mannitol and aspartame were mixed up using a mortar and pestle. The blends were lubricated with 1% magnesium stearate and 1% aerosil. The blends ready for compression were converted into tablets. Tablets were compressed at 3 mm size flat round punch to get tablet machine (ErwekaAR 4100, Germany). The compositions of experimental factorial design were shown in Table 1.

Methodology for isolation of Plantago ovata mucilage

For the isolation of mucilage, seeds of Plantago ovata were used. They were soaked in distilled water for 48 h and then boiled for 1 h for complete release of mucilage into water. The material was filtered by squeezing in a muslin cloth to remove marc. Then equal volume of acetone was added to filtrate to precipitate the mucilage. The mucilage was separated and dried in oven at a temperature less than 60°, powdered (#60 mesh), weighed and stored in desicator until further use (10).

3^2 full factorial design

Response surface methodology (RSM) was characteristically employed to relate a response variable to the levels of the input variables and to generate a design matrix to choose the optimal formulations. A statistical model, which consisted of interactive and polynomial terms, was utilized to evaluate the responses (11,12). The responses were analyzed using analysis of variance (ANOVA) and the individual response parameters were evaluated using F test and polynomial equation was generated for each response using multiple linear regression analysis.

$Y = b_0 + b_1X_1 + b_2X_2 + b_{12}X_1X_2 + b_{11}X_1^2 + b_{22}X_2^2$

Where, Y is the dependent variable, b_0 is the arithmetic mean response of the nine runs and b_1 is the estimated coefficient for the factor X_1. The main effects (X_1 and X_2) represent the average result of changing one factor at a time from its low to high value. The interaction terms (X_1 X_2) show how the response changes when two factors are simultaneously changed. The polynomial terms (X_1^2 and X_2^2) are included to investigate non-linearity. A 3^2 full factorial design was employed to study the effect of independent variables, i.e., amount of mucilage (X_1) and the amount of crospovidone (X_2) on dependent variables wetting time, disintegration time and Q_5 (cumulative amount of drug release after 5 minutes).

After application of full factorial design and with the help of produced polynomial terms, amount of two formulation variable was optimized. The optimized amount of the crospovidone and Psyllium mucilage were incorporated in the tablet which was used as the check point of the regression analysis model (Tables 1 and 2).

Evaluation of Mixed Powder Blend of Drug and Excipients

Evaluation of mixed blends of drug and excipients were carried out for all the formulations for angle of repose, bulk density, tapped density, Hausner's ratio and Carr's index.

Bulk density (D_b) and tapped density (D_t)

Both bulk density and tapped bulk density were determined. A suitable amount of powder from each formulation, previously lightly shaken to break agglomerates formed, was introduced into a 10 ml measuring cylinder. After initial volume was observed, the cylinder was allowed to fall under its own weight on to a hard surface from a height of 2.5 cm at 2 seconds intervals. The tapping was continued until no further change in volume was noted. Bulk density and tapped bulk density were calculated

Table 1. Factorial design batches

Ingredients	F_1	F_2	F_3	F_4	F_5	F_6	F_7	F_8	F_9
Rizatriptan benzoate	10	10	10	10	10	10	10	10	10
Crospovidone	3	6	9	3	6	9	3	6	9
Psyllium mucilage	6	6	6	9	9	9	12	12	12
Aerosil	1.5	1.5	1.5	1.5	1.5	1.5	1.5	1.5	1.5
Magnesium stearate	1.5	1.5	1.5	1.5	1.5	1.5	1.5	1.5	1.5
Aspartame	1.5	1.5	1.5	1.5	1.5	1.5	1.5	1.5	1.5
Avicel PH 102 up to	150	150	150	150	150	150	150	150	150

F: formulation

Table 2. Design and summary response data

Run	Independent variable in code form				Dependent variable		
	Coded form		Actual form				
	Factor A	Factor B	Psyllium mucilage (mg)	C.P (mg)	WT (S)	DT (s)	Q_5%
1	-1	-1	6	3	62	56	84
2	-1	0	6	6	59	54	93
3	-1	1	6	9	51	48	100
4	0	-1	9	3	49	45	90
5	0	0	9	6	44	41	97
6	0	1	9	9	41	37	101
7	1	-1	12	3	40	32	84
8	1	0	12	6	30	27	83
9	1	1	12	9	33	30	81

C.P: crospovidone, WT: Wetting time, DT: Disintegration time, Q_5: Drug release after 5 minutes

using following formula (13):

$$D_b = \frac{weight\ of\ the\ power}{volume\ of\ the\ packing}$$

$$D_t = \frac{weight\ of\ the\ power}{tapped\ volume\ of\ the\ packing}$$

Carr's index

The Compressibility Index of the powder blend was determined by Carr's compressibility index. It is a Simple test to evaluate the D_b and D_t of a powder and the rate at which it packed down. The formula for Carr's Index is as below:

$$Carr\ index = \frac{D_t - D_b}{D_t} \times 100$$

Where D_t is tapped density of the powder and D_b is bulk density of the powder.

Hausner's ratio

Hausner's ratio was calculated from bulk and tapped density of Rizatriptan blend powder formulation and it is expressed as:

$$Hausner's\ ratio = \frac{D_t}{D_t}$$

Where D_t is tapped density and D_b is bulk density.

Angle of repose

Angle of repose (θ) was determined using fixed funnel method. The height of the funnel was adjusted in such a way that the tip of the funnel just touched the apex of the heap of the granules. The granules were allowed to flow through the funnel freely onto the surface. The diameter of the granular cone was measured and angle of repose was calculated using the following equation:

$$\tan\theta = \frac{h}{r}$$

Where h and r are the height and radius of the cone (Table 3).

Evaluation parameters of orally disintegrating tablets

Weight variation

Randomly, 20 tablets were selected after compression and the mean weight was determined (14). None of the tablets deviated from the average weight by more than ±7.5%.

Table 3. Powder flow properties of the Rizatriptan formulations

Code	Angle of repose (θ)	Bulk density (gr/cm$^{3)}$	Tapped density (gr/cm$^{3)}$	Carr's index (I)	Hausner's ratio
F_1	31.4±0.02	0.37±0.06	0.41±0.02	10.15±1.13	1.11
F_2	31±0.03	0.32±0.07	0.35±0.02	09.10±1.01	1.10
F_3	30.6±0.02	0.34±0.04	0.37±0.02	07.94±0.35	1.08
F_4	30.1±.003	0.36±0.02	0.39±0.02	06.63±1.27	1.07
F_5	30.3±0.01	0.33±0.03	0.36±0.02	09.53±1.05	1.10
F_6	29.4±0.05	0.35±0.04	0.39±0.01	09.53±1.11	1,10
F_7	29±0.02	0.36±0.07	0.39±0.01	07.08±1.36	1.07
F_8	29.4±0.01	0.37±0.05	0.43±0.01	14.75±1.55	1.17
F_9	28.9±0.03	0.34±0.07	0.37±0.02	07.94±0.35	1.08

F: formulation

Tablet thickness

The thickness was measured by placing tablet between two arms of the Vernier calipers. 5 tablets were taken and their thickness was measured (15).

Tablet hardness

Hardness of tablet is defined as the force applied across the diameter of the tablet in order to break the tablet. The hardness of the tablets was determined by diametral compression using erweka Hardness Tester (16).

Friability Testing

This test was performed to determine the effects of friction and shock. Pre-weighed sample of 10 tablets was placed in the erweka friabilator and rotated at 25 rpm for about 4 min. The tablets were dedusted and reweighed, and the friability percentage was calculated. Compressed tablets should not lose more than 1% of weight (17).

$$Percentage\ friability = \frac{Initial\ weight - Final\ weight}{Initial\ weight} \times 100$$

Wetting time

The wetting time of the tablets was measured using a simple procedure. Five circular tissue papers of 10-cm diameter were placed in a petridish with a 10-cm diameter. Ten milliliters of water containing eosin, a water-soluble dye, was added to the petridish. A tablet was carefully placed on the surface of tissue paper. The time required for water to reach the upper surface of the tablets was noted as the wetting time. The wetting times were measured (18)

Water absorption ratio

A piece of tissue paper folded twice was placed in a small petridish (Internal Diameter = 6.5 cm) containing 6 ml of water. A tablet was placed on the paper and the time required for complete wetting was then measured. The water absorption ratio (R) was determined using the following equation (19).

$$R = \frac{W_a - W_b}{W_a} \times 100$$

Where, W_b is the weight of the tablet before water absorption and W_a is the weight of the tablet after water absorption.

In vitro disintegration test

The in vitro disintegration studies were carried out using a Digital Tablet Disintegration test Apparatus (Erweka ZT- Germany). One tablet was placed in each of the six tubes of the basket assembly and then disk was added to each tube. This assembly was then suspended in a one-liter beaker containing water with its temperature being maintained at 37±2 °C. The basket was then moved up and down through a distance of 5 to 6 cm, at the frequency of 28 to 32 cycles per minute. The time required for complete disintegration of the tablet was recorded (20).

Dissolution test

The release rate of Rizatriptan benzoate from orally disintegrating tablets was determined using United State Pharmacopoeia (USP) XXIV dissolution testing apparatus II (paddle method). The dissolution test was performed using 900 ml of 0.1N HCl pH 1.2 as a dissolution medium, at 37±0.5 °C and 50 rpm. A sample (5 ml) of the solution was withdrawn from the dissolution apparatus at 1, 2, 3, 4, 5, 10, 20 and 30 min. The samples were filtered through a 0.45 membrane filter. Absorbance of these solutions was measured at 280 nm using a Shimadzu spectrophotometer. Cumulative percentage of drug release was calculated using an equation obtained from a standard curve (21).

Content uniformity

Ten tablets of each batch were weighed and powdered. Aliquot of this powder containing Rizatriptan benzoate equivalent to 5 mg of Rizatriptan was accurately weighed, suspended in approximately 50 ml of 0.1 N HCl and shaken for 15 min. Final volume was adjusted to 100 ml with 0.1 N HCl and filtered (Whatmann No.1 filter paper). From this 10 ml was diluted to 100 ml. The final volume was made by taking 2 ml of above solution and diluted to

Table 4. Evaluation of the prepared orodispersible tablets of Rizatriptan

Tests	F_1	F_2	F_3	F_4	F_5	F_6	F_7	F_8	F_9
Weight variation (Mean±SD)	151±3.45	149±2.24	149±3.12	150±3.71	152±3.32	148±1.58	147±3.28	151±3.45	149±2.24
Hardness (kg/cm²)	3.81±0.25	3±0.27	3.8±0.22	3.8±.023	3.7±0.27	3.1±0.19	3.7±0.22	3±0.23	3.2±0.21
Friability	0.57±0.16	0.68±0.14	0.81±0.15	0.93±0.147	0.96±0.157	0.72±0.155	0.44±0.138	0.80±0.149	0.66±0.153
Thickness (mm)	3.2	2.9	3.00	3.1	3.1	3.2	2.9	3.3	3.4
Wetting time (s)	62	59	51	49	44	41	40	30	33
Water absorption ratio	78.12	80.25	82.34	85.74	86.64	88.57	90.47	93	91
In-vitro disintegration time (s)	56	54	48	45	41	37	32	27	30
Assay	98.3	97.2	98.7	96.7	98.2	95.8	99.4	97.2	97.3

F: formulation

10 ml with 0.1 N HCl. Absorbance of this solution was recorded at 280 nm using UV/Vis spectrophotometer against a reagent blank and the content was compared from a calibration curve prepared with standard Rizatriptan benzoate in the same medium (Table 4). The mean percent drug content was calculated as an average of three determinations (22).

Data analysis

Response surface model factorial designs with 2 independent formulation variables at 3 different levels were used to study the effect of dependent variables (23). All the batches of orally disintegration were statically (95% or $p<0.05$) evaluated with regard to disintegration time, wetting time and drug release after 5 minutes.

Optimization of formulation ingredients

After generating the polynomial equations relating the dependent and independent variables, the process was optimized for responses, optimization was performed to obtain the value of X_1 and X_2, which targeted disintegration time (DT)= 35 seconds; wetting time (WT)= 40 seconds; drug release after 5 minutes (Q_5) =99. The optimized amount of crospovidone and Psyllium mucilage was incorporated in the tablet which was also used as the check point of the regression analysis model (24). The optimized orally disintegrating tablet was prepared and evaluated for the physiochemical properties.

Results

Data analysis

A response surface model factorial design with 2 independents variable at 3 different levels was used to study the effects in dependent variables. All the batches if orally disintegrating time, wetting time and drug release after 5 minutes. Transformed values of the batches along their results are show in Table 5. the dependent variables (DT,WT,Q_5) obtained at various levels of the 2 independent variable (X_1 and X_2) were subjected to multiple regressions to yield a second-order polynomial equation, the obtained coefficient are shown in Table 5. The DT, WT and Q_5 values measured form different batches shows wide variation. These results clearly indicated the DT, WT and Q_5 are strong affected by the variables selected for the study. This was also reflected by the wide range of value for coefficients of the term equation the value of correlation coefficient (R^2) of polynomial regression equation was found to be greater than 0.99, indication good fit for all dependent variable shown in Table 5.

X_1 and X_2 represents the average result if changing one variable at a time from its low level to its high level. The interaction terms (X_1X_2, X_1X_2 and X_2X_2) show how the DT, Wt and Q_5 changes when 2 variables are simultaneously changed. Using the polynomial equations, the optimized formulations were obtained for the response parameters.

Polynomial equation for disintegration time

$$Y=43.56-14.5X_1-4X_2+1X_1X_2+1.17X_1^2+1.67X_2^2$$

Polynomial equation for wetting time

$$Y=40.56-13.5X_1-4X_2+1.5X_1X_2+0.17X_1^2+0.67X_2^2$$

Polynomial equation for drug release after 5 minutes

$$Y=96.67-5X_1+5.5X_2-4.75X_1X_2-8.5X_1^2+1X_2^2$$

Response surface counterplot

The relationship between the dependent and independent variable was further elucidate by constructing counter plots. The effects of X_1 and X_2 with their interaction on DT, WT and Q_5 at different levels (low, medium and high level) are displayed in Figures 1-3 .the interaction effect between X_1 and X_2 are shown in response surface plot Figures 4-6.

Optimization of orally disintegrating tablet

The optimization of the orally disintegrating tablet was decided to target DT= 35 sec, WT= 40 and drug release Q_5= 99%.

Optimized concentrations were obtained from the software and the counter plot shown in Figure 7. Comparative values of predicted and observed responses along with the

Table 5. Analysis of variance (ANOVA) response surface cubic model

	Source	Sum of squares	Df	Mean square	F value	Prob of P value< F value	R^2
For Wetting time	Model	945.78	7	135.11	304.00	0.0441	0.9995
	X_1	420.50	1	420.50	946.13	0.0207	
	X_2	32.00	1	32.00	72.00	0.0747	
	X_1X_2	4.00	1	4.00	9.00	0.2048	
	X_1^2	2.72	1	2.72	6.12	0.2445	
	X_2^2	5.56	1	5.56	12.50	0.1755	
	Residual	0.44	1	0.44			
	Cor total	946.22	8				
For Disintegration time	Model	872.44	7	124.63	280.43	0.0459	0.9995
	X_1	364.50	1	364.50	820.13	0.0222	
	X_2	32.00	1	32.00	72.00	0.0747	
	X_1X_2	9.00	1	9.00	20.25	0.1392	
	X_1^2	0.00	1	0.00	0.12	0.7837	
	X_2^2	0.00	1	0.00	2.00	0.3918	
	Residual	0.44	1	0.44			
	Cor total	872.89	8				
For Drug release after 5 minutes	Model	479.75	7	68.54	274.14	0.0465	0.9995
	X_1	50.00	1	50.00	200.00	0.0449	
	X_2	60.50	1	84.50	760.50	0.0231	
	X_1X_2	90.25	1	90.25	361.00	0.0335	
	X_1^2	144.50	1	144.50	578.00	0.0265	
	X_2^2	2.00	1	2.00	8.00	0.2163	
	Residual	0.25	1	0.25			
	Cor total	480.00	8				

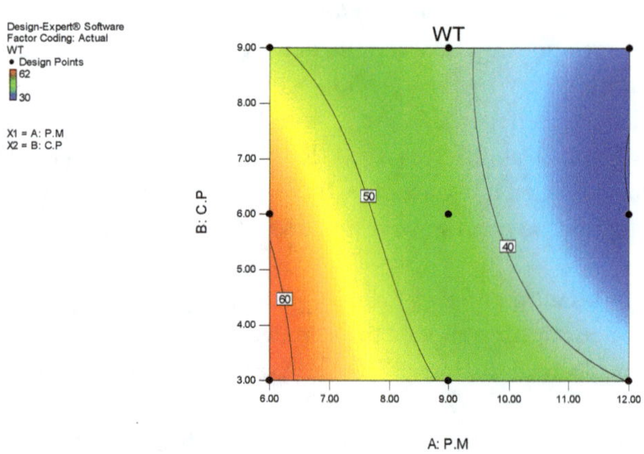

Figure 1. Counter plot for wetting time. WT: Wetting time, X1=A: P.M, X2=B:C.P, C.P: crospovidone, P.M: Psyllium mucilage.

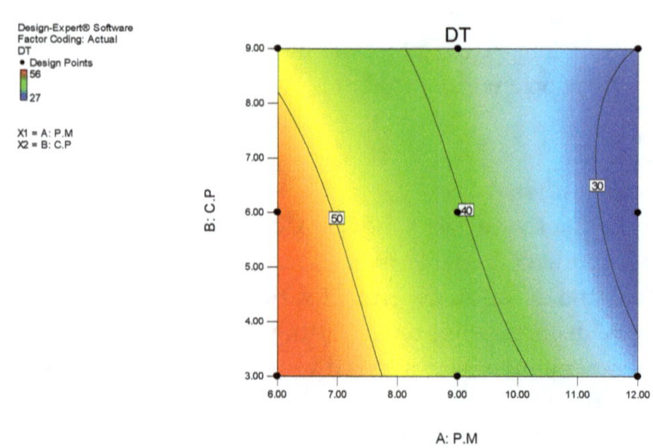

Figure 2. Counter plot for disintegration time. X1=A: P.M, X2=B:C.P; C.P: crospovidone, P.M: Psyllium mucilage, DT: disintegration time.

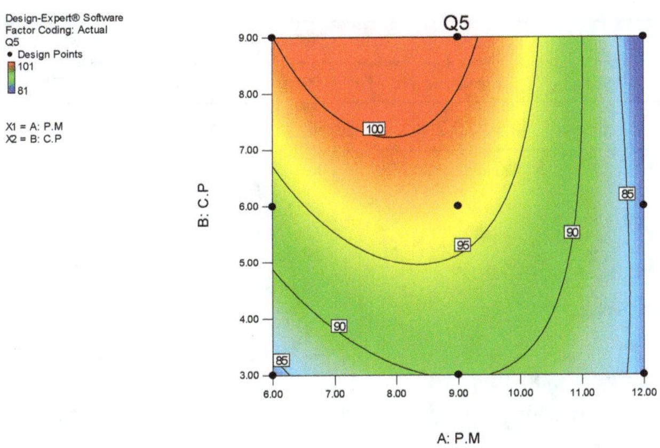

Figure 3. Counter plot for Q_5. X1=A: P.M, X2=B:C.P, C.P: crospovidone, P.M: Psyllium mucilage, Q_5: drug release after 5 minutes.

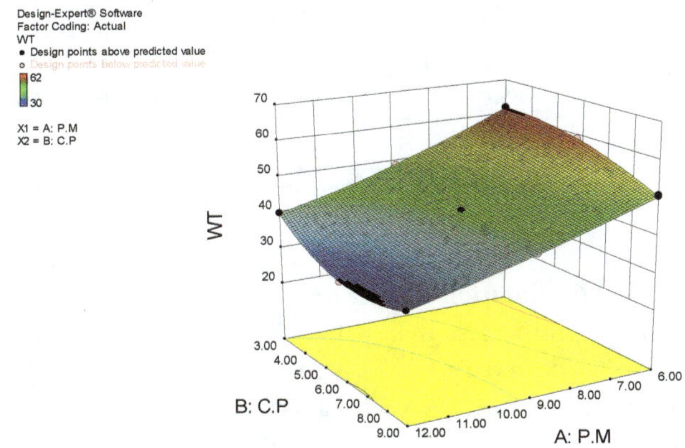

Figure 4. Response surface plot for wetting time. WT: Wetting time,X1=A: P.M, X2=B:C.P, C.P: crospovidone, P.M: Psyllium mucilage.

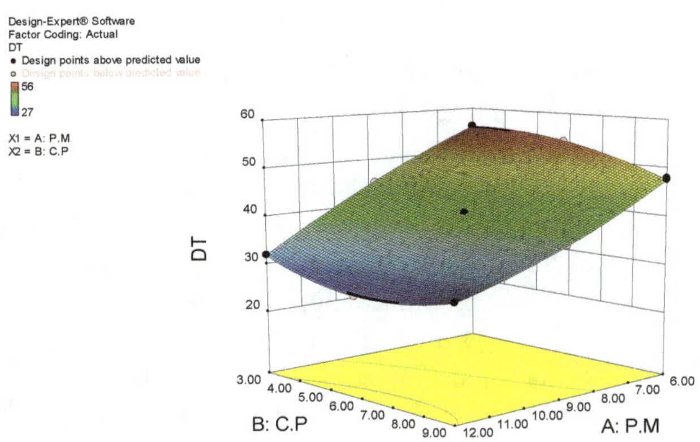

Figure 5. Response surface plot for Disintegration time. DT: Disintegration time, X1=A: P.M, X2=B:C.P, C.P: crospovidone, P.M: Psyllium mucilage.

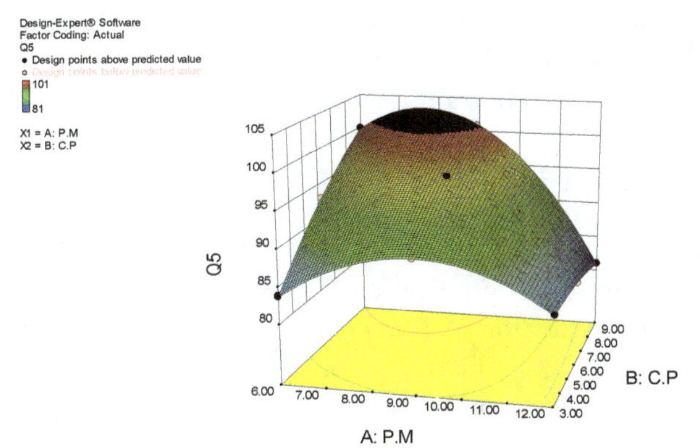

Figure 6. Response surface plot for Q_5. X1=A: P.M, X2=B:C.P, C.P: crospovidone, P.M: Psyllium mucilage, Q_5: drug release after 5 minutes.

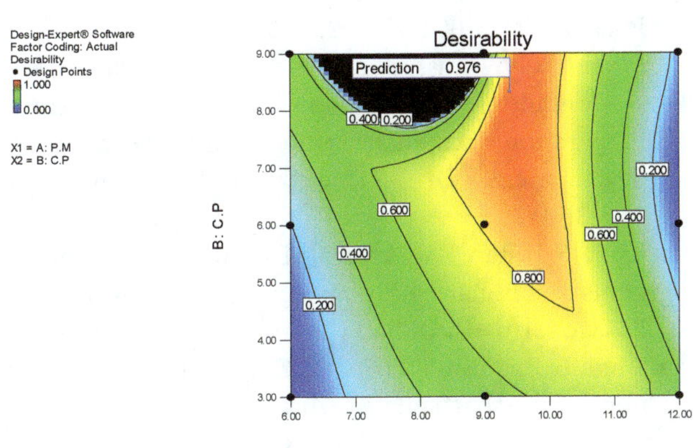

Figure 7. Counter plot for desirability. X1=A: P.M, X2=B:C.P, C.P: crospovidone, P.M: Psyllium mucilage.

formulation components are reported in Table 6.

Discussion

An optimized formulation of Rizatriptan orally disintegrating tablet was prepared in this study using the "Direct compression" method. Formulation and optimization procedures were facilitated using 3^2 full factorial designs.

About the WT and DT tests, it was observed that with increasing crospovidone and Psyllium mucilage DT and WT was both decreased; however, changes in the quantities of Psyllium mucilage had more significant effect than crospovidone (10).

On the other hand with increasing the percentage of Psyllium mucilage, speed of drug release was decreased, hence to create a suitable response, an optimum limit in usage Psyllium mucilage was found to have a proper amount of drug release.

Table 6. Comparative value of predicted and observed responses.

F_{NO}	Psyllium mucilage (mg)	crospovidone (mg)	DT (Sec)		WT		Q_5		Desirability
			Predicted	Observed	Predicted	Observed	Predicted	Observed	
O_1	9.40	8.32	36.47	36.3	39.99	39.2	99.00	99.12	0.976

WT: Wetting time, DT: Disintegration time, Q5: drug release after 5 minutes, O: Optimized batch

Effect of formulation vaiable on WT

Value of prob>f less than 0.05 show the model for WT is significant and Factor X_1 is found to be significant in this case. The negative coefficient for X_1 and X_2 indicate favorable effect on WT [increasing the amount of C.P and P.M (Psyllium mucilage) decrease the WT]. The results convey us that factor X_1 has significant effect on WT than that of X_2.

Effect of formulation vaiable on DT

Value of prob>f less than 0.05 show the model terms are significant and Factor X_1 is found to be significant in this case The negative coefficient for X_1 and X_2 indicate favorable effect on DT (increasing the amount of C.P and P.M decrease the DT). The results convey us that factor X_1 has significant effect on DT than that of X_2.

Effect of formulation vaiable on Q_5

Value of prob>f less than 0.05 show the model for Q_5 is significant and factor X_1, X_2, and X_1X_2 and X_1^2 are significant. The positive coefficient for X_2 indicates favorable effect on WT (increasing the amount of C.P increase the Q_5). The results convey us that factor X_2 has significant effect on Q_5 than that of X_1.

Conclusion

Overall, the results convey us that optimized orally disintegrating tablets of Rizatriptan containing 9.4 mg of C.P and 8.32 mg of P.M as a superdisntegrant by direct compression method showed responses as we desired.

Acknowledgments

Authors would like to thank the financial support offered by school of pharmacy and pharmaceutical science of Isfahan University of medical Sciences.

Authors' contributions

All contributed in the study, MT, MAS and ESh prepared the manuscript and Mk edited it.

Conflict of interests

The authors declared no competing interests.

Ethical considerations

Ethical issues (including plagiarism, data fabrication, double publication) have been completely observed by the authors.

Funding/Support

None.

References

1. Paramita D and Sabyasachi M. Orodispersible tablets: A new trend in drug delivery. J Nat Sci Biol Med 2010; 1(1): 2–5.
2. Lindgren S, Janzon L. Dysphagia: Prevalence of swallowing complaints and clinical finding. Med Clin North Am 1993;77:3–5.
3. Fu Y, Yang S, Jeong SH, Kimura S, Park K. Orally fast disintegrating tablets: Developments, technologies, taste-masking and clinical studies. Crit Rev Ther Drug Carrier Syst 2004; 21:433–76.
4. Bandari S, Mittapalli RK, Gannu R, Rao YM. Orodispersible tablets: An overview. Asian Journal of Pharmaceutics 2008;2:2–11.
5. Behnke K, Sogaard J, Martin S, Bauml J, Ravindran AV, Agren H. Mitrazapine orally disintegrating tablet versus sertraline: A prospective onset of action study. J Clin Psychopharmacol 2003; 23:358–64.
6. Krymchantowski AV, Bigal ME. Rizatriptan versus Rizatriptan plus rofecoxib versus rizatriptan plus tolfenamic acid in the acute treatment of migraine. BMC Neurol 2004;4:10.
7. Sanders-Bush E, Mayer SE. 5-hydroxytryptamine (Serotonin): Receptor agonists & antagonists. In: Brunton LL, Lazo JS, Parker KL, editors. Goodman & Gilman's The Pharmacological Basis of Therapeutics. 11th ed. New York: McGraw Hill; 2006:305–9.
8. Mahajan HS, Kuchekar BS, Badhan AC. Mouth dissolve tablets of Sumatriptan succinate. Indian J Pharm Sci 2004;66(2):238-40.
9. Mohan GV, Prassad DS, Kumar NR, Murty KV. Nimesulide Modified gum karaya solid mixture: Preparation, characterization, and formulation development. Drug Develop Ind Pharm 2003; 855:864-29.
10. Aveja SK, Rao KV, Arora J. Examination of natural gums and mucilages as sustaining materials in tablet dosage forms-II. Indian J Pharm Sci 1989; 51:115–8.
11. Singh B, Bhatowa R, Tripathi CB, Kapil R. Developing micro-/nanoparticulate drug delivery systems using "design of experiments". Int J Pharm Investig 2011;1:75–87
12. Bi Y, Sunada H, Danjo K, Yonezawa Y. Evaluation of rapidly disintegrating tablet prepared by a direct compression method. Drug Dev Ind Pharm 1999; 25:

571-58.

13. Lieberman HA, Lachman L. Pharmaceutical dosage forms tablets. 2nd edition. New York: Marcel Dekker;1989. p. 198-9.
14. Indian Pharmacopoeia, Vol-2. The Controller of Publication Delhi;1996. p. 735.
15. Banker GS, Anderson NR. In: Lachman L, Lieberman HA, Kanig JL, editors. The Theory and Practice of Industrial Pharmacy. 3rd ed. Mumbai:Varghese Publishing House;1987. p. 293-399.
16. Arora P, Arora V. Orodispersible tablets: A comprehensive review. International Journal of Pharmaceutical Sciences and Research 2013;2(2): 270-84.
17. Nawale RB, Mohite KP. Formulation and evaluation of domperidone orodispersible tablet. International Journal of Pharmaceutical Sciences and Research 2013; 4(9):3670-7.
18. Bandari S, Mittapalli RK, Gannu R, Rao YM. Orodispersible tablets: An overview. Asian Journal of Pharmaceutics 2008;2(1):2-11.
19. Kundu S, Sahoo PK. Recent trends in the developments of orally disintegrating technology. Pharma Times 2008; 40:11-5.
20. United States Pharmacopeia, National Formulary USP29/NF24. Rockville: The United States Pharmacopeia Convention; 2006.
21. United State Pharmacopoeia. Convention. NF Asian edition. 2004, p. 74-75.
22. Indian Pharmacopoeia. 4th ed. New Delhi: The Controller of Publications; 1996. p. 735–6.
23. Gohel M, Patel M, Amin A, Agrawal R, Dave R, Bariya N. Formulation design and optimization of mouth dissolve tablets of nimesulide using vacuum drying technique. AAPS Pharm Sci Tech 2004; 5(36):1-6.
24. Shimizu T, Sugaya M, Nakano Y. Formulation study for lansoprazol fast disintegrating tablet, III.design rapidly disintegrating tablets. Chem pharm Bull 2003;51:1121-7.

2

Effects of Chrysin plant flavonoid on proliferation and apoptosis of gastric cancer cell line (AGS)

Narges Askarian Dehkordi[1], Hedayatollah Shirzad[2*], Loghman Salimzadeh[3*], Behnam Zamanzad[2], Rezvan Meshkate[1], Mahbube Kiyani[1]

[1]Department of Immunology, Shahrekord University of Medical Sciences, Shahrekord, Iran
[2]Cell and Molecular, Research Center, Shahrekord University of Medical Sciences, Shahrekord, Iran
[3]Medical Plants Research Center, Shahrekord University of Medical Sciences, Shahrekord, Iran

ARTICLE INFO

Keywords:
Chrysin
Gastric cancer
Apoptosis

ABSTRACT

Introduction: Chrysin is a natural flavonoid antioxidant which its role in tumor cell death has been reported. The aim of this study was to investigate the mechanism of Chrysin effect on proliferation and apoptosis of gastric cancer cell line (AGS).
Methods: Cells were cultured and treated with different concentrations of Chrysin (90, 80, 70, 60, 50 μM) for 48 h and evaluated for cell viability. To examine the cytotoxic effect of drug in inducing apoptosis, staining with fluorescein isothiocyanate (FITC) and propidium iodide (PI) was used. The cells were treated for 48 h with different concentrations of Chrysin (50 of 90 μM) and examined for the morphological changes. The one-way analysis of variance (ANOVA) and the Excel software were used for data analysis.
Results: Different concentrations of Chrysin significantly inhibited the growth and proliferation of AGS cells ($p<0.05$). The IC_{50} dose was determined to be 67.5±0.66. Apoptosis induced by 50 and 70 μM of Chrysin was significantly greater than in untreated cells ($p<0.05$). Cells treated with high concentration of Chrysin (90 μM) showed more prominent growth inhibition and cell shrinkage compared to cells treated with the lower concentrations of Chrysin.
Conclusion: The results of this study showed that Chrysin effects on AGS cell line were significantly high and dose-dependent and might be helpful in the treatment of gastric cancer. Chrysin may therefore be considered a potential candidate for both cancer prevention and treatment. Further investigation is needed to validate the contribution of chrysin in tumor therapy *in vivo*.

Implication for health policy/practice/research/medical education:
Chrysin might be considered as a potential candidate for cancer prevention and treatment. Further investigation is needed to validate the contribution of chrysin in tumor therapy *in vivo*.

Introduction

Stomach cancer is one of the most important causes of cancer-related deaths worldwide and a major cause of cancer death in Asia (1). Treatment options for these patients include chemotherapy and surgery. But, therapeutic effects of chemotherapeutic drugs are not good enough and these drugs have many side effects (2). In recent years, a lot of researches have been done on drugs that might have protective or therapeutic effects against stomach cancer (3). Various flavonoids have been found to inhibit the development of cancer. Epidemiological studies have also shown that consumption of dietary flavonoids in fruits and vegetables may help reduce the incidence of cancer. This issue has been confirmed on *in vivo* and *in vitro* studies (4). Several mechanisms of action have been proposed for the effect of flavonoids including carcinogens inactivation, inhibition of angiogenesis and elimination of drug resistance or a combination of these mechanisms. Damage to healthy cells and development of cellular resistance to anticancer drugs restrict the use of chemotherapy drugs. All of these suppose the use of flavonoids for future clinical studies (5). Chrysin is a natural flavonoid compound extracted from honey, plants and propolis and been shown to possess anti-

***Corresponding authors**: Hedayatollah Shirzad; Email: shirzadeh@yahoo.com
& Loghman Salimzadeh; Email: Loghman_salim@yahoo.com

inflammatory and antioxidant properties (6). The potential apoptotic effect of chrysin has been reported in human cervical cancer, esophageal squamous cancer, malignant glioma, leukemia, breast, prostate and colon cancers, in vitro (7). The aim of this in vitro experimental study was to investigate the antiproliferative and apoptotic effects of Chrysin on gastric cancer cell line (AGS).

Materials and Methods

Cell culture and MTS assay

The AGS cell line (Pasture Institute, Iran) was cultured in DMEM medium and supplemented with 10% FBS, 100 U/ml penicillin, 100 µg/ml streptomycin and glutamine. The cells were harvested from the culture medium using trypsin (0.25%)-EDTA (0.1%). After washing, the number of viable cells was determined by trypan blue dye exclusion using a hemocytometer. Cells with viability greater than 95% were used for the experiment. MTS assay test was performed to determine the effect of chrysin in AGS cells. IC_{50} value which is the drug concentration required to kill 50% of the cells was obtained, too. Briefly, appropriate numbers of cells (10,000 cells) were cultured in 96-well plates. After 24 h incubation, different doses of Chrysin (90, 80, 70, 60, 50 µM) were added to each well. At least three wells were allocated for each concentration. Wells with cells but without drugs served as controls and 3 wells were used to assess the drug-free control. After 48 h, MTS test was performed. Cell Titer 96® AQueous One Solution Cell Proliferation Assay Kit was used for MTS assay according to the manufacturer's protocol. For this purpose, 20 µl of MTS working solution were added to each well. When MTS solution was absorbed by living cells a formazan product that had an absorbance maximum at 450 nms was produced, thus optical density (OD) would be the number of cells per well. The absorbance (optical density, OD) of formazan was measured using spectrophotometry. IC_{50} value was calculated as the sample concentration that caused 50% cell death as compared to the control cells (no drug added).

Assessment of apoptosis

To examine the cytotoxic effect of drug and its mechanisms in inducing apoptosis FITC Annexin V Apoptosis Detection Kit (BD) was used according to the manufacturer's protocol. Cancer cells were added in each well of 6-well plate. After 24 h, cells were treated at dose levels higher and lower than the IC_{50} value of chrysin (50 and 70 µM). After 24 h incubation, cells were rinsed with cold PBS and re-suspended in 100 µl of binding buffer. Then, stained with 5 µl FITC Annexin V and 10 µl Propidium iodide and incubated for 15 min at room temperature in the dark. The cells were examined by flow-cytometer. Cells that are FITC Annexin V positive and PI negative are in early stage of apoptosis; cells that are FITC Annexin V and PI positive are in late stage of apoptosis or already dead, cell that are FITC Annexin V negative and PI positive are considered necrotic.

Morphological study

The morphological changes of the cells and cells death were observed by using a normal inverted microscope. Cells were treated for 48 h with different concentrations of Chrysin (50 of 90 µM) and then morphological changes were examined and recorded.

Statistical analysis

In the present study, AGS cells were divided into two groups: Control group that did not receive any treatment and a group that received a drug. All experiments were carried out in triplicate. All results were expressed as mean ± SEM. Data were analyzed statistically using the SPSS 16 software. The one-way analysis of variance (ANOVA) was used to determine whether there were any significant differences between the means. A probability level of $p<0.05$ was considered statistically significant.

Results

Effects of different concentrations of Chrysin on the cell growth and proliferation

Results of the Chrysin effect on the growth and proliferation of AGS cell was reported as the average of several independent experiments (Figure 1). Different concentrations of Chrysin significantly inhibited the growth and proliferation of gastric carcinoma cells ($p<0.05$). The IC50 dose was determined to be 67.5±0.66.

Inducing apoptosis in cancer cells treated with Chrysin

In control group (untreated) 0.94% necrosis and 2.48% early apoptosis was observed. Induced necrosis, early apoptosis and late apoptosis in AGS cells treated with 50 µM Chrysin respectively were 2.91, 2.21 and 19.3. In cells treated with 70 µM Chrysin they were 1.26, 4.23 and 22.9, respectively, (Figures 2 and 3). Apoptosis induced by 50 and 70 µM of Chrysin was significantly greater than in untreated cells ($p<0.05$).

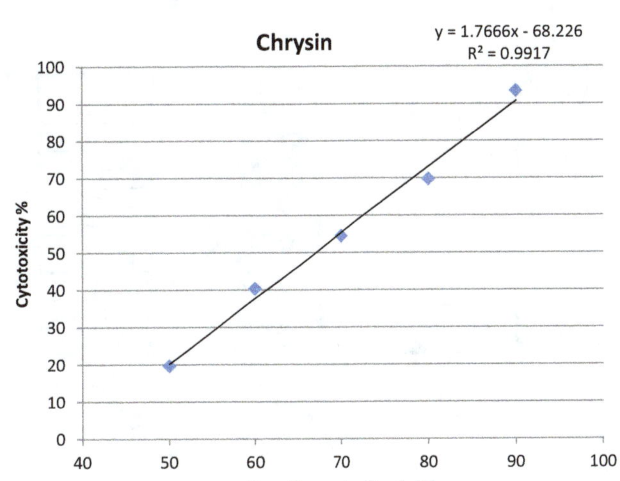

Figure 1. Effect of chrysin on the cell growth and proliferation. The cytotoxicity of AGS was increased significantly with increasing the concentration of chrysin.

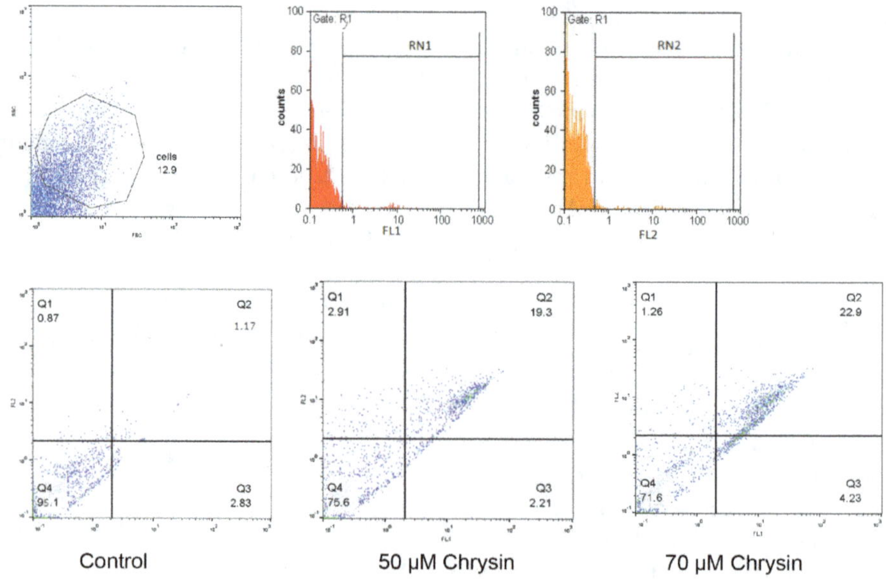

Figure 2. Flow-cytometry analysis using Annexin V-FITC/PI double staining depicting apoptosis. The cells were treated with 50 and 70 μM chrysin for 48 h or media only (control), and apoptosis was examined by flow-cytometry after Annexin V-PI double staining. Necrotic cells lose membrane integrity, permitting PI entry. Viable cells exhibited Annexin V (-)/PI (-); early apoptotic cells exhibited Annexin (+)/PI (-); late apoptotic cells or necrotic cells exhibited Annexin V (+)/PI (+).

Morphological Evaluation

There were no significant morphological changes after 24 h of incubation with the low concentration of Chrysin (50 μM), but after 48 h of incubation with 50 and 90 μM of Chrysin, significant changes in morphology were observed (Figure 4). Cells treated with high concentration of Chrysin (90 μM) compared to cells treated with the lower concentrations showed more prominent growth inhibition and cell shrinkage.

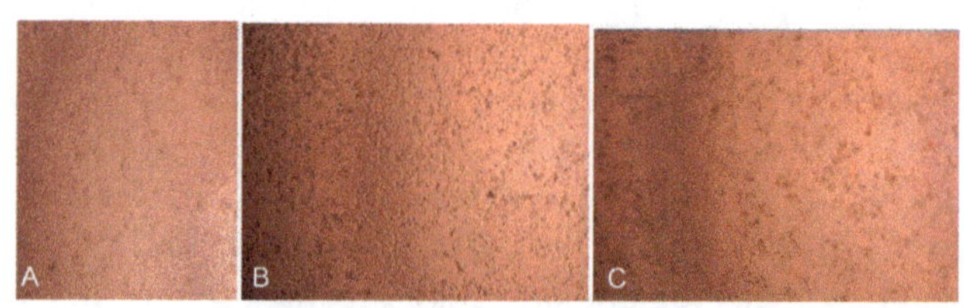

Figure 4. Morphological changes of cells after treatment with different concentrations of chrysin 48 hours post-treatment. A) Normal cells; B) 50 mM; and C) 90 mM. Cells treated with high concentration of Chrysin (90 μM) compared to cells treated with the lower concentrations showed more prominent growth inhibition and cell shrinkage.

Discussion

In recent years, considerable efforts have been done to identify naturally occurring compound and related synthetic agents that can prevent the development and recurrence of cancer. Several natural compounds have been found to induce apoptosis in various tumor cells and there are clear evidences that these compounds are potent inhibitors of cancer cell proliferation (8). Chrysin is a natural flavonoid extracted from honey, propolis (a wax) and various plants. It has been reported to have potent antioxidant and anti-inflammatory properties and promotes cell death by perturbing cell cycle progression. In order to determine the effect of Chrysin on gastric cancer, its effects on growth and proliferation of human gastric adenocarcinoma cell line were assessed in vitro using a MTS assay test. The results of this study showed that different concentrations of Chrysin markedly inhibit growth and proliferation in AGS cells in a dose-dependent manner. Inhibition of growth in cancer cells by minimum and maximum concentrations of Chrysin (50 and 90 μM) were 19.6 and 93.2, respectively. Our results showed that Chrysin had significant cytotoxic activity against human gastric cancer cells. This is the first report on chrysin-induced cytotoxicity and apoptosis in human gastric adenocarcinoma cell line.

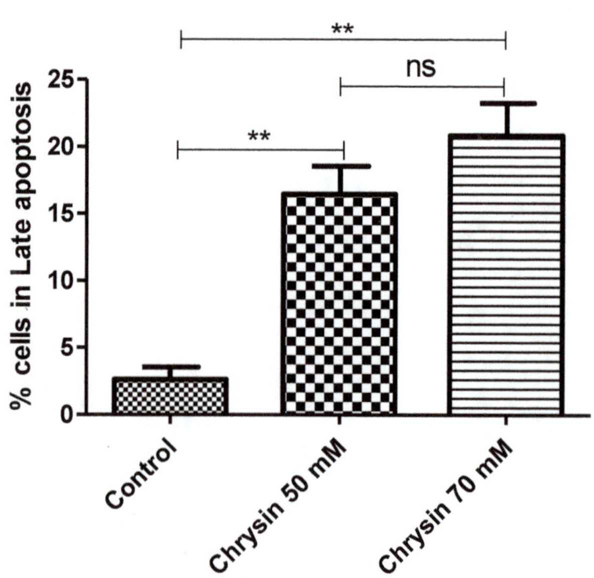

Figure 3. Induction of apoptosis in AGS cells after 48-hour treatment with chrysin. Statistical analysis performed by ANOVA followed by post hoc Tukey,S test. Value of **p<0.001 was assumed statistically significant. (ns: not significant and p>0.05)

Xue *et al* investigated the cytotoxic and antiproliferative effects of Chrysin on prostate cancer cell line which is in agreement with our results. Their results showed that Chrysin exhibited inhibitory effects on angiogenesis in mouse model, the critical step of tumor growth and metastasis (9). Hong *et al* reported the anticancer effect of Chrysin on MDA-MB231 breast cancer cells. In their study, the effect of Chrysin on cells was determined 24 and 48 h after treatment. 24 h after treatment no significant effect was observed, but after 48 h treatment with concentrations of 20 and 40 μM respectively 73.9 and 73.1 viability were observed. Thus, 20 μM Chrysin for 48 h was reported as the effective concentration (4). In Zhang *et al* study anticancer effects of Chrysin on a human esophageal adenocarcinoma cell line (OE33) was investigated and reported IC_{50} value of Chrysin was 90 μM. In our study IC_{50} value of Chrysin was 66 μM and it seems that cytotoxic effects of Chrysin on gastric cancer cells were much more than those on esophageal adenocarcinoma OE33 cells (10).

In the present study, types of cell death (apoptosis or necrosis) induced by Chrysin in AGS cells were determined by flow-cytometry. Chrysin induced early and late apoptosis and necrosis in gastric cancer cells, but the rate of late apoptosis was significantly higher. Thus secondary apoptosis seems to be the major mechanism of tumor cell killing. Therefore, apoptosis plays an important role in the anticancer activity of Chrysin. Zheng *et al* reported that Chrysin induces apoptosis human myeloid leukemia cell lines by induction of caspases and inactivation of Akt (11). In another study, anticancer effects of this drug and its derivatives on human gastric cancer cell lines (SGC-7901) and human colon carcinoma cell lines (HT-29) have been reported (12).

Conclusion

The results of our study showed that Chrysin could inhibit gastric cancer cells. Further researches are needed to fully understand the mechanism of action, in order to use in modern therapies as chemotherapy adjuvant in the treatment of gastric cancer. Because chemotherapy drugs that are used to treat cancer often cause unwanted side-effects, simultaneous use of various compounds derived from medicinal plants may increase effectiveness of other drugs in treatment of cancer.

Acknowledgments

We would like to thank the Research deputy of Shahrekord University of Medical Sciences for providing financial support. We also would like to thank the staff of the Central Research Laboratory who helped us.

Authors' contributions

All authors contributed to research design. NAD performed the experiment and prepared the first draft of the manuscript. HS edited the final version of the paper. All authors read and confirmed the final draft of the manuscript.

Conflict of interests

The authors declared no competing interests.

Ethical considerations

Ethical issues (including plagiarism, misconduct, data fabrication, falsification, double publication or submission, redundancy) have been completely observed by the authors.

Funding/Support

It has been supported by Isfahan Pharmaceutical Sciences Research Center, Isfahan University of Medical Sciences.

References

1. Hundahl SA, Phillips JL, Menck HR. The National Cancer Data Base report on poor survival of US gastric carcinoma patients treated with gastrectomy. Cancer 2000; 88(4): 921-32.
2. Treasure T, Fallowfield L, Lees B. Pulmonary metastasectomy in colorectal cancer: the PulMiCC trial. J Thorac Oncol 2010; 5(6): S203-S6.
3. Cragg L, Fox A, Nation K, Reid C, Anderson M. Neural correlates of successful and partial inhibitions in children: An ERP study. Dev Psychobiol 2009; 51(7): 533-43.
4. Hong TB, Rahumatullah A, Yogarajah T, Ahmad M, Yin KB. Potential effects of chrysin on MDA-MB-231 cells. Int J Mol Sci 2010; 11(3): 1057-69.
5. Li-Weber M. Targeting apoptosis pathways in cancer by Chinese medicine. Cancer Lett 2013; 332(2): 304-12.
6. Weng MS, Ho YS, Lin JK. Chrysin induces G1 phase cell cycle arrest in C6 glioma cells through inducing p21Waf1/Cip1 expression: Involvement of p38 mitogen-activated protein kinase. Biochem Pharmacol 2005; 69(12): 1815-27.
7. Khoo BY, Chua SL, Balaram P. Apoptotic effects of chrysin in human cancer cell lines. Int J Mol Sci 2010; 11(5): 2188-99.
8. Schilling T, Kairat A, Melino G, Krammer PH, Stremmel W, Oren M, *et al.* Interference with the p53 family network contributes to the gain of oncogenic function of mutant p53 in hepatocellular carcinoma. Biochem Biophys Res Commun 2010; 394(3): 817-23.
9. Fu B, Xue J, Li Z, Shi X, Jiang BH, Fang J. Chrysin inhibits expression of hypoxia-inducible factor-1α through reducing hypoxia-inducible factor-1α stability and inhibiting its protein synthesis. Mol Cancer Ther 2007; 6(1): 220-6.
10. Zhang Q, Zhao XH, Wang ZJ. Flavones and flavonols exert cytotoxic effects on a human oesophageal adenocarcinoma cell line (OE33) by causing G2/M arrest and inducing apoptosis. Food Chem Toxicol 2008; 46(6): 2042-53.
11. Zheng X, Meng WD, Xu YY, Cao JG, Qing FL. Synthesis and anticancer effect of chrysin derivatives. Bioorg Med Chem Lett 2003; 13(5): 881-4.
12. Xie ZH, Quan MF, Liu F, Cao JG, Zhang JS. 5-allyl-7-gen-difluoromethoxychrysin enhances TRAIL-induced apoptosis in human lung carcinoma A549 cells. BMC Cancer 2011; 11: 322.

3

Catecholamines are active plant-based drug compounds in *Pisum sativum*, *Phaseolus vulgaris* and *Vicia faba* Species

Mahdi Khozaei[1*], Fatemeh Ghorbani[2], Gashtasb Mardani[3], Rahman Emamzadeh[1]

[1]Department of Biology, University of Isfahan, Isfahan, Iran
[2]Department of Science, Islamic Azad University, Olom Tahghighat Branch, Tehran, Iran
[3]Medical Plants Research Center, Shahrekord University of Medical Sciences, Shahrekord, Iran

ARTICLE INFO

Keywords:
L-DOPA
Dopamine
HPLC
Herbal medicine
Catecholamines

ABSTRACT

Introduction: Catecholamines (L-DOPA and dopamine) are the key metabolites found in nervous system and their endogenous deficiency is associated with different patho-physiological disorders. Therefore, it is important to screen the new herbal sources of catecholamines for drug preparation. In this study, the amount of L-DOPA and dopamine were investigated in the leaves and roots of three species from legume family such as *Pisum sativum* (garden pea), *Phaseolus vulgaris* (haricot bean) and *Vicia faba* (broad bean); using TLC and HPLC.
Methods: The seeds of *P. sativum, P. Vulgaris* and *V. faba* were treated and cultured under the glasshouse conditions. The extraction from 1 gram of each plant sample was obtained and assayed for L-DOPA and dopamine using thin layer chromatography (TLC) and reversed-phase HPLC.
Results: The results indicated that all cultivars accumulated different levels of L-DOPA and dopamine in leaves and roots. The quantitative results showed that the metabolites concentrations were high in the leaves of *P. Sativum* and *V. faba* compared to that in roots.
Conclusion: The present study may provide a new avenue for preparation and estimation of L-DOPA and dopamine from plant sources and may be used for further analysis and therapeutic studies.

Implication for health policy/practice/research/medical education:
The results of the study may provide a new avenue for preparation and estimation of L-DOPA and dopamine from plant sources and may be used for further analysis and therapeutic studies.

Introduction

High-tech herbal medicine is a growing field of biotechnology for screening and development of plant components, both for the quality evaluation of crude therapeutic compounds found in plants and understanding of their mechanism of action (1,2). There are different types of herbal drugs to treat pathophysiological disorders. Among them, a number of important herbal-based drugs such as Menoherb, Diacimi and Diablack cohosh tablets have been introduced to treat nervous system. Moreover, it is important to find other valuable herbal sources for drug preparation, each of which may have new opportunities for pharmaceutical industry.

L-DOPA and dopamine are the crucial metabolites found in the brain as well as the rest of the nervous system. These metabolites play the critical role in the control of movement; and different physiological impacts such as stimulating effect on the heart, the circulation and the rate of metabolism (3). L-DOPA and dopamine, moreover, help to modulate brain activity, control coordination and movement, and regulate the flow of information to different areas of the brain. Biochemically, dopamine is a derivative of the tyrosine. Tyrosine is modified by tyrosine hydroxylase to form L-DOPA. L-DOPA decarboxylase then removes carbon dioxide from L-DOPA to for dopamine family (4,5) (Figure 1).

***Corresponding author**: Dr Mahdi Khozaei, Department of Biology, University of Isfahan, Isfahan, P.O. box 81746-73441, Iran.
Email: m.khozaei@sci.ui.ac.ir

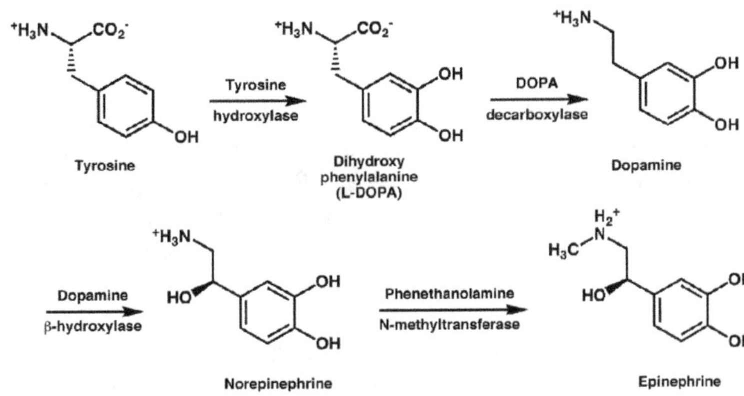

Figure 1. The L-DOPA and dopamine metabolic pathways

Although a number of crops such as beets and bananas contain amino acids, phenylalanine and tyrosine the precursor for synthesis of L-DOPA and dopamine but the occurrence of these compounds have been directly reported in a number of plants (6,7). It was shown that *Prurient mucuna* (the Indian pea) has large amount of dopamine (8). Therefore, the presence of catecholamines in other species of legume including *Pisum sativum* (garden pea), *Phaseolus vulgaris* (haricot bean) and *Vicia faba* (broad bean) was questioned. In Iran, *Pisum sativum* and *Phaseolus vulgaris* are used as herbal drugs due to their medicinal properties, to control the nervous irritability and restlessness in traditional medicine. *V. Faba*, moreover, is recommended for Parkinson's disease (9).

Up to date, there is no more evidence for detection and quantification of dopamine and l-DOPA in legume family particularly, *P. sativum*, *P. Vulgaris* and *V. faba* which are used as cultivars in agriculture. In this study, attempts have been made to discover a new source of L-DOPA and dopamine in legume family. In this study, therefore, the amount of L-DOPA and dopamine were investigated in the leaves and roots of three species from legume family such as *Pisum sativum* (garden pea), *Phaseolus vulgaris* (haricot bean) and *Vicia faba* (broad bean); using TLC and HPLC methods.

Materials and Methods

Materials and chemicals

The RP- TLC plates and analytical grade solvents such as ethyl acetate, n-propanol and acetic acid were purchased from Sigma (Sigma-Aldrich, St. Louis, MO, USA). L-DOPA and dopamine were obtained from Merck. The HPLC grade water was prepared by a Millipore type water purifier instrument.

Sample preparation

The seeds of *P. sativum*, *P. Vulgaris* and *V. faba* were obtained from the Agricultural Research Center, Isfahan, Iran. Seeds were placed according to the method of Martin *et al.* (10) in a moistened environment at 25 °C in the dark condition. After 24 h, germinated seeds were transferred into pots and kept under the glasshouse conditions until the four-leaf stages. Then, the plant materials from the roots and leaves in the four-leaf stages were collected and kept away from light, heat and moisture until use.

Extraction of metabolites

Briefly, 1 gram of each plant sample was grinded to powder and was extracted by floating in the extraction solution containing water-ethanol (1:1) and keeping at dark for five days. Then, each sample was subjected to ultrasonication for three minutes, centrifuged at 2000 rpm for 10 min and filtered at 0.22 μm to remove any remaining cell debris.

Preliminary studies by thin layer chromatography

The TLC plates were run as described by Hossaina and Beckerb (11) in ethyl acetate-n-propanol-water-acetic acid (19:2:10:1) at pH 6.2 and spots were visualized by ninhydrin reagent (0.3%). About 10 mg/ml of L-DOPA and dopamine (Merck) were run as standard to detect the place of catecholamines. Moreover, to estimate the concentration of analytes in samples, densitometry–based analysis of each spot was carried out using the GelBandFitter package.

Quantitative studies by high performance liquid chromatography (HPLC)

The spectra from high-resolution reversed-phase HPLC system with a RP C18 column was used to perform the analyses (12) Detection was done using a photodiode array detector and the detector was operated at 280 nm. Chromatographic software Chromoquest 30 was applied for data collection and processing.

Standard stock solutions of L-DOPA and dopamine were prepared with water to a concentration 10 mg ml^{-1} and stored at 4 °C. The working concentration ranges from 0.25-25 mg ml^{-1} were prepared by diluting with water to obtain the calibration curves. Then, the standard graphs were prepared using peak area versus concentrations of working solutions in mobile phase. The concentrations of L-DOPA and dopamine in the plant samples were calculated by comparison with peak intensity obtained from standard solutions.

Statistical analysis and data mining

The ANOVA analysis was performed using Statgraphics Centurion plus 5. The statistical difference between means of variables were tested using Dancan test (Statgraphics Centurion plus 5).

Results

Sample Preparation and Extraction of Bio-component

The cultured seeds of *P. sativum*, *P. Vulgaris* and *V. faba* were fallowed until the four-leaf stage, under the glasshouse condition. The extracted compounds from 1 g of leaves and roots with the extraction solvent including water-ethanol (1:1) were compared at 280 nm in order to estimate the extraction conditions (data was not shown). The UV-visible spectroscopy analysis showed a reliable increase in OD absorption at 280 nm, when compared with the control. The increase in absorbance at 280 nm was attributed to the increase of the active compounds such as dopamine and L-DOPA. The extracted bio-components were used for further analysis to assay the dopamine and L-DOPA.

TLC of Extracted bio-components

As the preliminary studies, the plants extracted from the roots and leafs were separated on TLC plates (Merck) and process using ninhydrin. The content of L-DOPA and dopamine metabolites were studied by comparing the Rf obtained from both the standard and the sample spots on chromatography (Figure 2) and semi-quantitative study was performed using the GelBandFitter software (data not shown). It has been reported that in *M. purient*, which belongs to the legume family, the catecholamine compounds synthesis actively. Due to the close phylogenetic relationship between *M. purient* and *P. sativum*, *P. Vulgaris* and *V. faba*, the presence of the catecholamine in these species is interesting. As it can be seen in Figure 2, the amount of L-DOPA and dopamine on the leaves of all plants is greater than the roots.

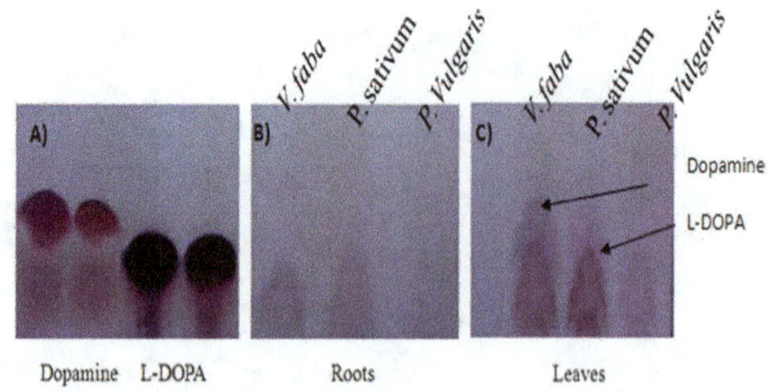

Figure 2. TLC analysis of L-DOPA and dopamine. A. Standard spots of catecholamines. B and C). The amount of L-DOPA and dopamine in roots and leaves of plant samples.

Quantitative Studies by HPLC

The HPLC-based methods for the determination and evaluation of bioactive compounds from plants have been taken into consideration in recent years. To determine the amount of L-DOPA and dopamine in plant samples, the chromatographic approaches were used. Briefly, the mobile phase was consisting of HPLC grade water and the presence of each analyte was studied at 280 nm. The retention time was 1.8 min and 2.3 min for dopamine and L-DOPA, respectively, at a flow-rate of 1 ml min^{-1}. A good separation (with symmetry peak) from the HPLC was achieved using the RP C18 column for the standard concentrations of L-DOPA and dopamine (Figure 3A).

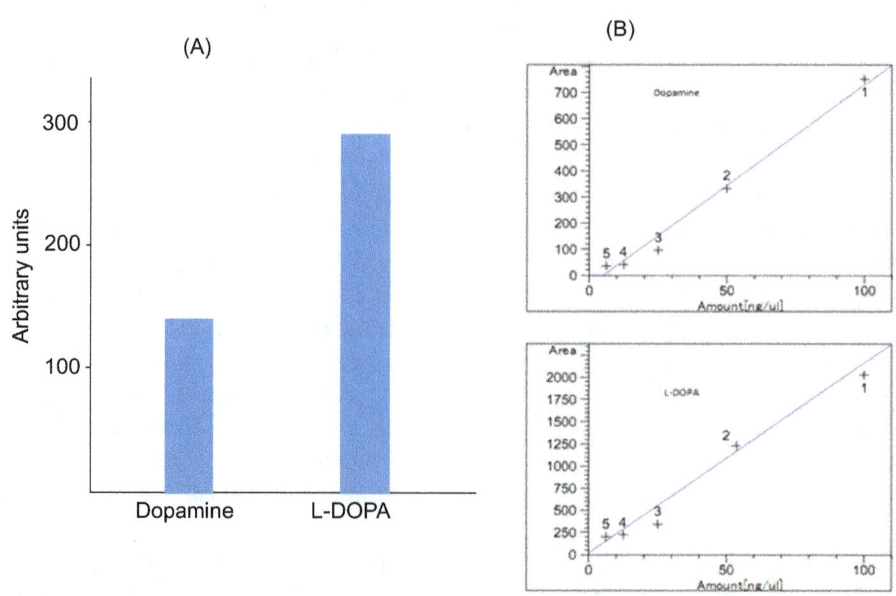

Figure 3. Figure 3A shows a typical signal obtained from the analysis of a standard and solution of commercial L-DOPA and dopamine using the proposed method. Data are the average results of three independent experiments. Figure 3B shows the regression equation and correlation coefficient (r) for L-DOPA and dopamine. The HPLC-based assays show a good level of linearity.

Furthermore, observed retention times (1.8 min and 2.3 min) allowed a rapid assay of L-DOPA and dopamine.
The linearity of the HPLC method was assayed using the calibration standard solutions of L-DOPA and dopamine. The linear ranges of concentration were found to be 1-100 mg ml^{-1} for both the L-DOPA and dopamine. The regression equation and correlation coefficient (r) were y=7.7x+38.99 (y: peak area, x: concentration) and 0.9925 for L-DOPA and y=21.47x+21.24 and 0.9926 for dopamine, respectively. The linearity of the HPLC assays was evaluated by the high correlation coefficients (r) for the regression equations, and the curves showed a reliable intensity consistent with the standard concentrations of analytes (Figure 3B). Therefore, the method was supposed as a fast and reliable way for preparation and quantitative assay of L-DOPA and dopamine in both leaves and roots of *P. sativum*, *P. Vulgaris* and *V. faba*.
The amount of L-DOPA and dopamine in each extraction solution from *P. sativum*, *P. Vulgaris* and *V. Faba* were analysed using the validated HPLC method. About 10 ml of each extract assayed using HPLC and the concentration of analytes was calculated using the standard regression equation (Table 1 and 2).
The data, which are obtained from HPLC, are consistent with the results obtained with TLC. The concentration of both the L-DOPA and dopamine in leaves are more than the concentrations in roots. The overall content of L-DOPA, the precursor of dopamine was obtained more than dopamine in roots and leaves of *P. sativum*, *V. faba* and *P. vulgaris*, respectively. Therefore, it seems that the L-DOPA is imported not only in the dopamine biosynthesis but also in other metabolic pathways (13,14). Finally, the results showed significant levels for L-DOPA and dopamine in *P. sativum*, *V. Faba* and *P. Vulgaris* which may be used in further studies to examine the effects of these plants in neurological disorders such as Parkinson's disease.

Table 1. The amount of L- DOPA in leaves and roots of *P. sativum*, *P. Vulgaris* and *V. faba*. The Mean values and analysis of variance. Values followed by different capital letters are significantly different per P < 0.01. n = 4

Species	L-dopa in the leaves (ng.g FW^{-1})	L-dopa in the root (ng.g FW^{-1})
P. sativum	67.93A	64.16A
P. Vulgaris	20.33C	14.05C
V. faba	63.41B	20.52B

Table 2. The amount of dopamine in leaves and roots of *P. sativum*, *P. Vulgaris* and *V. faba*. The Mean values and analysis of variance. Values followed by different capital letters are significantly different per P < 0.01. n = 4.

Species	Dopamine in the leaves (ng.g FW^{-1})	Dopamine in the root (ng.g FW^{-1})
P. sativum	19.21A	4.131A
P. Vulgaris	9.67C	3.86B
V. faba	15.21B	3.63C

Discussion

In this paper, the extraction and extermination of dopamine and L-DOPA from *P. sativum*, *P. Vulgaris and V. faba* from the roots and leaves was carried out. The results may be used for further therapeutic studies.
L-DOPA and dopamine are important metabolites found in the nervous system. It was suggested that *Prurient mucuna* (the Indian pea) contains a high content of L-DOPA in the seeds, roots and leaves (14). In this study, the amounts of catecholamines in the roots and leaves of three other species from legume family including *P. sativum* (garden pea), *P. vulgaris* (haricot bean) and *V. faba* (broad bean), were investigated. The fractionation procedure was carried out and samples were subjected to spectroscopy studies. A significant increase in OD absorption was obtained when extracted fractions were assayed at 280 nm. An increase in ultraviolet wavelength was discussed which resulted in increasing of the concentration of bio-active compounds such as dopamine and L-DOPA. Furthermore, it can be assumed that the extraction conditions were effective enough to obtain the aromatic components.
The TLC studies confirmed the presence of L-DOPA and dopamine on the leaves and roots in all samples (Figure 2). Interestingly, the accumulation of L-DOPA and dopamine in leaves was more than roots. Therefore, although the metabolism pathway of catecholamines in legume family is not clear in details, it can be proposed that the metabolic pathway might be active in the production of catecholamine compounds on the leaves (13,14). Furthermore, the results confirmed that the leaves are more appropriate than the roots for the purposes of therapeutic treatment. The quantitative studies to assay the amount of L-DOPA and dopamine in each extraction solution from *P. sativum*, *P. Vulgaris* and *V. Faba* were done using the HPLC method (Table 1 and 2). The results were consistent with the data from TLC and showed that the extraction from *P. sativum*, *P. Vulgaris and V. faba* contained both L-DOPA and dopamine and the concentrations of these metabolites in leaves were more than that was detected in roots. The data provided in this study suggested that TLC was a reliable method for detection of catecholamines and the data obtained from this technique was matched from that gained from HPLC. Furthermore, the results were in consist with the previous reports in embryo of velvet bean and *V. faba* (broad beans) (*Mucuna pruriens*) in which, the catecholamines actively metabolism by plant (8,13,15). In conclusion, the present study may provide a new and reliable protocol for extraction of L-DOPA and dopamine from *P. sativum*, *P. Vulgaris and V. faba* for further analysis and therapeutic studies.

Author' contributions

MK designed the project; MK, FG, GM performed the experiments; MK provided expertise and access to analysis of metabolites; MK, FG, GM analysed the data; MK, RE wrote the paper; all authors read it.

Conflict of interests

The authors declared no competing interests.

Ethical considerations

Ethical issues (including plagiarism, misconduct, data fabrication, falsification, double publication or submission, redundancy) have been completely observed by the authors.

Funding/Support

The work described here was founded by University of Isfahan (grant number 910813).

References

1. Corpa N, Pendrya B. The role of Western herbal medicine in the treatment of gout. J Herb Med 2013; 3(4):157-170.
2. Li L, Sing P. Use of herbal medicines and natural products: an alternative approach to overcoming the apoptotic resistance of pancreatic cancer. The International Journal of Biochemistry & Cell Biology, In Press.
3. Meiser J, Weindl D, Karste H. Complexity of dopamine metabolism. J Cell Commun Signal 2013;11:34.
4. Smith TA. Plant amines. In: EA Bell, BV Charlwood, editors. Secondary Plant Products, Encyclopedia of Plant Physiol. New Series Vol 8. Berlin: Springer Verlag;1980. p. 433-460.
5. Endress RA, Jager A, Kreis W. Catecholamine biosynthesis dependent on the dark in betacyanin-forming Portulaca callus. J Plant Physiol 1984; 11(5): 291-295.
6. Tretyn A, Kendrick RE. Acetylcholine in plants: presence, metabolism and mecha-nism of action. Bot Rev 1991;57:33–73.
7. Kuklin AI, Conger BV. Catecholamines in plants. J Plant Growth Regul 1995;14:91–97.
8. Wichers HI, Pras N, Huizing HI. Mucuna pruriens: in vitro production of L-DOPA. Biotechnol Agric For 1989 ; 7: 349-366.
9. Blumenthal M, Busse WR, Goldberg A, Grenwald J, Hall T, Riggins CW, *et al.* The Complete German Comission E Monographs-Therapeutic Guide to Herbal Medicines. Boston: American Botanical Council;1998. p. 157.
10. Martin RE, Miller RL, Cushwa CT. Germination response of legume seeds subjected to moist and dry heat. Ecology 1975; 56(6):1441-1445.
11. Hossaina MA, Beckerb K. Nutritive value and antinutritional factors in different varieties of Sesbania seeds and their morphological fractions. Food Chem 2001;73(4):421–431.
12. Wichers HJ, Visser JF, Huizing HJ, Pras N. Occurrence of L-DOPA and dopamine in plants and cell cultures of Mucuna pruriens and effects of 2,4-D and NaCI on these compounds. Plant Cell Tissue Organ Cult 1993;33:259-264.
13. Mohseni MSM, Golshani B. Simultaneous Determination of Levodopa and Carbidopa from Fava Bean, Green Peas and Green Beans by High Performance Liquid Gas Chromatography. J Clin Diagn Res 2013;7:1004–1007.
14. Harris NN, Javellana J, Davies KM, Lewis DH, Jameson PE, Deroles SC, *et al.* Betalain production is possible in anthocyanin-producing plant species given the presence of DOPA-dioxygenase and L-DOPA. BMC Plant Biol 2012;12:34.
15. Burbano C, Cuadrado C, Muzquiz M, Cubero JI. Variation of favism-inducing factors (vicine, convicine and L-DOPA) during pod development in Vicia faba L. Plant Foods Hum. Nutr 1995; 47: 265–274.

The effect of feeding with soybean on serum levels of TSH, T_3 and T_4 in male mice

Mehrdad Modaresi[1]*, Hormat Khorrami[2], Majid Asadi-Samani[3]

[1]Biology Faculty, Khorasgan (Isfahan) Branch, Islamic Azad University, Isfahan, Iran
[2]Payam-e-Noor University, Isfahan Center, Isfahan, Iran
[3]Medical Plants Research Center, Shahrekord University of Medical Sciences, Shahrekord, Iran

ARTICLE INFO

Keywords:
Isoflavone
Soybean
Thyroid stimulating hormone
Triiodothyronine
Thyroxine
Male mice

ABSTRACT

Introduction: Soybean possesses isoflavones and might, therefore, cause problem in thyroid hormone synthesis. The purpose of this study was to study the effect of soybean on serum levels of Thyroid stimulating hormone (TSH), Triiodothyronine (T_3), and Thyroxine (T_4) in male mice.
Methods: In this experimental study, 24 Balb/C male mice were randomly assigned to three groups of eight including control or base diet-fed group and treatment groups 1 and 2 receiving respectively 30% and 50% soybean-containing diet. After nine weeks, the blood sample was taken from the animals' heart and serum levels of TSH, T_3, and T_4 were measured. The data were analyzed by SPSS software using one-way ANOVA and Duncan's test.
Results: In 50% soybean group, a significant decrease was observed in T_4 serum level compared to the control group ($p<0.05$). On the other hand, this hormone level non-significantly decreased in the group fed by 30% soybean compared to the control group ($p<0.05$). TSH serum level increased significantly in 30% soybean group compared to the control group ($p<0.05$). But, serum level of T_3 was not significantly different between 30% or 50% soybean groups and control group ($p>0.05$).
Conclusion: In view of the findings, it is estimated that the effect of addition of soybean into meal on thyroid function is dose-dependent, so that the diet containing 30% and 50% soybean might cause increased TSH release in thyrotrope cells and hence variation in pituitary-thyroid axis function.

Implication for health policy/practice/research/medical education:
Feeding with soybean can have a dose-dependent effect on thyroid function and might cause increased TSH release in thyrotrope cells and variation in pituitary-thyroid axis function.

Introduction

Soybean (*Glycine max*) has been of interest as an effective herbal compound to treat osteoporosis and reduce menopausal symptoms (1). Soybean could inhibit peroxidase enzyme thanks to containing various isoflavones and therefore causes inhibition of thyroid hormones synthesis (2).

Soybean contains minerals, protein, vitamin, and various carbohydrates. 60% of the dried soybean weight consists of fat (17.20%) and protein (40-67.30%). Since soybean protein is rich in vitamins B1 and B2, pantothenic acid, colin, niacin, and all essential amino acids for the body, it is undoubtedly considered as a main source of nutrients for human (3).

One of the other important compounds found in soybean which is today the main reason for tendency toward its consumption worldwide is phytoestrogen. Phytoestrogens are plant derivatives of estrogens with diphenolic structure found in fruits, vegetables, peas, and particularly seeds like cotton, alfalfa, clover, and soybeans. Phytoestrogens enjoy all physiological, physical, and chemical specifications of estrogens. The main isoflavone of soy is genistein (4).

By recent works, administration of estrogen-containing drugs causes increased risk of breast and endometrial cancers in postmenopausal women. Use of estrogen-like compounds particularly plant types (phytoestrogens)

*__Corresponding author__: Mehrdad Modaresi,
Email: mehrdad_modaresi@hotmail.com

abundantly found in soy foods including soy milk and protein not only satisfies postmenopausal women's need for estrogen, but also is free from any side effect and decreases the risk of cancer development (5).

Some studies indicated that soy consumption could lead to suppression of thyroid activity and goiter incidence (6). Also, the reported effects for soy on cancer, osteoporosis, and cardiovascular diseases have led to increased interest in soy consumption. Although the US Food and Drug Administration IN 1999 mentioned soy as contributing to cholesterol decrease and containing numerous bioactive elements, soy isoflavones are still attracting public attention. On the other hand, genistein found in soy causes dilation of blood vessels, improvement of blood vessel elasticity, and decrease in blood pressure by increasing nitric oxide release.

All these contribute positively to heart and decrease systolic and diastolic pressure (6); however, some studies have indicated that phytoestrogens causes decreased quality of sperm in men. Empirically, the diet rich in phytoestrogen compounds such as soy could cause change in pituitary–hypothalamic–gonadal axis in men as with diethyl acetyl nisterol compounds (7).

Since thyroid is considered as one of the most important endocrine glands and contributes to regulating general metabolism of the body including its most fundamental constituent, that is oxygen, growing of fetal nervous system, and functioning of most body's organs such as cardiovascular, digestive, and reproductive systems, any disturbance in function of thyroid leads to disturbance in function of other body organs, and genistein found in soy could cause disorder effects on pituitary-hypothalamic axis, we aimed to investigate soy effects on concentrations of Thyroid stimulating hormone (TSH), Triiodothyronine (T_3), and Thyroxine (T_4).

Materials and Methods

In this study, 24 Balb/C male mice with mean weight of 35±5 g were enrolled. The study samples were maintained in appropriate laboratory at 25±3 °C, with normal light period, and in sterilized cages. The mice were provided with enough water and food.

The mice were randomly assigned to three groups of eight each including control group (fed with base diet) and intervention groups 1 and 2 (fed with the diet containing respectively soy 30% and soy 50%).

As this study was based on feeding of mice with soy protein, the consumed food by each mouse was calculated by the difference in weight of the given food per day during a week. Livestock concentrate for feeding the mice was pulverized by an electric mortar and then the food mixture containing soy 30% and 50% was prepared based on the treatment dose. The mixture was again pelleted and made available to the mice. The duration of treatment was considered nine weeks for each animal.

After nine weeks treatment, the blood was taken to investigate the levels of TSH, T_4, and T_3. For this, experimental samples were partially anesthetized by ether and the blood was taken directly from the heart. The samples were collected and were hormonally measured. Hormonal measurement was done by immunoenzymatic methods in the solid-phase by Eliza reader.

Results

In the group treated with soy 30% in the diet, mean serum level of TSH hormones increased significantly compared to the control group and group treated with soy 50% in the diet ($p<0.05$); However, the increase in the group treated with the diet containing soy 50% was not significant compared to the control group ($p>0.05$) (Figure 1).

In the group treated with soy 50% in the diet, mean serum level of T_4 hormones decreased significantly compared to the control group ($p<0.05$). However, the corresponding decrease was not significant in the group treated with the diet containing soy 30% compared to the control group ($p>0.05$; Figure 2).

In the group treated with soy 30% in the diet, mean serum level of T_3 hormones decreased and in the group treated with soy 50% in the diet T_3 hormones increased (Figure 3). However, these variations were not significant compared

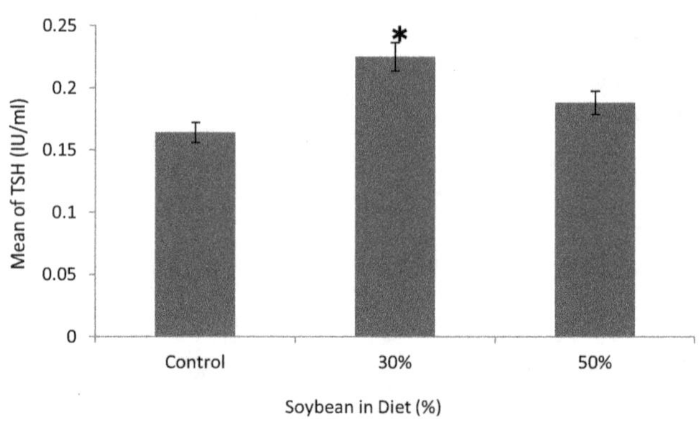

Figure 1. Comparison of serum TSH hormones in the groups of study; *Significant difference from control group ($p<0.05$)

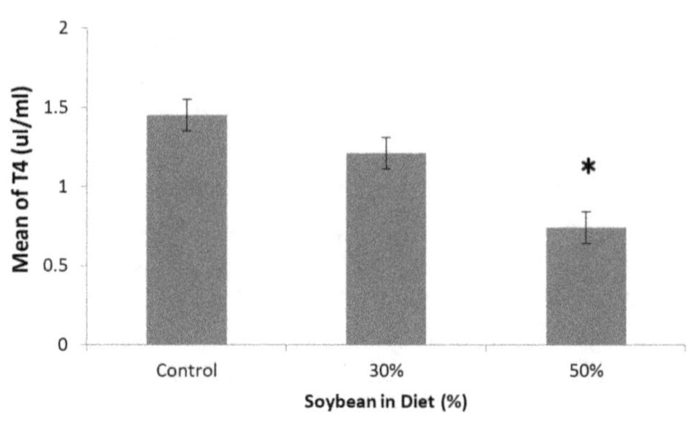

Figure 2. Comparison of serum T_4 hormones in the groups of study; *Significant difference from control group ($p<0.05$)

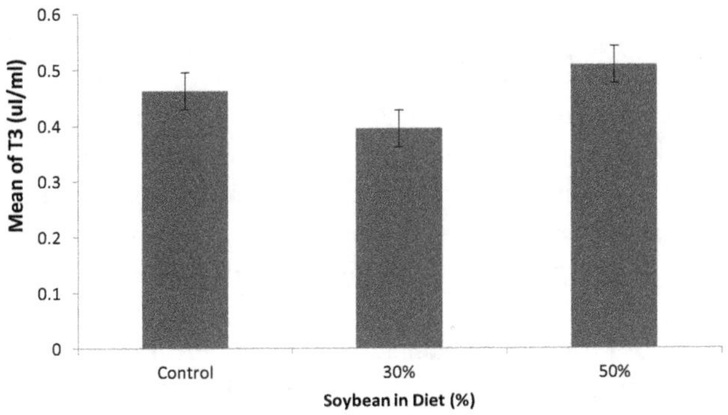

Figure 3. Comparison of serum T_3 hormones in the groups of study

to the control group (p>0.05).

Discussion

In this study, the effects of the diet containing soy 30% and 50% on serum levels of TSH, T_3, and T_4 were investigated in laboratory male mice and the results indicated mean serum level of TSH hormones increased significantly in the group treated with soy 30% compared to the control group. Isoflavones found in soy, particularly genistein, prevent thyroid peroxidase which is vital to thyroid hormones synthesis. This primary decrease in thyroid hormones stimulates pituitary-thyroid axis and hence the serum level of this hormone increases (8). But, this increase was non-significant in the group treated with soy 50%.

Other studies have reported risk of developing hypothyroidism due to consuming soybean and its products. This is another explanation for inhibitory effect of soy's estrogen-like compounds on hypothalamic-pituitary-thyroid axis. Since increased serum level of TSH normally causes increase in thyroglobulin proteolysis and thyroid hormones release in the blood, increase in T_3 and T_4 is expected. However, the phytoestrogens found in soy caused decreased susceptibility of pituitary-thyroid glands axis in normal feedback mechanism and function (8). As noted, T_4 serum level decreased significantly in the group treated with 50% soy. T_4 serum level decreased in 30% soy group non-significantly, but the decrease was still noted. General course and mechanism of soy's isoflavone effect on thyroid-pituitary axis is still unknown. Isoflavones are fundamentally known as anti-thyroid compounds (9,10), as they prevent the function of thyroid peroxidase, which is the key enzyme for synthesis of thyroid hormones. However, other works have also demonstrated an extensive thyroid hyperplasia by treatment with soy (11,12). Studies also highlighted that the children and individuals fed with greater amounts of soy needed more iodine, even up to twice more than that required by other individuals (13,14).

Conclusion

The foods rich in soy phytoestrogens are found abundantly in Southeast Asian populations' meal and are likely to contribute greatly to thyroid function. Therefore, it is recommended to pay attention to dose-dependent consumption of soy and its components as pharmaceutical compounds with plant origin.

Acknowledgments

Appreciate and thanks to all persons in biology department of Payam-Noor University of Isfahan who helped us in implementing this project.

Authors' contributions

All the authors wrote the manuscript equally.

Conflict of interests

The authors declared no competing interests.

Ethical considerations

Ethical issues (including plagiarism, misconduct, data fabrication, falsification, double publication or submission, redundancy) have been completely observed by the authors.

Funding/Support

This project was financially supported by Payam-Noor University of Isfahan.

References

1. Chang HC, Doerge DR. Dietary genistein inactivates rat thyroid peroxidasein Vivo without an apparent hypothyroid effect. Toxicol Appl Pharmacol 2000; 168(3):244-52.
2. Doerge DR, Sheehan DM. Goitrogenic and estrogenic activity of soy isoflavones. Environ Health Perspect 2002; 110 (Suppl 3): 349-53.
3. Zargari A. Medicinal plants. Tehran: Tehran University Publication; 2004. p. 352-56.
4. Vandenplas Y, Castrellon PG, Rivas R, Gutiérrez CJ, Garcia LD, Jimenez JE, *et al.* Safety of soya-based infant formulas in children. Br J Nutr 2014; 111(08): 1340-60.
5. Evans B, Griffiths K, Morton M. Inhibition of 5α-reductase in genital skin fibroblasts and prostate tissue by dietary lignans and isoflavonoids. J Endocrinol 1995; 147(2):295-302.
6. Crouse JR, Morgan T, Terry JG, Ellis J, Vitolins M, Burke GL. A randomized trial comparing the effect of casein with that of soy protein containing varying amounts of isoflavones on plasma concentrations of lipids and lipoproteins. Arch Int Med 1999; 159(17):2070-6.
7. Malloy MJ, Kane JP. Agents used in hyperlipidemia. In: Katzung BG editor. Basic & clinical Pharmacology. 8th ed. New York: Mc Graw- Hill; 2001. p. 588–95.
8. Greco D, Stabenfeldt GH. Endocrinology. In: Cunningham JG, editor. Textbook of Veterinary Physiology. 4th ed. Philadelphia: Elsevier Saunders Inc;2007.

9. Messina M, Redmond G. Effects of soy protein and soybean isoflavones on thyroid function in healthy adults and hypothyroid patients: a review of the relevant literature. Thyroid 2006; 16(3):249-58.
10. Borradaile N, De Dreu L, Wilcox L, Edwards J, Huff M. Soya phytoestrogens, genistein and daidzein, decrease apolipoprotein B secretion from HepG2 cells through multiple mechanisms. Biochem J 2002; 366:531-9.
11. Divi RL, Chang HC, Doerge DR. Anti-thyroid isoflavones from soybean: isolation, characterization, and mechanisms of action. Biochem Pharmacol 1997; 54(10):1087-96.
12. Chen H, Walfish P. Effects of estradiol benzoate on thyroid-pituitary function in female rats. Endocrinology 1978; 103(4):1023-30.
13. Ikeda T, Nishikawa A, Imazawa T, Kimura S, Hirose M. Dramatic synergism between excess soybean intake and iodine deficiency on the development of rat thyroid hyperplasia. Carcinogenesis 2000; 21(4):707-13.
14. Van Ruth SM, Shaker ES, Morrissey PA. Influence of methanolic extracts of soybean seeds and soybean oil on lipid oxidation in linseed oil. Food Chem 2001;75(2):177-84.

5

Microbial quality of some medicinal herbal products in Kashan, Iran

Navid Mazroi Arani[1], **Reza Sharafati Chaleshtori**[2*], **Mahmoud Rafieian-kopaei**[3]

[1]Food and Hygiene Control Laboratory, Deputy of Food and Drug, Kashan University of Medical Sciences, Kashan, Iran
[2]Research Center for Biochemistry and Nutrition in Metabolic Diseases, Kashan University of Medical Sciences, Kashan, Iran
[3]Medical Plants Research Center, Shahrekord University of Medical Sciences, Shahrekord, Iran

ARTICLE INFO

Keywords:
Herbal waters
E. coli
Clostridia
Enterococcus
Pseudomonas

ABSTRACT

Introduction: The use of medicinal plants has risen worldwide. In Iran, herbal waters and rose waters are of traditional medicinal products and as a result, they are widespreadly consumed. Therefore, diagnosis of microbial quality of these products is important. The aim of this study was to evaluate microbial quality of herbal extracts distributed in Kashan, Iran.

Methods: In this descriptive study, 256 samples of herbal waters and 191 samples of rose waters (total samples of 447) distributed in Kashan during 2012 to 2013 were purchased and transferred to laboratory. Then microbial tests such as total aerobic bacterial count, mold and yeast count, total *coliforms*, and detection of *Enterococcus, Pseudomonas* and *sulphite-reducing Clostridia* were evaluated based on national standard of Iran.

Results: Contamination with *Pseudomonas* and *Enterococcus* was observed in the herbal water samples. 196 cases (43.84%) of the total samples, 113 cases (44.15%) of the herbal waters and 83 cases (43.45%) of the rose waters were usable based on the national standard of Iran. Neither herbal waters nor rosewater samples were contaminated by *E.Coli* and *Sulphite-reducing clostridia*. Additionally, none of the rosewater samples was contaminated by *Coliforms* and *Pseudomonas.*

Conclusion: Based on the findings and due to the fact that these products are contaminated with aerobic mesophilic bacteria, mold and yeast, to minimize the risks we recommend to apply pasteurized temperature, high-quality packaging material and hygiene observance in processing time of herbal waters and rose waters.

Implication for health policy/practice/research/medical education:
The herbal products such as the ones distributed in Kashan might be contaminated with aerobic mesophilic bacteria, mold and yeast, therefore, it is suggested that manufacturers of herbal waters pay attention to the hygiene observance, Good Hygiene Practice, the use of pasteurization temperatures, observance of condition of the manufactory and appropriate packaging in the manufacturing processes to reduce secondary contamination and enhance the quality of the final product.

Introduction

Medicinal plants are of the most valuable natural resources found in a wide range in Iran. The use of herbs to treat diseases has a long history in many countries, especially in Iran (1). Herbal waters and rose waters are used for nutritional purposes in many foodstuffs like sweets and ice creams as well as in treating rheumatic and heart pain, and strengthening the stomach. In addition, rose waters are also used in religious ceremonies and pilgrimage places (1,2).

Nowadays, the herb therapy and drugs of plant origin are increasingly used; in a way that about one-third to half of medicinal products found in the United States enjoy herbal origin (3). Besides, herbal products and lots of

***Corresponding author**: Reza Sharafati Chaleshtori, Research Center for Biochemistry and Nutrition in Metabolic Diseases, Kashan University of Medical Sciences, Kashan, Iran.
E- mail: sharafati33@yahoo.com

supplements are produced in the United Kingdom in a safe and risk-free form (3,4). In addition to public people, clinical microbiologists tend highly to use these drugs in the treatment of infections in that comparatively the side effects of these drugs are significantly lower than chemical drugs. In a study it was shown that consumption of medicinal plants increased 38% in 1990 and 1997, and revenue from the sale of these products was about 5.1 billion dollars in 1997 (5).

Bacteria are of the major causes of microbial infections and food borne poisoning. Over the past decade, the incidence of food borne microbial diseases in the developing and developed countries has been overwhelming, while there is no exact statistics of incidence and the occurrence of infections and food borne poisoning, especially in developing countries (6). The evaluation of existence of a variety of the microorganisms in herbal extracts is a mean to determine their hygienic status of this product. Also, pathogenic microbes such as enterobacter, enterococcus, shigella and streptococcus have been shown to grow on herbal materials (2). Therefore, of the most important evaluation of these products is the existence of coliforms indicating its fecal contamination (1).

Escherichia coli is a normal flora in the intestines of humans and many warm-blooded animals and they are reported to be 10^9 CFU/g. Thus, it was suggested as the specific indicator of fecal contamination in 1982. In microbial tests, searching for *coliforms* spp. are utilized as an important indicator of health products such as herbal extracts (7).

Enterococcus is resistant bacteria to bile salts and sodium azide and these bacteria can confirm fecal contamination of food material through the presence or absence of *Coliform*. Hence, these are used as a secondary indicator of fecal contamination in foodstuffs (8).

Regarding to the spending too much time and money in identifying different types of foodborne pathogens, identification of indicator microorganisms was carried out. As an example, *sulphite-reducing Clostridia* are anaerobic bacteria, producing spores and belong to genus *Clostridia* and *Bacillaceae* family. Spores of *sulfite-reducing Clostridia* are widely distributed in the environment. They are found in human and animal faeces as well as in sewage and soil. Unlike coliforms and *E. coli*, they remained alive in water for a long time and are more resistant against chemical and physical agents compared to vegetative forms and can indicate the presence of defects in the refining process of the products and are presented as an indicator of intermittent contamination (7,9). In a study in Birjand, the microbial contamination of herbal waters was reported to be 80% (1).

So far, a few studies on microbial and hygienic quality of herbal waters and rosewaters have been done in Iran. According to the consumption approach to this product in raw as a medicinal herbal product, this study was carried out to examine the microbial quality of herbal waters and rose waters distributed in Kashan, Iran.

Materials and Methods

Sample collection

This is a descriptive study carried out on 256 samples of herbal waters and 191 samples of rose waters (totally 447 samples) distributed in Kashan during the 2012 to 2013. Food samples were taken to Kashan University of Medical Sciences for laboratory tests. Then microbial tests were performed according to Iranian national standards with the code numbers as follow: 3270, 3545, 5272, 7724-2, 7725-1, 5353, 4207 and 8869 (10-17).

Total aerobic bacterial count

The total bacteria were counted by pour plate method in the plate count agar (Merck ink, Darmstadt, Germany). Then they were incubated for 72 h in the temperature of 30±1 °C (10).

Mold and yeast count

To count mold and yeast, 100 ml of sample passed through a sterile filters (0.22 μm) and through using a forceps, filter was placed onto the surface of the Yeast Extract Glucose Chloramphenicol Agar (YGCA; Merck Ink, Darmstadt, Germany) and then, the media were incubated at 25 °C for 3 to 5 days (11).

Detection of coliforms spp. and E.coli

In order to detect *coliforms* spp. and *E.coli*, 100 ml of the sample was passed through sterile filter (0.22 μm). The filter was placed on the surface of MacConkey agar medium (Merck ink, Darmstadt, Germany) by means of a sterile forceps. It was incubated at 37 °C for 24 to 48 h at 37 °C. In the case of colonies growth, they were counted and reported in the samples of 100 ml. The grown colonies were used for differential diagnosis of *E. coli* by TSI, SIM, MR-VP and urea Tests (Merck ink, Darmstadt, Germany) (16).

Detection of Enterococcus spp.

To detect *Enterococcus* spp., 100 ml of the sample was passed through sterile filter (0.22 μm). The filter was placed on the KF *Enterococcus* (Merck ink, Darmstadt, Germany) specific culture using sterile forceps. The plates were incubated at 37 °C for 48 h. The Formation of colonies with red, cherry and pink color demonstrated the existence of *Enterococcus* (15).

Detection of Pseudomonas

Pseudomonas presence was monitored by passing 100 ml of samples through sterile filter (0.22 μm), cultivating the filter retentive on the surface of cetrimide agar (Merck ink, Darmstadt, Germany) using sterile forceps. Then plates were incubated for 24 to 48 h at 37 °C. The formation of colonies with green color indicates the presence of

Pseudomonas (14).

Detection of sulfite-reducing Clostridia

Samples were put into water bath to monitor *sulfite-reducing Clostridia* presence. Heating at 70 °C for 20 min causes heat shock and spores transformation to vegetative form. After cooling, 100 ml of the sample was passed through a membrane filter. By means of sterile forceps, filter was placed on specific Sulfite Polymyxin Sulfadiazine culture (SPS). Then the medium was incubated in an anaerobic jar at 42 °C for 48 h. If sulfite- reducing *Clostridia*, are present in the sample, black colonies will be observed (17).

Statistical analysis

The data were analyzed using SPSS software version 11.5 through Fisher's exact test.

Results

Based on the results gained from the total sample, 43.84 percent (196 cases) of the herbal waters and rosewaters were usable according to national standards of Iran and 56.16% (251 cases) were non-usable. 108 cases (42.18%) of herbal water samples were uncountable regarding to the total count of mesophilic bacteria and total bacteria count for 116 (45.32%) cases was less than 100 cfu/ml. Also, 32 cases (12.5%) of samples had total bacterial count between 10^2 to 6 $\times 10^3$ cfu/ml which had an average of $1.153\times10^3\pm1.738\times10^3$ cfu/ml. Nine cases (3.5%) of samples shown contamination combined to mold and yeast and high contamination count to mesophilic bacteria. Only one case (0.3%) of samples had contamination of combined with high counts of mesophilic bacteria and identified *Enterococcus*. Besides, one sample (0.3%) associated with high count of contamination of mesophilic bacteria, mold, yeast and *Pseudomonas* was observed. Of rose water samples, 72 (37.7%) of the total count of mesophilic bacteria were uncountable and 85 (44.5%) of their total bacteria counts were less than 100. Total bacterial counts were between 10^2 to 6×10^3 cfu/ml for 34 (17.8%) of samples, which had an average of $1.656\times10^3\pm2.031\times10^3$ cfu/ml. The comparative distribution of contamination of herbal water and rose water samples based on microbial tests are presented in Table 1.

Based on the obtained results, there was no significant difference between usability and non-usability of distributed herbal waters and rose waters ($p>0.05$). The results gained from the microbial tests presented as acceptability and unacceptability of herbal water and rosewater samples based on the national standard of Iran are shown in Table 2.

Also, there was significant difference between usability and non-usability conventionally herbal water samples and the industrially herbal water samples ($p<0.05$). 24.68% conventionally herbal waters and 52.52% industrially herbal water samples were usable.

The comparative distribution of herbal water samples which were consumable based on traditional and industrial process are presented in Table 3. The maximum permitted number of bacteria, based on the national standards of Iran, can be seen in Table 4.

Table 1. Comparative distribution of contamination of herbal water and rose water samples based on Microbiological tests

	Microbiological tests							Total
	Total bacteria count (cfu/ml)*	*Coliforms*	*Enterococcus*	*Pseudomonas*	*Sulfite-reducing Clostridia*	Mold	Yeast	
Kind of herbal products								
Herbal waters	$1.153\times10^3\pm1.738\times10^3$	0.35% (1)	0.7% (2)	0.35% (1)	0% (0)	10.5% (27)	12.9% (33)	100% (256)
Rose waters	$1.656\times10^3\pm2.031\times10^3$	0% (0)	0.53% (1)	0% (0)	0% (0)	5.76% (11)	9.43% (18)	100% (191)

*Average ± SD for Total bacteria count

Table 2. Comparative distribution of consumability of herbal water and rose water samples based on Iranian national standards

Microbiological tests	Usable		Unusable	
	Herbal waters	Rose waters	Herbal waters	Rose waters
Total bacterial count	48.82%	44.5%	51.18%	55.5%
Mold	89.5%	94.24%	10.5%	5.76%
Yeast	87.1%	90.57%	12.9%	9.43%
Coliforms	99.7%	100%	0.3%	0%
Enterococcus	99.3%	99.47%	0.7%	0.53%
Pseudomonas	99.7%	100%	0.3%	0%
Sulfite-reducing Clostridia	100%	100%	0%	0%

Table 3. Comparative distribution of consumability of herbal water samples based on traditional and industrial process

Kind of process	Usable	Unusable	Total number
Traditional	19 (24.68%)	58 (75.32%)	77
Industrial	94 (52.52%)	85 (47.48%)	179

Table 4. microbiological properties of herbal waters and rose waters based on Iranian national standards

Maximum limit in 100 cc	Microbiological properties						
	Total bacterial count	Mold	Yeast	*Coliforms*	*Enterococcus*	*pseudomonas*	*sulfite-reducing Clostridia*
Herbal waters	200 cfu/ml	0	0	0	0	0	0
Rose waters	100 cfu/ml	0	0	0	0	0	0

Discussion

Based on the obtained results, 113 cases of herbal water (44.15%) and 83 rosewater (43.45%) samples were non-usable based on the national standards of Iran. That was due to the excessive existence of aerobic mesophilic bacteria, mold and yeast, *coliforms* detection, identification of *Pseudomonas* and *Enterococcus* in them. However, in none of the samples, *E. coli* and *sulfite reducing Clostridia* was observed. Given that none of the health indicator microorganisms, especially fecal contamination (18) was isolated from the samples, it might be indicated that compliance of employees with the terms of individual hygiene and cross contamination are during production and post-production of herbal waters and rose waters. However, the presence of one case of *Pseudomonas* and one case of *Enterococcus* in herbal waters caused it to be non-usable. As mentioned above, the samples was diagnosed as non-usable according to the total count of mesophilic bacteria by pour plate method and mold and yeast count based on membrane filtration based on the national standard of Iran. In a way that, out of 246 cases (55.03 %) of the samples, the total amount of bacterial count exceeded the standard level and 37 (8.27%) and 51 (11.4%) cases of the samples have been out of standard limit according to the mold and yeast count.

These infections can be due to the lack of pasteurization, the use of contaminated glass and plastic bottles and lack of proper cap-packaging of herbal waters and rose waters (19).

According to the National Public Health Service (NHS), pour plate method of counting bacteria alone cannot be used to show the dangers threatening food safety, such as water. The method is more appropriate to evaluate the healthiness of groundwater resources and to determine the efficiency of water refining processes such as coagulation, filtration and disinfection and can indicate the health and cleanliness of the water distribution system (7,19).

The present study was consistent with the study of Soltan Dallal *et al.* (7). In this study, the application of membrane filtration technique to detect *Coliforms* and *E. coli*, along with other microorganisms such as *pseudomonas aeruginosa, Enterococcus, sulfite-reducing Clostridia* was diagnosed as appropriate.

In a way that, for example, most probable number method (MPN) can increase application of medium membrane filtration technique to detect mentioned microorganisms in liquid foods such as herbal waters and rose waters for the detection of *Coliforms* and *E.coli* due to the time-consumability, hard labor of workforce needs to a large area for culture (7). So far, a few studies have been done for the microbial quality of herbal waters and rose waters. In a study in 2005, microbial quality of rose waters distilled by conventional and industrial methods by production manufactory in Kashan showed that 63.97% of all the samples were non-usable from Iranian national standards point of view. In a way that, all conventionally distilled samples were non-usable and 35.41% of the industrial rosewater samples were usable. It is also suggested that the traditional manufactory of rosewaters be converted to industrial plants (19). In the present study, the 43.45% of distributed rosewaters were usable. Also, 75.32% conventionally herbal waters and 47.48% industrially herbal water samples were non-usable. In a study by Khodadi *et al.*, 80% of traditional herbal waters in Birjand were microbial contaminated, but this contamination was observed in 60% of industrially herbal waters. In addition, in another study by Fazl Ara *et al.*, in 14.81% of the traditionally herbal waters *Enterococcus* spp. were identified by impedance method (1,20).

The results of this study indicate the microbial contamination of both herbal waters and rose waters but in none of the samples, microbial indicators of fecal contamination was detected.

Despite the antibacterial properties of various medicinal plants and herbal waters prepared from them, one of the reason for bacterial activity observed in the understudy herbal waters may be to due lack of hygiene practices during their collection and distillation. It may also be due to their antibacterial effects reduction as they are diluted.

Conclusion

Based on the results of this study, it is suggested that manufacturers of herbal waters pay attention to the hygiene observance, Good Hygiene Practice (GHP), the use of pasteurization temperatures, observance of condition of the manufactory and Good Manufacturing Practices

(GMP) and appropriate packaging in the manufacturing processes to reduce secondary contamination and enhance the quality of the final product.

Acknowledgments
Thanks to the personnel of the deputy of food and drug affiliated to the Kashan University of Medical Sciences for the cooperation in the implementation of this research.

Authors' Contributions
All authors had equal role in design, work, statistical analysis and manuscript writing.

Conflict of interests
The authors declare no conflict of interests.

Ethical considerations
Ethical issues (including plagiarism, misconduct, data fabrication, falsification, double publication or submission, redundancy) have been completely observed by the author.

Funding/Support
This research was financially supported by Kashan University of Medical Sciences, Kashan, Iran.

References

1. Khodadadi M, Motamed Rezaei O, Jahani M, Dorri H. The survey on Bacterial and fungi contamination of herbaceous distillates that distributed in Birjand city. J Birjand Univ Med Sci 2012; 19: 51-8.
2. Zhang J, Wider B, Shang H, Li X, Ernst E. Quality of herbal medicines: challenges and solutions. Complement Ther Med 2012; 20:100-6.
3. Sharafati-Chaleshtori R, Rokni N, Razavilar V, Rafieian-Kopaei M. Evaluation of antibacterial and antioxidant activity of Tarragon (Artemisia dracunculus L.) essential oil and its chemical composition. Jundishapur J Microbiol 2013; 6: doi: 10.5812/jjm.7877
4. Safavi F, Ebrahimi P, Mighani H. In vitro anti-bacterial activity of root and aerial parts of scrophularia striata bioss on escherichia coli, staphylococcus aureus and bacillus cereus. Armaghane-danesh 2013; 18: 603-14.
5. Alkhateeb FM, Doucette WR, Ganther-Urmie JM. Influences on consumer spending for herbal products. Res Social Adm Pharm 2006; 2: 254-65.
6. Zolfaghari MR, Gaeini R, Kalhor N, Khalilian M, Razavian MH, Soleimani Sasani M. Study of microbial contamination of milk and pasteurization dairy products in Qom province. J Microbial World 2012; 5: 47-57.
7. Soltan Dallal MM, Khaksar R, Tabatabaei Bafroei A, Norozizan S, Fazelifard P, Fakharian F, *et al*. Evaluation of contamination in available bottled potable water by filtration method. J Microbial Biotech 2009; 1:14-7.
8. Safari R, Yaghoubzadeh Z. Bacterial Bioindicators in Shirood River in Mazandaran Province. J Mazandaran Univ Med Sci 2013; 23: 289-99.
9. Lee FC, Hakim SL, Kamaluddin MA, Thong KL. Clostridium perfringens and sulphite reducing clostridia densities in selected tropical Malaysian rivers. Southeast Asian J Trop Med Public Health 2012; 43:129-35.
10. Institute of standards and industrial research of Iran. Microbiology of food and animal feeding stuffs-Horizontal method for the enumeration of microorganisms – Colony count technique at 30°C. ISIRI Number. 5272, 2007.
11. Institute of standards and industrial research of Iran. Water quality - Enumeration of microorganisms in water by culture - Guideline. ISIRI Number 4207, 2007.
12. Institute of standards and industrial research of Iran. Microbiology of herbaceous distillates – Specifications. ISIRI Number 3545, 2007.
13. Institute of standards and industrial research of Iran. Microbiology of rose water–Specifications. ISIRI Number 3270, 2007.
14. Institute of standards and industrial research of Iran. Water quality – Detection and enumeration of pseudomonas aeruginosa by membrane filtration method. ISIRI Number 8869, 2006.
15. Institute of standards and industrial research of Iran. Water quality- Detection and enumeration of intestinal enterococci. ISIRI Number 7724-2, 2004.
16. Institute of standards and industrial research of Iran. Water quality- Detection and enumeration of Escherichia coli and coliform bacteria. ISIRI Number 7725-1, 2004.
17. Institute of standards and industrial research of Iran. Detection and Enumeration of the Spores of Sulfite - reducing Anaerobes (clostridia) - Method by Membrane filteration. ISIRI Number 5353, 2002.
18. Jayakody P, Parajuli PB, Brooks JP. Evaluating spatial and temporal variability of fecal coliform bacteria loads at the pelahatchie watershed in Mississippi. Hum Ecol Risk Assess 2014; 20: 1023-41.
19. Peymaneh Abedi Mohtasab T, Heidarzadeh H, Doulati M, Hossieni A. Evaluation of the microbial quality of traditional rose water and industrial rose water in Kashan, 2005. 9th Iranian Nutrition Congress. Tabriz: Tabriz University of Medical Sciences; 2006.
20. Fazlara A, Tuiserkani A. Hygienic evaluation of herbal waters from the aspect of enterococci with using impedance-splitting method. 10th Iranian Congress of Microbiology. Ilam: Ilam University of Medical Sciences; 2009.

6

Evaluation of antidepressant-like effect of hydroalcoholic extract of *Passiflora incarnata* in animal models of depression in male mice

Nima Jafarpoor[1], Saeid Abbasi-Maleki[1*], Majid Asadi-Samani[2], Mir Hadi Khayatnouri[3]

[1]Department of Pharmacology, Urmia Branch, Islamic Azad University, Urmia, Iran
[2]Medical Plants Research Center, Shahrekord University of Medical Sciences, Shahrekord, Iran
[3]Department of Pharmacology, Tabriz Branch, Islamic Azad University, Tabriz, Iran

ARTICLE INFO

Keywords:
Passiflora incarnata
Hydroalcoholic extract
Forced swim test
Tail suspension test
Mice

ABSTRACT

Introduction: *Passiflora incarnata* (PI) is one of the commonest herbal anti-anxiety and sedative agents. The aim of the present study was to investigate the antidepressant effect of hydroalcoholic extract of PI in forced swim test (FST) and tail suspension test (TST) in male mice.
Methods: In this experimental study, 48 male mice were randomly divided into 6 groups of 8: Negative and positive control groups received normal saline (10 ml/kg), fluoxetine (20 mg/kg) and imipramine (30 mg/kg), respectively and treatment groups received extracts of PI (200, 400 and 800 mg/kg). Immobility, swimming and climbing behaviors were recorded during 6-min.
Results: All doses of PI extract compared to control group significantly reduced the duration of immobility time in both of two tests ($p<0.001$). Also, these extracts increased swimming time ($p<0.001$) without significant change of climbing time.
Conclusion: PI has considerable antidepressant-like effect in animal models of depression. However, further studies are needed to determine its exact mechanism of action.

Implication for health policy/practice/research/medical education:
considerable antidepressant-like effect in animal models of depression and its usage might be useful in depressive patients.

Introduction

Depression is a prevalent psychiatric dysfunction that is identified with depressed mood, loss of interest or pleasure, feelings of guilt or low value, disturbance of sleep and appetite, low power and poor centralization, interfering with normal function, and often has problems at work, community and family. According to the World Health Organization (WHO), depression will become the second factor contributing to disability of disease in 2020 (1,2). It has been shown that various factors such as psychological-social, genetic and biological factors play a role as causing depression. However, one of the major biological causes of depression is reduction in the amount of neurotransmitters such as serotonin (5-hydroxytriptamine, 5HT), dopamine (DA) and noradrenalin (NA) (3,4).

Nowadays, various pharmacological treatments, including tricyclic antidepressants, selective serotonin reuptake inhibitors, monoamine oxidase inhibitors and selective serotonin-noradrenalin inhibitors are used (5). These drugs exert their effects by increasing the amount of brain monoamines (6). However, most of these drugs cause some unwanted symptoms and their mechanism of action has not been very satisfactory. Therefore, it is essential to search new, strong and especially healthy drugs (7).

*__Corresponding author__: Saeid Abbasi Maleki, Pharmacology Department, Urmia Branch, Islamic Azad University, Urmia, Iran.
Email: dr.s.a.maleki@gmail.com

Passionflower is an herbaceous plant with the scientific name of *Passiflora incarnate* (PI). This plant is a perennial herb and has a climbing or trailing stem with alternate and lobed leaves. It shows individual blue flowers. Fruits are green and after ripening will be orange. This plant is cultivated in different countries and even in northern Iran as an ornamental plant. It has been shown that passion flower has a number of compounds including flavonoids, the cyanogenic glycosides, indole alkaloids and other alkaloids, such as the passiflorine, harmaline, harmine and harmalol in its building. Studies have reported that passion flower has different effects such as analgesic, anticonvulsant, anti-bacterial, anti-anxiety, hypnotics, sedatives, etc. (8,9). Considering that no study already has been done on anti- depression effects of passionflower; the purpose of the present study was to investigate the effect of passionflower hydroalcoholic extract in the forced swim test and the tail suspension test as two animal models of depression in male mice.

Materials and Methods

In this experimental study, 48 male albino mice NMRI (weighing 20 to 30 g) were randomly divided into 6 groups of 8. Animals were housed in cages of 5 at 22 ± 1 °C in a 12-h light/dark cycle, and had free access to water and food. Each animal was evaluated only once. Animals were transferred laboratory to adapt to the lab environment for 48 hours before testing. All procedures in this study were performed in accordance with the NIH Guide for the Care and Use of Laboratory Animals. The experimental protocol was approved by the Committee on Animal Research; Urmia Medical University.

In this study, fluoxetine hydrochloride (Arya Pharmaceutical Co., Iran), imipramine hydrochloride (medicine Pars Co., Iran) and PI hydroalcoholic extract (Iran Darouk Pharmaceutical Co., Iran); all in powder form were used. All drugs and extracts were dissolved in normal saline (NS 0.9%) and administered intraperitoneally (i.p.) at a constant volume of 10 ml/kg.

The negative control group or normal saline group received normal saline (10 ml/kg, i.p). Positive control groups received fluoxetine (20 ml/kg, i.p) and imipramine (30 ml/kg, i.p). The other three groups were treated with different doses of 200, 400 and 800 mg/kg of PI hydroalcoholic extract, respectively.

In the forced swim test (FST), mice were separately placed in cylindrical containers, with dimensions of 8 × 12 × 25 cm, containing water at 25 °C, 30 min after injection of extracts or drugs. Each mouse was judged to be immobile when it ceased struggling and remained floating motionless in the water, making only those movements necessary to keep its head above water. The whole test was 6 minutes, 2 minutes to match the animal to the environment, and next 4 minutes were recorded as immobility time, swimming time and climbing time in seconds by the chronometer (10). In the forced swim test, immobility time and its reduction were recorded as depression and anti-depression effect, respectively. Swimming is equivalent to active movements of the hands and feet of the animal and the rotation around the cylinder, and climbing is also equivalent to active movements of animal hands on the walls of the cylinder (11). Tail suspension test (TST) is also an additional common animal model for estimating depression in animals. In this test, the metal legs with a height of 70 cm were used and a string of 50 cm was longitudinally stretched between two metal legs. Mice tail was closed by a clause and the animal was hung on the tail. In this part also the test began with a rush mice, 30 min after drug or extract administration. The immobility time was considered when the animal was completely immobile, disabled and had no response. The period of this test, the same as the previous method, was 6 minutes, again first 2 minutes to match the animal to the environment and next 4 minutes were recorded as immobility time in seconds by the chronometer. In both tests, all the samples were recorded by a person who did not know which sample belonged to which group. The test was performed 30 min after drug or extract injection (12).

In this study, one-way analysis of variance (one-way ANOVA) and Tukey test were used. The statistical analysis was performed using SPSS, version 19, and in each case the $p<0.05$ was considered as the significance level.

Results

The results of this study showed that normal saline injection caused no significant change in the immobility, swimming and climbing times compared with the situation before the injection. Therefore, all experimental groups were compared with saline as a negative control.

Results showed that all three doses of hydroalcoholic extract of PI in the forced swim test (128.83±9.34, 114.14±6.64 and 99.73±9.15 respectively; $p<0.001$) and tail suspension test (120.03±10.49, 97.98± 8.51 and 76.72± 6.05 respectively; $p<0.001$) significantly reduced the immobility time compared with control groups (189.11±7.25 and 197.55±3.86 respectively) (Figure 1 and 2).

Fluoxetine and imipramine in comparison with the control group significantly decreased the immobility time (73.55± 7.03 and 23.79±5.36 respectively; $p<0.001$) (Figure 1). Both drugs also reduced immobility time in the tail-supension test (128.6± 6.02 and 27.08±3.73 respectively; $p<0.001$) (Figure 2).

Doses of hydroalcoholic extract of passion flower (107.67±9.67, 120.84±5.69 and 138.21±10.41 respectively; $p<0.001$) compared with the control group (44.56±6.84) significantly increased the swimming time (Figure 1). Climbing behavior did not increase significantly by any of the doses of extract (Figure 1). In this section, fluoxetine increased swimming behavior compared to the control group (153.85±11.3; $p<0.001$), without significant change of climbing behavior ($p>0.05$) (Figure 1). But conversely, imipramine increased the climbing behavior (105.66±11.39; $p=0.000$), but was not observed a

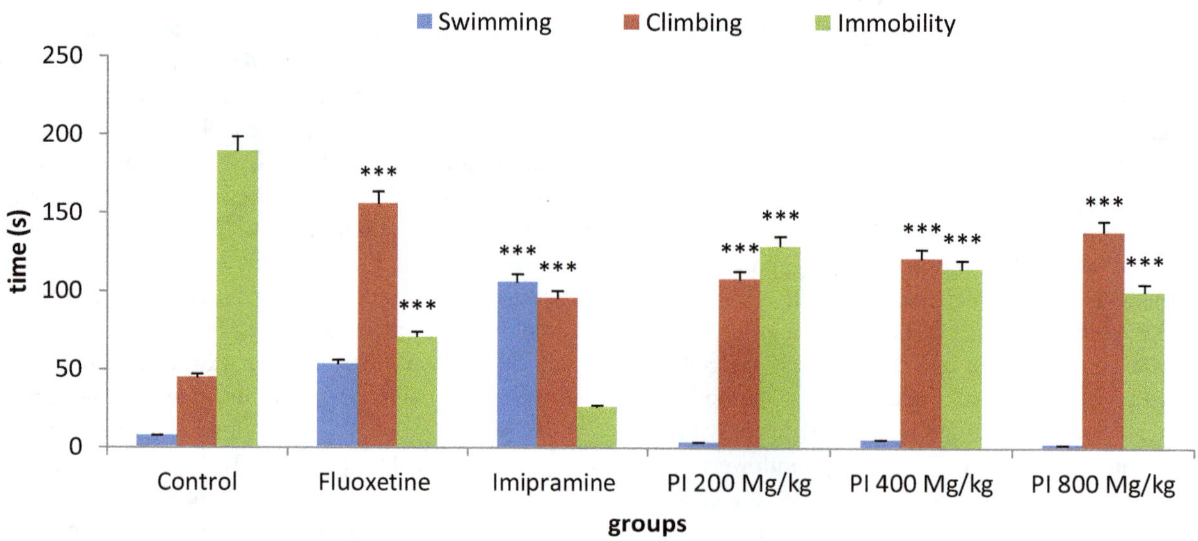

Figure 1. The effect of different doses of hydroalcoholic extract of *Passiflora incarnata* (PI; 200, 400, and 800 mg/kg; i.p), fluoxetine (20 mg/kg; i.p), and imipramine (30 mg/kg; i.p) on immobility, swimming and climbing in the forced swimming test in mice. The data are shown as Mean±SEM; ***significant at $p<0.05$ compared with control group.

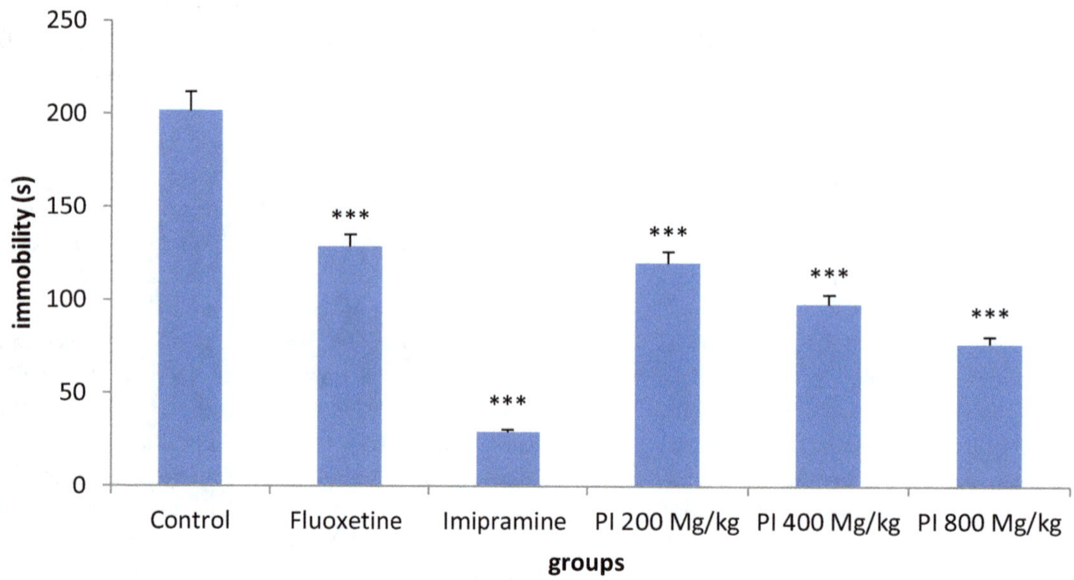

Figure 2. The effect of different doses of hydroalcoholic extract of *Passiflora incarnata* (PI; 200, 400, and 800 mg/kg; i.p), fluoxetine (20 mg/kg; i.p), and imipramine (30 mg/kg; i.p) on immobility time in the tail-supension test in male mice. The data are shown as Mean±SEM; ***significant at $p<0.05$ comparison with control group.

significant increase in the swimming behavior ($p<0.05$) (Figure 1).

Discussion

In this study, the antidepression effects of hydroalcoholic extract of PI were studied in mice by using FST and TST as an animal models of depression. Forced swim test is one of the most commonly used animal models for estimating the anti-depression effects of chemical and herbal agents in mice and rats. This model is sensitive to the effects of all medications and extracts (13). Tail suspension test is also among other animal models to estimate the effect of antidepressants. This test unlike the FST, does not lead to a stress and reduction in body temperature that usually is caused by the forced swim test (14). The results of this study demonstrated that different doses of PI extract compared with the control group decreased immobility time in both the FST and TST. On the other hand, the extract increased swimming time, but climbing behavior did not significantly enhance. The results of the present in accordance with other findings. The effects of fluoxetine and imipramine were demonstrated in the FST and TST (15,16). In other words, previous studies have reported that the drugs with serotonergic mechanism (e.g. fluoxetine) reduce the time immobility, increase the swimming time, without any significant change of climbing time. On the hand, drugs with noradrenergic mechanisms reduce the immobility time, increase the climbing time and the changes are not significant in the swimming time (17,18). Although the exact mechanism of antidepression effect of PI has not been established, but consistent with other findings and conclusions of this study, the effects of the PI extract is similar to fluoxetine. In support of these findings, studies have shown that PI has several compounds in its building, but among them, the beta-carboline alkaloids such as harmaline, harmine and harmalol have anti-depression properties (19). In this regard, it has been shown that these alkaloids are irreversible monoamine oxidase-A inhibitors (20). There are two isoforms (MAO-A and MAO-B) for the monoamine oxidase enzyme. MAO-A inhibits reduce the degeneration of adrenaline and serotonin in the brain, but MAO-B inhibits reduce the degeneration of dopamine. Thus, MAO-A inhibitors are used in depression and MAO-B inhibitors are applied in diseases such as Parkinson's (21,22). Therefore, inhibition of MAO-A by the passion flower alkaloids increases the amount of adrenaline and serotonin in the brain of animals treated with it (19). In agreement with these findings, it has been shown that the harmine binds to MAO-A and many cell surface receptors, including the serotonin receptor 2A (5HT2A) that are involved in pharmacotherapy for depression (23-25). On the other hand, other studies have reported that harman and other beta-carbolines can cause a wide range of antagonistic effects against benzodiazepines via binding to inverse agonist sites of GABA-A receptors. Unlike benzodiazepines that bind to benzodiazepine receptor sites (BZ1 and BZ2) and reduce norepinephrine and serotonin release, beta-carbolines bind to inverse agonist sites and increase catecholamines and serotonin release (26,27). In support of these findings, flumazenil (antagonist of benzodiazepine receptors and an inverse agonist) antagonized the beta-carboline effect (28). Thus, it seems that serotonergic and GABAergic systems involved in PI antidepressant effects.

Conclusion

According to the results of this study, PI has considerable antidepressant-like effect in animal models of depression. However, concomitant use of serotonin and GABA antagonists along with the PI extract, and isolation of each of its components and evaluation of them on depression is recommended in order to determine the exact mechanism of PI antidepression effects.

Acknowledgements

This study is the result of DVM thesis, (No. 10310501861064), Urmia branch, Islamic Azad University. Authors of this article thank Iran Darouk Pharmaceutical Co. for delivering PI powder. The assistance of Dr. Abolhassan Tash is gratefully acknowledged.

Authors' contributions

All the authors wrote the manuscript equally.

Conflict of interests

The authors declared no competing interests.

Ethical considerations

Ethical issues (including plagiarism, misconduct, data fabrication, falsification, double publication or submission, redundancy) have been completely observed by the authors.

Funding/Support

None.

References

1. Onasanwo SA, Chatterjee M, Palit G. Antidepressant and anxiolytic potentials of dichloromethane fraction from *Hedranthera barteri*. Afr J Biomed Res 2010; 13(1): 76–81.
2. Frey BN, Lord C, Soares CN. Depression during menopausal transition: a review of treatment strategies and pathophysiological correlates. Menopause Int 2008; 14:123–128.
3. Moallem SA, Hosscinzadeh H, Ghoncheh F. Evaluation of antidepressant effect of aerial parts of Echium vulgare on mice. Iran J Basic Med Sci 2007; 10:189-196.
4. Berton O, Nestler EJ. New approaches to antidepressant drug discovery: beyond monoamines. Nat Rev 2006; 7:137–151.
5. Nemeroff CB. Stress, menopause and vulnerability for psychiatric illness. Expert Rev Neurother 2007; 7: S11–13.
6. Jithan A, Chinnalalaiah R. Synthesis and evaluation of antidepressant activity of some curcumin-like compounds. Int Pharm Communique 2009; 2:38-41.
7. Nasri H, Shirzad H. Toxicity and safety of medicinal plants. J HerbMed Plarmacol 2013; 2(2): 21-22.
8. Salehi Surmaghi MH. Medicinal Plants and Phytotherapy. 3rd edition. Tehran: Doniaie Taghzieh press;2010. p. 333-335.
9. Dhawan K, Dhawan S, Sharma A. Review Passiflora: a review update. J Ethnopharmacol 2004; 94:1–23.
10. Hosseinzadeh H, Motamedshariaty V, Hadizadeh F. Antidepressant effect of kaempferol, a constituent of saffron (*Crocus sativus*) petal, in mice and rats. Pharmacologyonline 2007; 2:367-370.
11. Potdar VH, Kibile SJ. Evaluation of antidepressant like-effect of citrus maxima leaves in animal models of depression. Iran J Basic Med Sci 2001; 14(5):478-483.
12. Li-Qin S. Information on research and application of ginseng, the king of traditional and herbal medicines. Asian J Drug Metab Pharmacokinetic 2004;

4:261-284.

13. Petit-Demouliere B, Chenu F, Bourin M. Forced swimming test in mice: a review of antidepressant activity. Psychopharmacol (Berl) 2005; 177(3):245-255.
14. Cryan JF, Mombereau C, Vassout A. The tail suspension test as a model for assessing antidepressant activity: review of pharmacological and genetic studies in mice. Neurosci Biobehav Rev 2005; 29(4-5):571-625.
15. Dhingra D, Sharma A. Evaluation of antidepressant-like activity of glycyrrhizin in mice. Indian J Pharmacol 2005;37(6):390-394.
16. Emamghoreishi M, Talebianpour. Antidepressant effect of Melissa officinalis in the forced swimming test. DARU 2009;17(1):42-47.
17. Detke MJ, Rickels M, Lucki I. Active behaviors in the rat forced swimming test differentially produced by serotonergic and noradrenergic antidepressants. Psychopharmacology (Berl) 2005;121:66-72.
18. Page ME, Detke MJ, Dalvi A, Kirby JG, Lucki I. Serotoninergic mediation of the effects of fluoxetine, but not desipramine, in the rat forced swimming test. Psychopharmacology (Berl) 1999;147:162-167.
19. Abourashad E, Vanderplank J, Khan I. High-speed extraction and HPLC fingerprinting of medicinal plants. II. Application to harman alkaloids of genus Passiflora. Pharmaceutica Biol 2003;41:100–106.
20. Callaway JC, McKenna DJ, Grob CS, Brito GS, Raymon LP, Poland RE, *et al.* Pharmacokinetics of Hoasca alkaloids in healthy humans. J Ethnopharmacol 1999; 65;243–256.
21. Ulus IH, Maher TJ, Wurtman RJ. Characterization of phentermine and related compounds as monoamine oxidase (MAO) inhibitors. Biochem Pharmacol 2000; 59: 1611–1621.
22. Mickey BI, Ducci F, Hodgkinson CA, Langenecker SA, Goldman D, Zubieta JK. Monoamine oxidase a genotype predicts human serotonin 1A receptor availability in vivo. J Neurosci 2008;28(44):11354–11359.
23. Kim DH, Jang YY, Han ES, Lee CS. Protective effect of harmaline and harmalol against dopamine- and 6-hydroxydopamine-induced oxidative damage of brain mitochondria and synaptosomes, and viability loss of PC12 cells. Eur J Neurosci 2001; 13(10): 1861-1872.
24. Glennon RA, Dukat M, Grella B, Hong SS, Costantino L, Teitler M, *et al.* Binding of β-carbolines and related agents at serotonin (5-HT2 and 5-HT1A), dopamine (D2) and benzodiazepine receptors. *Drug Alcohol Depend* 2000; 60(2):121–132.
25. Preskorn SH, Baker B, Kolluri S, Menniti FS, Krams M, Landen JW. An innovative design to establish proof of concept of the antidepressant effects of the NR2B subunit selective n-methyl-d-aspartate antagonist, CP-101,606, in patients with treatment-refractory major depressive disorder. J Clinic Psychopharmacol 2008;28(6):631–637.
26. Verheij R, Timmerman L, Passchier J, Fekkes D, Pepplinkhuizen L. Trait anxiety, coping with stress, and norharman. Psychol Rep 1997; 80(1):51-59.
27. Buckholtz NS, Boggan WO. Monoamine oxidase inhibition in brain and liver produced by betacarbolines: structure-activity relationships and substrate specificity. Biochem Pharmacol 1977;26(21):1991-6.
28. Farzin D, Mansouri N. Antidepressant-like effect of harmane and other β-carbolines in the mouse forced swim test. Eur Neuropsychopharmacol 2006; 16(5): 324–328.

Evaluation of the effect of Chrysin and Caffeic acid phenethyl ester on eIF4E expression in AGS cell line

Marziyeh Abolhasani[1], Morteza Hashemzadeh-Chaleshtori[2], Abbas Doosti[1], Nematolah Amini Sarteshnizi[3], Mostafa Gholami-Arjenaki[4], Hossein Teimori[2*]

[1]Department of Biology, Islamic Azad University, Shahrekord Branch, Shahrekord, Iran
[2]Cellular and Molecular Research Center, Shahrekord University of Medical Sciences, Shahrekord, Iran
[3]Department of Biology, University of Mohaghegh Ardabili, Ardabil, Iran
[4]Clinical Biochemistry Research Center, Shahrekord University of Medical Sciences, Shahrekord, Iran

ARTICLE INFO

Keywords:
Gastric cancer
AGS cell line
eIF4E
Chrysin
CAPE

ABSTRACT

Introduction: The Ras/Akt/mTORC1 signal transduction pathways play a critical role in regulating translation and converge on initiation factor eukaryotic translation initiation factor 4E (eIF4E) which is overexpressed in various malignancies. In the current study we aimed to assess the effect of chrysin and caffeic acid phenethyl ester (CAPE) on eIF4E expression level in human stomach cancer AGS cell line.
Methods: AGS cells were treated with 15, 20, 30 and 40 µM concentration of chrysin and CAPE separately, then eIF4E expression was evaluated in treated cells using real time-PCR method.
Results: A significant decrease in eIF4E expression in the cells following 40 µM chrysin treatment was observed ($p<0.05$). There was a significant decrease in CAPE-treated cells in a dose dependent manner. Indeed the cells treated with 30 and 40 µM concentrations of CAPE, showed a significant decline in eIF4E expression ($p<0.05$).
Conclusion: Our results suggest that CAPE and chrysin may be useful as a potential therapeutic agent for treatment of gastric cancers with an elevated eIF4E expression level.

Implication for health policy/practice/research/medical education:
Chrysin and caffeic acid phenethyl ester – two components of propolis decreases eukaryotic translation initiation factor 4E (eIF4E) gene expression and might be useful in developing chemotherapeutic agents for treating human gastric cancer.

Introduction

Gastric cancer is the cause of cancer-related mortality in the world. It is the fourth most frequent cancer while is the second most common cause of cancer death (1). However, American Cancer Society has estimated that stomach cancer affects 21,600 new cases in the USA in 2013 (2). This disease had more prevalence in Asian populations, including Korea, Japan, and China (3). Despite considerable improvements in surgical, chemo, radio and other adjuvant therapies, the five-year survival rate of patients at the advanced stage remains less than 20 to 25% (4,5). Recently, regulation of oncogenesis that is grip of eukaryotic translation initiation factor 4E (eIF4E), has been considered by many researchers. eIF4E is one of the subunits of eIF4F complex which recognizes the 5′ cap structure of spectrum mRNAs involving in angiogenesis, metastasis and cell growth (6) which is activated via PI3K/AKT signaling pathway (7,8). Recently, there have been many reports on the elevated levels of eIF4E in various human cancers such as human gastric cancer cell lines (9). Hence, expression of this factor may be a potential target for therapeutic purpose for cancer.

***Corresponding author**: Hossein Teimori, Cellular and Molecular Research Center, Shahrekord University of Medical Sciences, Shahrekord, Iran. Email: hosseintimm@yahoo.com

Chrysin and Caffeic Acid Phenyl Ster (CAPE) are two components of propolis. This components have important biological roles. It has been proposed that propolis components such as chrysin and CAPE could be potential candidate agents in treatment of cancer due to their beneficial anticancer properties (10-12). It has been demonstrated before that Chrysin and CAPE may have an anti-cancer properties because of apoptotic induction and inactivation of PI3K/Akt pathways effects (13-15).
Many studies have reported an elevated activity of PI3K/Akt pathways and expression of eIF4E in cancer cells (9,16) and it has been proposed that chrysin may inactive PI3K/Akt signaling pathway through down-regulation of NF-kB pathway and conversely, activating of IAP. Thus, it might play an important role in apoptosis induction by promoting caspase-3 activity (15). Moreover, U937 cells treated by chrysin have shown an increased cytochrome c release from the mitochondria into cytosol (15).
CAPE and Chrysin activate several caspases, they inhibit PI3K/Akt signal pathway, IAP, c-FLIP (anti-apoptotic proteins), and lead to suppress in the activity of IKK and NF-kB (11,12). Considering multiple beneficial effects of CAPE and Chrysin in apoptosis and down-regulating of eIF4E, we conducted an experiment to evaluate eIF4E mRNA expression with this component in gastric cancer AGS cell line.

Materials and Methods

Cell culture and treatment

In this experimental study, the human AGS cell line was obtained from Royan institute and was cultured in DMEM supplemented with 10% FBS and 1% Penicillin-streptomycin.
IC50 was determined in AGS cells following incubation a serial dilutions of chrysin (Sigma Aldrich cat#:C80105) and CAPE (Sigma Aldrich cat#:C8221) separately for 48 h. Then AGS cells were treated with Chrysin and CAPE in four concentration 15, 20, 30 and 40 μM for 48 h in triplicate.

RNA extraction and cDNA synthesize

Total RNA was extract using Biozol (cat# BSC51M1) according Kit protocol. RNA concentration was measured by NanoDrop1000 UV-Vis spectrophotometer (Thermo Scientific Inc., USA). Then, cDNA was synthesized according to the manufacturer's instructions (Thermo Scientific Inc., USA).

Real time PCR assay

Real time-PCR was performed using Rotor-Gene 3000 (Corbett Robotics, Australia), Maxima SYBR Green/Rox qPCR Master Mix (Thermo Scientific Inc., USA) and specific primers. Primer sequences for eIF4E were: sense 5′-CCTACAGAAC AGATGGGCACTC-3′, antisense 5′-GCCCAAAAGTCTTCAACAGTATCA-3' (6) and for GAPDH was sense: 5′-TTCACCACCATGGAGA-AGGC-3′ RW: 5′-CCCTTTTGGCTC CACCCT-3′.
Each reaction was performed in a final 25 μl mixture containing 12.5 μl of Maxima SYBR Green/Rox qPCR Master Mix, 2 μl of each primers, 11.1 μl of DEPC Treated Water and 1 μl cDNA. Thermal cycling was performed as described herein: initial denaturation for 10 min at 95 °C; followed by 40 cycles of 95 °C for 30 s, 57 °C for 30 s and 72 °C for 30 s.
The melting carve plot profile of real time PCR product was: Ramp from 72 degrees to 95 degrees, Rising by 1 degree(s) each step, Wait for 45 s on first step, then Wait for 5 s on for each step after wards Acquire to Melt A on FAM/ SYBR. eIF4E expression was normalized with GAPDH mRNA and relative expression analyzed using $\Delta\Delta$Ct method.

Statistics analysis

The results were expressed as mean ± SD and statistical analyses were done using GraphPad Prism software (v5.01, USA) and Kruskal-Wallis tests followed by post hoc comparisons, Dunn's multiple comparison.

Results

Effect of Chrysin on eIF4E

Different chyrsin concentrations ranging around IC50 dose were used to evaluate the effect of chyrsin on expression of eIF4E.
As it is shown in Figure 1 expression of eIF4E was not significantly altered by 15, 20 and 30 μM concentrations of chrysin, whereas concentration of 40 μM markedly decreased eIF4E expression in AGS cells (3.84-fold, $p \leq 0.05$).

Effect of CAPE on eIF4E

The effect of CAPE on AGS cells is shown in Figure 2, expression of eIF4E was not significantly altered by 10, 15, and 20 concentrations of CAPE, whereas concentration of 30 and 40 μM noticeable decreased eIF4E expression in CAPE treated AGS cells (3.03-fold, $p \leq 0.05$ for

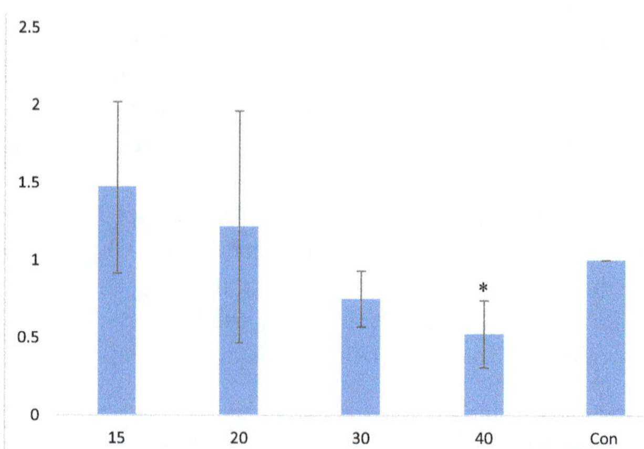

Figure 1. The effect of chrysin on eIF4E expression in AGS cells. The data are expressed as means ± SD and (*) $p \leq 0.05$ compared with the corresponding value of control group.

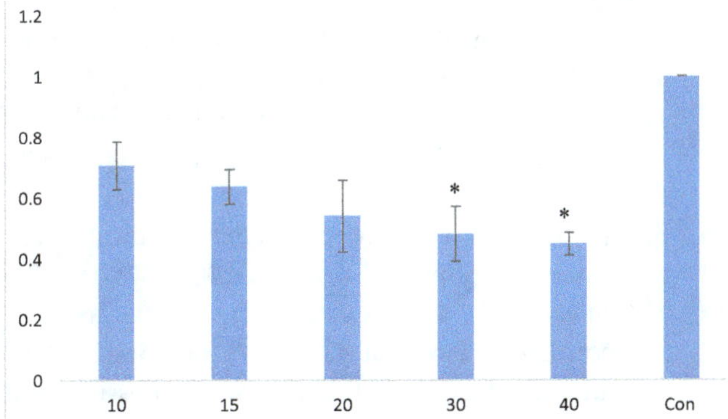

Figure 2. The effect of CAPE on eIF4E expression in AGS cells. The data are expressed as means ± SD and (*) p≤ 0.05 compared with the corresponding value of control group.

30 μl concentration and 2.85-fold, p≤0.05 for 40 μl concentration).

Discussion

Here we showed that eIF4E mRNA was down-regulated in AGS cells after chrysin or caffeic acid treatment. Many studies have shown the eIF4E up-regulation in various cancers such as gastric, prostate, breast, colon, lung and skin cancers (9,17-24). However, eIF4E regulates a set of oncogenes which control proliferation including CMYC, CDK2, Cyclin D1 or oncogenes that involved in metastasis such as MMP9 and Heparanase or oncogenes that play roles in invasion and angiogenesis like Mcl-1, Bcl-2, Survivin ,VEGF and FGF2 (7,8).

A previous study by Liang *et al* has shown that eIF4E was increased in different gastric cancer cells including AGS cell line which may involve in vascular invasion (9).

Furthermore, recent studies have provided evidence that chrysin activates Bax, p53, p21 caspases and p38 MAPK and conversely deactivates NF-κB pathway. Therefore, inhibition of IAP, c-FLIP and Akt activity derived by chrysin and caffeic acid may induce extrinsic pathway of apoptosis (11,12).

Targeting of eIF4E by ribavirin which compete with eIF4E for coupling to the m7G cap and therefore blocks eIF4E activity, led to a relative improvement in patients with acute myeloid leukemia (25). Considering the fact that Bcl2 and several capases are downstream targets of eIF4E and suppressing effects of chrysin and caffeic acid on eIF4E expression, our results support the notion that chrysin and caffeic acid may have anti-cancer effects by inducing apoptosis in cancer cells.

It has been previously shown that chrysin significantly suppressed migration and invasion of triple-negative breast cancer cells (26). Moreover, it was previously demonstrated by Samarghandian *et al* that chrysin restrain the development of lung cancer cells. They notify that chrysin induces apoptosis in cancer cells via regulation of the Bcl-2 family, caspase-3 and -9 (27).

A previous report by Lirdprapamongkol *et al* indicated a remarked over expression of VEGF in mouse T14 breast cancer cells led to resistance of these cells to apoptosis. This study showed that antimetastsic activity of DR5mAb was increased when it used with chrysin (28).

In one study that was performed by Chung *et al,* they suggest that the antimetastatic and anti-tumor effects of CAPE are mediated through the selective suppression of MMP-9 enzyme activity and transcriptional down-regulation by the dual inhibition of NF-κB as well as MMP-9 catalytic activity (29). The MMP-9 is one of eIF4E targets therefore our results that show decline of eIF4E expression in CAPE treatment cells, confirm the antimetastatic role of this companant.

Two other studies was shown that CAPE inhibits the NF-κB factor which Augments the susceptibility of intestinal epithelial cells to anticancer drugs. So, these studies present CAPE to be an effective assistant of chemotherapy and augment therapeutic efficacy therefore it can decline chemotherapy-induced toxicities (30,31).

Murtaza *et al* suggest that CAPE is an effective inhibitor of NF-κB and a stimulator of the functions of glutathione S-transferase, it drains GSH levels. Subsequently, tumor cells are radiosensitized due to this drainage (32).

With regards the co-relation of eIF4E expression with cancer incidence and our observations suggest that chrysin and caffeic acid might be promising treatments for cancer which may improve many aspects of cancer such as angiogenesis and metastasis derived by down-regulating of eIF4E expression. Moreover, since eIF4E as a key components of AKT pathway, was down-regulated by both chrysin and caffeic acid, this suggests that chrysin and caffeic acid could be useful in cancer treatment due to their suppressive effect on AKT signaling. The exact mechanism underlying the down-regulating effects of chrysin and caffeic acid on eIF4E expression remained to be elucidated. To the best of our knowledge, there are no previous report about the down-regulating effects of chrysin or caffeic acid on eIF4E.

Authors' contributions

MA and NAS performed the project. HT was the supervisor and MHC and AD were the Advisors. NAS and MGA analyzed the data and MA wrote the article.

Conflict of interests

The authors declared no competing interests.

Ethical considerations

Ethical issues (including plagiarism, misconduct, data fabrication, falsification, double publication or submission, redundancy) have been completely observed by the authors.

Funding/Support

None.

References

1. Ferlay J, Shin H, Bray F, Forman D, Mathers C, Maxwell Parkin D. Estimates of worldwide burden of cancer in 2008: GLOBOCAN 2008. Int J Cancer. 2010; 127(12): 2893-917
2. American Cancer Society. Stomach Cancer Overview. [updated 2013 march 18; cited 2013 oct 5]. Available from: http://www.cancer.org/acs/groups/cid/documents/webcontent/003077-pdf
3. Jemal A, Bray F, Center MM, Ferlay J, Ward E, Forman D. Global cancer statistics. CA Cancer J Clin 2011; 61(2): 69-90.
4. Avdulov S, Li S, Michalek V, Burrichter D, Peterson M, Perlman D, *et al.* Activation of translation complex eIF4F is essential for the genesis and maintenance of the malignant phenotype in human mammary epithelial cells. Cancer Cell 2004; 5: 553-63.
5. Chen CN, Hsieh FJ, Cheng YM, Lee PH, Chang KJ. Expression of eukaryotic initiation factor 4E in gastric adenocarcinoma and its association with clinical outcome. J Surg Oncol 2004; 86: 22-7.
6. Mamane Y, Petroulakis E, Rong L, Yoshida K, Ler LW, Sonenberg N. eIF4E – from translation to transformation. Oncogene 2004; 23: 3172–9.
7. De Benedetti A, Graff JR. eIF-4E expression and its role in malignancies and metastases. Oncogene 2004; 23: 3189-99.
8. Dong K, Wang R, Wang X, Lin F, Shen JJ, Gao P, *et al.* Tumor-specific RNAi targeting eIF4E suppresses tumor growth, induces apoptosis and enhances cisplatin cytotoxicity in human breast carcinoma cells. Breast Cancer Res Treat 2009; 113: 443-56.
9. Liang S, Guo R, Zhang Z, Liu D, Xu H, Xu Z, *et al.* Upregulation of the eIF4E signaling pathway contributes to the progression of gastric cancer, and targeting eIF4E by perifosine inhibits cell growth. Oncol Rep 2013; 29(6): 2422-30
10. Williams CA, Harborne JB, Newman M, Greenham J, Eagles J. Chrysin and other leaf exudate flavonoids in the genus Pelargonium. Phytochemistry 1997; 46: 1349-53.
11. Wua J, Omeneb C, Karkoszkaa J, Boslanda M, Eckarda J, Kleina C, *et al.* Caffeic acid phenethyl ester (CAPE), derived from a honeybee product propolis, exhibits a diversity of anti-tumor effects in pre-clinical models of human breast cancer. Cancer lett 2011; 308(1): 43-53.
12. Sawicka D, Car H, Halina Borawska M, Nikliński J. The anticancer activity of propolis. Folia Histochem Cytobiol 2012; 50(1): 25-37.
13. Lapidot T, Walker MD, Kanner J. Antioxidant and prooxidant effects of phenolics on pancreatic beta-cells in vitro. J Agric Food Chem 2002; 50: 7220-5.
14. Cho H, Yun CW, Park WK, Kong JY, Kim KS, Park Y, *et al.* Modulation of the activity of pro-inflammatory enzymes, COX-2 and iNOS, by chrysin derivatives. Pharmacol Res 2004; 49: 37-43.
15. Woo KJ, Jeong YJ, Park JW, Kwon TK. Chrysin-induced apoptosis is mediated through caspase activation and Akt inactivation in U937 leukemia cells. Biochem Biophys Res Commun 2004; 325: 1215-22.
16. Bielak-Zmijewska A. Mechanisms of tumor cell resistance to apoptosis. Kosmos 2003; 52: 157–71.
17. McClusky DR, Chu Q, Yu H, Debenedetti A, Johnson LW, Meschonat C, *et al.* A prospective trial on initiation factor 4E (eIF4E) overexpression and cancer recurrence in node-positive breast cancer. Ann Surg 2005; 242(4): 584-90.
18. Li BD, Gruner JS, Abreo F, Johnson LW, Yu H, Nawas S, *et al.* Prospective study of eukaryotic initiation factor 4E protein elevation and breast cancer outcome. Ann Surg 2002; 235(5): 732-8.
19. Jacobson BA, Alter MD, Kratzke MG, Frizelle SP, Zhang Y, Peterson MS, *et al.* Repression of cap-dependent translation attenuates the transformed phenotype in non-small cell lung cancer both in vitro and in vivo. Cancer Res 2006; 15; 66(8): 4256-62.
20. Seki N, Takasu T, Mandai K, Nakata M, Saeki H, Heike Y, *et al.* Expression of eukaryotic initiation factor 4E in atypical adenomatous hyperplasia and adenocarcinoma of the human peripheral lung. Clin Cancer Res 2002; 8(10): 3046-53.
21. Rosenwald IB, Hutzler MJ, Wang S, Savas L, Fraire AE. Expression of eukaryotic translation initiation factors 4E and 2alpha is increased frequently in bronchioloalveolar but not in squamous cell carcinomas of the lung. Cancer 2001; 15; 92(8): 2164-71.
22. Matthews-Greer J, Caldito G, de Benedetti A, Herrera GA, Dominguez-Malagon H, Chanona-Vilchis J, *et al.* eIF4E as a marker for cervical neoplasia. Appl Immunohistochem Mol Morphol 2005; 13(4): 367-70.
23. Lee JW, Choi JJ, Lee KM, Choi CH, Kim TJ, Lee JH, *et al.* eIF-4E expression is associated with histopathologic grades in cervical neoplasia. Hum Pathol 2005; 36(11): 1197-203.
24. Furic L, Rong L, Larsson O, Koumakpayi IH, Yoshida K, Brueschke A, *et al.* eIF4E phosphorylation promotes tumorigenesis and is associated with prostate cancer progression. Proc Natl Acad Sci U S A 2010; 107(32): 14134-9.
25. Assouline S, Culjkovic B, Cocolakis E, Rousseau C, Beslu N, Amri A, *et al.* Molecular targeting of the oncogene eIF4E in acute myeloid leukemia (AML): a proof-of-principle clinical trial with ribavirin. Blood 2009; 114(2): 257-60.
26. Yang B, Huang J, Xiang T, Yin X, Luo X, Huang J, *et al.* Chrysin inhibits metastatic potential of human triple-negative breast cancer cells by modulating matrix metalloproteinase-10, epithelial to mesenchymal

transition, and PI3K/Akt signaling pathway. J Appl Toxicol 2014; 34(1): 105-12.

27. Samarghandian S, Delkhosh MB, Mohammadi G. Role of Caspases, Bax and Bcl-2 in Chrysin-Induced Apoptosis in the A549 Human Lung Adenocarcinoma Epithelial Cells. Anticancer Agents Med Chem 2014; 14(6): 901-9.
28. Lirdprapamongkol K, Sakurai H, Abdelhamed S, Yokoyama S, Maruyama T, Athikomkulchai S, *et al.* A flavonoid chrysin suppresses hypoxic survival and metastatic growth of mouse breast cancer cells. Oncol Rep 2013; 30(5): 2357-64.
29. Chung TW, Moon SK, Chang YC, Ko JH, Lee YC, Cho G, *et al.* Novel and therapeutic effect of caffeic acid and caffeic acid phenyl ester on hepatocarcinoma cells: complete regression of hepatoma growth and metastasis by dual mechanism. FASEB J 2004; 18(14): 1670-81.
30. Kizilay A, Kalcioglu MT, Ozerol E, Iraz M, Gulec M, Akyol O, *et al.* Caffeic acid phenethyl ester ameliorated ototoxicity induced by cisplatin in rats. J Chemother 2004; 16(4): 381-7.
31. van't Land B, Blijlevens NM, Marteijn J, Timal S, Donnelly JP, de Witte TJ, *et al.* Role of curcumin and the inhibition of NF-KB in the onset of chemotherapy-induced mucosal barrier injury. Leukemia 2004; 18(2): 276-84.
32. Murtaza G, Karim S, Akram MR, Khan SA, Azhar S, Mumtaz A, *et al.* Caffeic Acid Phenethyl Ester and Therapeutic Potentials. Hindawi Publishing Corporation. Biomed Res Int 2014; 2014: 145342.

8

Hepatoprotective and Hypolipidemic Effects of *Carthamus tinctorius* oil in Alloxan-induced Type 1 Diabetic Rats

Parivash Rahimi[1], Sedigheh Asgary[2*], Najmeh Kabiri[3]

[1]Department of Biology, Faculty of Sciences, Isfahan University, Isfahan, Iran
[2]Isfahan Cardiovascular Research Center, Isfahan Cardiovascular Research Institute, Isfahan University of Medical Sciences, Isfahan, Iran
[3]Shahrekord University of Medical Sciences, Shahrekord, Iran

ARTICLE INFO

Keywords:
Carthamus tinctorius
Safflower oil
Hepatoprotection
Hypolipidemia

ABSTRACT

Introduction: Hepatoprotective and hypolipidemic effects of *Carthamus tinctorius* Linn. (Safflower) seed oil was investigated in diabetic rats.
Methods: Diabetes was induced by administration of 120 mg/kg alloxan monohydrate. The seed oil of safflower at dose of 200 mg/kg was administered as single dose per day to diabetic rats for a period of 28 days. The effect of oil on blood glucose level was measured in the diabetic rats. Serum lipid profile [total cholesterol (TC), triglycerides (TGs), low density (LDL) and high density lipoprotein (HDL) and enzymes such as alanine aminotransferase (ALT), aspartate aminotransferase (AST) and alkaline phosphatase (ALP) were also determined.
Results: Levels of blood glucose, TC, TGs, LDL, ALT, AST and ALP decreased and HDL increased in alloxan induced diabetic rats after treatment with 200 mg/kg safflower seed oil for 28 days.
Conclusion: The present study demonstrates that seed oil of safflower seems to be useful for the prevention of diabetes complications.

Implication for health policy/practice/research/medical education:
The present study demonstrates that safflower seed oil might to be useful for the prevention of diabetes complications including hepatotoxicity and hyperlipidemia.

Introduction

Diabetes mellitus is a disease in which homeostasis of carbohydrate, protein and lipid metabolism is improperly regulated by hormone insulin resulting in elevation of fasting and postprandial blood glucose levels (1). The major chronic complications associated with diabetes include retinopathy, neuropathy, nephropathy, and atherosclerotic coronary artery disease and peripheral atherosclerotic vascular disease (2). According to recent estimation, the global population is approaching the midst of a diabetes pandemic. By the year 2010 the total number of people worldwide with diabetes is predicted to reach 239 million (3). Besides hyperglycemia, several other factors like hyperlipidemia and enhanced oxidative stress play a major role in diabetic pathogenesis. Despite the great strides that have been made in the understanding and management of this disease, the graph of diabetes-related mortality is rising unabated. Although a numbers of synthetic drugs are available in the market diabetes and its related complications still remain uncontrolled. On the other hand, traditional medicinal plants have been used successfully since ancient times by physicians and laymen to treat diabetes and its related complications, presenting a stirring prospect for the expansion of an alternative way of treatment of diabetes (4,5). Liver is a big organ that its main function is managing and controlling carbohydrates,

***Corresponding author**: Sedigheh Asgary, Isfahan Cardiovascular Research Center, Isfahan Cardiovascular Research Institute, Isfahan University of Medical Sciences, Isfahan, Iran. E-mail: sasgary@yahoo.com lipids, and proteins metabolism. Maintaining normal blood glucose levels by taking and storing glucose in form of glycogen (glycogenesis), cleavage of glycogen into glucose (glycogenolysis), and forming glucose from non-carbohydrate sources such as amino acids (gluconeogenesis) are some other functions of liver (6). Various studies have shown that alloxan has deleterious effects on liver and kidney (7). Disruption in livers function that is demonstrated with increasing in alanine and aspartate aminotransferases (ALT & AST) have been reported one week after alloxan injection. These enzymes are measured for investigating livers function (8). Aminotransferases are the markers of the healthy hepatocytes. ALT is mainly found in the liver but AST, other than liver, is found in some other organs, so it is a less-specific marker for liver. Liver has a major role for maintaining post-prandial normal glucose concentration and it is the main site of insulin clearance (9).

Carthamus tinctorius, commonly known as safflower, false saffron or dyers saffron belongs to the family asteraceae and since centuries it has been grown from China to Mediterranean regions, but now is grown for commercial purposes in Pakistan, India, USA, Ethiopia, Mexico, Kazakhstan, Argentina, Australia, Spain, Turkey, Canada and Iran (10). Safflower is an oilseed crop in the Compositae that is valued for its oils rich in unsaturated fatty acids The major fatty acid in safflower oil is linoleic acid (80%) (11). Carthamus tinctorius L extracts and oil are important in drug development with numerous pharmacological activities in the world. It is a useful plant in painful menstrual problems, post-partum hemorrhage and osteoporosis. C. tinctorius has recently been shown to have antidiabetic activities. Caryophyllene, p-allyltoluene, 1-acetoxytetralin and heneicosane were identified as the major components for C. tinctorius flowers essential oil (12). This study was designed to investigate the Hepatoprotective and Hypolipidemic effects of *Carthamus tinctorius* Linn seed oil in diabetic rats.

Material and Methods

Preparation of safflower oil

The seed of safflower was collected during September 2013 from Isfahan province.

The plant was identified by Dr. L. Ghaem Maghami of Isfahan University of Medical Sciences and a voucher specimen (No. 2338) was kept in the herbarium of the Sciences Faculty. Seeds of Carthamus tinctorius (800 g) were hydrodistilled for 3 h in a Clevenger type apparatus. Five percent v/v of the resulting oil was prepared using saline solution of dimethylsulfoxide (DMSO) (13).

Preparation of diabetic rats

Alloxan monohydrate, dissolved in saline, was injected to rats intra-peritoneally at dose of 120 mg/kg body weight. After 4 days, rats with marked hyperglycemia (serum glucose more than 200 mg/dl) were selected and used for the study (14).

Experimental design

Eighteen male Wistar rats with (200±20 g) were purchased from Pasteur Institute, Iran and were kept in animal house of Isfahan University. They were kept at 20±5 °C, relative humidity of 30±5% and light/dark cycle for 12 h. All animals were fed with rodent pellet diet and water was allowed ad-labium under strict hygienic conditions. These rats were randomly divided into 3 groups with 6 rats per group, as follows: The rats in group 1 (C: controlled group) were administrated 0.5 ml saline, group 2 (D: diabetic rats), group 3 (D+SO) diabetic rats receiving safflower oil at 200 mg/kg in saline. Treatment period was 28 days.

Collection of samples

At the end of experiment, rats were sacrificed and their fasting blood was collected for the estimation of blood parameters. Serum was obtained immediately by centrifugation (15 min at 4000 rpm), which was used for the measurement of various biochemical parameters. All analyses were carried out within 24 h of blood collection.

Statistical analysis

The results are expressed as the mean±standard deviation (SD) of triplicate analyses. All statistical comparisons were performed using a one-way analysis of variance (ANOVA) followed by a two-tailed t-test. Differences were considered significant at a p level of 0.05 or lower.

Results

Effect of safflower oil on FBG and serum lipid profile

Diabetes significantly increased serum FBG, TG, Cholesterol, VLDL and LDL concentrations in comparison with the control group. Treatment of diabetic animals with safflower oil significantly inhibited the increase in serum FBG, TG, Cholesterol, VLDL and LDL with the untreated diabetic animals. The treatment of diabetic animals with safflower oil also significantly inhibited decrease of serum HDL concentrations in comparison with the untreated diabetic animals ($p<0.05$; Table 1).

Effect of safflower oil on serum ALT, AST and ALP activity

Serum ALT, AST and ALP activity as markers of liver function significantly ($p<0.05$) were increased in the untreated diabetic animals in comparison with the control group. Treatment of the diabetic animals with SO could significantly inhibit an increase of serum ALT and ALP activity in comparison with the untreated diabetic animals. Treatment by SO could maintain serum ALT and ALP activity of the treated animal at the same level as that of the control group (Table 2).

Discussion

Alloxan administration produces diabetes status by destruction of pancreatic β-cells with changes in metabolic

Table 1. The effects of safflower oil (SO) on FBG, TC, TG, LDL-C, HDL-C and VLDL-C in experimental rats

Parameter	Control	Diabetic	Diabetic + SO
FBG (mg/dL)	88 ± 21*	356 ± 61	288 ± 46*#
TG (mg/dL)	76.01 ± 15.56*	102.02 ± 21.01	72.02 ± 22.87*
TC (mg/dL)	73.00 ± 16.01*	117.09 ± 24.15	86.66 ± 23.24*#
HDL (mg/dL)	36.64 ± 6.90*	29.57 ± 10.09	34.55 ± 9.46*
LDL (mg/dL)	19.61 ± 3.78*	71.58 ± 14.24	38.42 ± 9.91*#
VLDL (mg/dL)	13.43 ± 4.33*	21.41 ± 5.05	13.90 ± 4.65*

Values are represented as mean ± SEM

*Significant change in comparison with diabetic without treatment at $p<0.05$.

#Significant change in comparison with control at $p<0.05$.

Table 2. The effects of safflower oil (SO) on ALT, AST and ALP levels in experimental rats

Parameter	Control	Diabetic	Diabetic + SO
ALT (U/L)	37.72 ± 1.36	50.13 ± 3.80*	38.± 4.59**
AST (U/L)	65.86 ± 1.81	122.02 ± 1.01*	108.02 ± 2.87**
ALP (U/L)	143.12 ± 1.21*	179.79 ± 2.15**	118.23 ± 2. 4**

Values are represented as mean ± SEM

*Significant change in comparison with diabetic without treatment at $p<0.05$.

**Significant change in comparison with control at $p<0.05$.

variables as well liver functions (15). In the alloxan-induced diabetes mellitus, the rise in blood glucose is also accompanied by an increase in plasma cholesterol, triglycerides cholesterol, AST, and ALT levels (16,17). The diabetogenic effects of alloxan are partly attributed to the specific cytotoxic action mediated by reactive oxygen species generation leading to the damage of large number of β-cells accompanied by a decrease in endogenous insulin release. However, alloxan-administered rats became hyperglycaemic in a short period of time, followed by a hepatic glucose overproduction (18).

Medicinal plants and natural antioxidants with hypolipidemic effects could prevent or be helpful in reducing the complications of lipid profile seen in diabetic patients (19). The mechanism of hypolipidemic action of medicinal plants may also be due to the inhibition of glycation lipoproteins, enzymes and proteins that involve lipid and lipoprotein metabolism (20,21).

Safflower is especially attractive as an oilseed crop, given that its seed oils are rich in mono- and polyunsaturated fatty acids (22). The major fatty acid in safflower oil is linoleic acid (80%). Linoleic acid is a polyunsaturated essential fatty acid called omega-6 fatty acid. In physiological literature, it has been used in the biosynthesis of prostaglandins and reported to be rich in the lipids of cell membranes. There is evidence that free fatty acids play an important role in regulating animal insulin secretion response and glucose homeostasis. It was recognized in a previous study that elevated plasma free fatty acids had both stimulatory and inhibitory effects on insulin secretion. Elevated free fatty acids were proved to enhance glucose-stimulated insulin secretion in fasted rats. Prolonged exposure to elevated fatty acids induced an impairment of animal insulin secretion in β-cells secretion function, whereas an acute exposure was found to enhance insulin secretion (23). In addition, saturated fatty acids induced lipoapoptosis in human β-cells, whereas unsaturated fatty acids had no effect. The insulinotropic effect of free fatty acids was profoundly influenced by the chain length and degree of saturation of individual fatty acids under certain circumstances. Long-chain and saturated fatty acids were more effective than medium-chain and unsaturated fatty acids (24).

C. carthamus oils may be exert their antihyperglycemic effect by potentiating plasma insulin action, secretion or its release from bound form. In diabetic status, lipoprotein lipase is not activated due to insulin deficiency resulting in hypertriglyceridemia and hypertriglyceridemia. This is in agreement with the fact that the glycemia level is the major determinant of total and very low-density lipoprotein cholesterol concentrations (25).

The liver is an important insulin-dependent tissue, which plays a pivotal role in glucose and lipid homeostasis and is severely affected during diabetes. The increase in the activities of serum glutamic pyruvic transaminase (SGPT) (ALT), serum glutamic oxaloacetic transaminase (SGOT or AST) and ALP indicated that diabetes might be induced due to liver dysfunction. Therefore, increase in the activities of SGPT, SGOT and ALP, may be mainly due to the leakage of these enzymes from the cytosol of hepatic cells into the blood stream (26).

Treatment of alloxan diabetic groups with safflower oil for 28 consecutive days could restore the activities of the above enzymes to their normal levels. A possible explanation for effects of safflower oil on the activities of AST, ALT and ALP in plasma and liver is that these treatments may inhibit the liver damage induced by alloxan.

Conclusion

Findings of the present study clearly indicate that treatment with safflower oil is effective in its hepatoprotection and hypolipidemia in diabetic rats. It is very difficult to comment on the mechanism of hepatoprotective and hypolipidemic activities of safflower oil, since the study was not designed accordingly.

Acknowledgements

We thank all the team of Isfahan Cardiovascular Research Center Laboratory for all their help.

Authors' contributions

All the authors wrote the mamuscript equally.

Conflict of interests

The authors declared no competing interests.

Ethical considerations

Ethical issues (including plagiarism, misconduct, data fabrication, falsification, double publication or submission, redundancy) have been completely observed by the authors.

Funding/Support

This research was financially supported by the grant number 4041 from Isfahan Cardiovascular Research Center (ICRC).

References

1. Tiwari AK, Rao JM. Diabetes mellitus and multiple therapeutic approaches of phytochemicals: Present status and future prospects. Curr Sci 2002; 83:30-8.
2. Ediriweera ER, Ratnasoori WD. Review on Herbs Used in treatment of Diabetes Mellitus by Sri Lankan Ayurvedic and Traditional Physicians. AYU 2009 30(4):373-91
3. Rao KN, Krishna MB, Srinivas N. Effect of chronic administration of Boerhaavia diffusa Linn leaf extract on experimental diabetes in rats. Trop J Pharma Res 2004; 3:305-9.
4. Ocvirk S, Kistler M, Khan S, Talukder SH, Hauner H. Traditional medicinal plants used for the treatment of diabetes in rural and urban areas of Dhaka, Bangladesh an ethnobotanical survey. J Ethnobiol Ethnomed 2013,9:43
5. Kavishankar GB, Lakshmidevi N, Mahadeva-Murthy S, Rakash HS, Niranjana SR. Diabetes and medicinal plants-A review. Int J Pharm Biomed Sci 2011; 2(3):65-80.
6. Aja PM, Nwafor EJ, Ibiam AU, Orji OU, Ezeani N, Nwali BU. Evaluation of Anti-diabetic and Liver Enzymes Activity of Aqueous Extracts of Moringa oleifera and Bridelia ferruginea Leaves in Alloxan Induced Diabetic Albino Rats. Int J Biochem Res Rev 2013; 3(3): 248-58.
7. Giannini EG, Testa R, Savarino V. Liver enzyme alteration: a guide for clinicians. CMAJ 2005;172:367-79.
8. Zafar M, Naqvi S, Kaimkhani MA. Altered Liver Morphology and Enzymes in Streptozotocin Induced Diabetic Rats. Int J Morphol 2009;27:719-25.
9. Pratt DS, Kaplan MM. Evaluation of abnormal liver enzyme results in asymptomatic patients. N Engl J Med 2009;342:1266-71.
10. Parisa Z, Jinous A, Mehrnaz K. The essential oil composition of Carthamus tinctorius L. flower growing in Iran. African J Biotech 2012;11(65): 12921-4.
11. Pearl SA, Bowers JE, Reyes-Chin-Wo S, Michelmore RW, Burke JM. Genetic analysis of safflower domestication. BMC Plant Biol 2014;14(43):1471-2229.
12. Asgarpanah J, Kazemivash N. Phytochemistry, pharmacology and medicinal properties of Carthamus tinctorius L. Chin J Integr Med 2013;19(2):153-9.
13. Lahlou M. Methods to study the phytochemistry and bioactivity of essential oils. Phytother Res 2004;18:435-8.
14. Kazerooni T, Mousavizade K, Abdollahee A, Sarkarian M, Sattar A. Aborifacient effect of Prangos ferulacea on pregnant rats. Contraception 2006,73: 554-6.
15. Szkudelski T. The mechanism of alloxan and streptozotocin action in b-cells of the rat pancreas. Physiol Res 2001;50:536-46.
16. Adeneye AA. Hypoglycemic and hypolipidemic effects of methanol seed extract of Citrus paradisi Macfad (Rutaceae) in alloxan-induced diabetic Wistar rats. Nig QJ Hosp Med 2008;18(4):211-5.
17. Pari L, Saravanan G. Antidiabetic effect of cogent db, a herbal drug in alloxan induced diabetes. Comp Biochem Physiol 2002;131:19-25.
18. Martinez JA, Milagro FI. Effects of the oral administration of a β3-adrenergic agonist on lipid metabolism in alloxan-diabetic rats. J Pharm Pharmacol 2000; 52:851-6 .
19. Garjani A, Fathiazad F, Zakheri A, Akbari NA, Azarmie Y, Fakhrjoo A, *et al.* The effect of total extract of Securigera securidaca L. seeds on serum lipid profiles, antioxidant status,and vascular function in hypercholesterolemic rats. J Ethnopharmacol 2009; 126:525-32.
20. Jayasooriya AP, Sakono M, Yukizaki C, Kawano M, Yamamoto K, Fukuda N. Effects of Momordica charantia powder on serum glucose levels and various lipid parameters in rats fed with cholesterol-free and cholesterol-enriched diets. J Ethnopharmacol 2000; 72:331-6.

21. Harris CS, Beaulieu LP, Fraser MH, McIntyre KL, Owen PL, Martineau LC, *et al.* Inhibition of advanced glycation end product formation by medicinal plant extracts correlates with phenolic metabolites and antioxidant activity. Planta Med 2011;77:196-204.
22. Ibrahim A, Natrajan S, Ghafoorunissa R. Dietary trans-fatty acids alter adipocyte plasma membrane fatty acid composition and insulin sensitivity in rats. Metabolism 2005;54(2):240-6.
23. Mellouk Z, Hachimi Idrissi T, Louchami K, Hupkens E, Sener A, Yahia DA, *et al.* The metabolic syndrome of fructose-fed rats: effects of long-chain polyunsaturated ω3 and ω6 fatty acids. II. Time course of changes in food intake, body weight, plasma glucose and insulin concentrations and insulin resistance. Int J Mol Med. 2012;29(1):113-8.
24. Rivellese AA, Lilli S. Quality of dietary fatty acids, insulin sensitivity and type 2 diabetes. Biomed Pharmacother. 2003. 57: 84–87.
25. Momo CE, Oben JE, Tazoo D, Dongo E. Antidiabetic and hypolipidaemic effects of a methanol/methylene-chloride extract of Laportea ovalifolia (Urticaceae), measured in rats with alloxan-induced diabetes. Ann Trop Med Parasitol 2006; 100(1): 69-74.
26. Ohaeri OC. Effect of garlic oil on the levels of various enzyme in the serum and tissue of streptozotocin diabetic rats. Bioscience Reports 2001; 21: 19-24.

9

Therapeutic and pharmacological potential of *Foeniculum vulgare* Mill

Wesam Kooti[1], Maryam Moradi[1], Sara Ali-Akbari[1], Naim Sharafi-Ahvazi[1], Majid Asadi-Samani[2*], Damoon Ashtary-Larky[3]

[1]Member of Student Research Committee, Kurdistan University of Medical Sciences, Sanandaj, Iran
[2]Medical Plants Research Center, Shahrekord University of Medical Sciences, Shahrekord, Iran
[3]Member of Student Research Committee, Ahvaz Jundishapur University of Medical Sciences, Ahvaz, Iran

ARTICLE INFO

Keywords:
Foeniculum vulgare Mill
Pharmacology
Phytochemical compounds
Therapeutic uses
Traditional medicine

ABSTRACT

Introduction: Fennel (*Foeniculum vulgare* Mill) is one of the oldest spice plants which, due to its economic importance and significant pharmaceutical industry applications, is considered as one of the world's most important medicinal plants. The purpose of this study is to investigate and collect scientific reports such as morphological characteristics, phytochemical compounds and evaluation of the therapeutic properties of this valuable medicinal plant that have been published.
Methods: In order to gather the information the keywords Fennel and Foeniculum vulgare mill, therapeutic, and pharmacology have been searched until January 1, 2015 from journals accessible in databases such as ScienceDirect, Scopus, EBSCO, Medline, PubMed, Embase, SID and Iran Medex.
Results: The results showed that this plant has various pharmacological properties including antioxidant, anti-cancer activity, anti-inflammatory, antifungal, anti-bacterial and estrogenic effects which are probably due to the presence of aromatic compounds such as anethole, estragole and fenshon.
Conclusion: Fennel possesses various pharmacological properties and the fennel bioactive molecules play an important role in human health, hence, it might be used for different drug productions.

Implication for health policy/practice/research/medical education:
Fennel (*Foeniculum vulgare* Mill) has different pharmacological properties such as anti-allergic, analgesic, anti- inflammatory, antioxidant, antibacterial, anti-cancer, anti-stress, cytotoxicity, etc. The fennel bioactive molecules play an important role in human health and can be used for different drug productions.

Introduction

The use of herbs to treat diseases has been common since ancient times. Also the use of plants different parts is common in public health. Using natural remedies and herbal medicines is beneficial cost-effective method for treating diseases (1,2).

Nowadays medicinal herbs are good alternative to chemical drugs, one of the major reason for this is low side effect compared to chemical drugs (3,4). Plants have always played an important role in the health and treatment of human society (5). Medicinal herbs have fewer side effects than synthetic drugs and due to their antioxidant properties they reduce drugs toxicity (6,7). Also, the natural effective ingredients cause biological balance and prevent drug accumulation in body (8). So medicinal plants can be used in the treatment of various diseases (9)

From 422 000 flowering plants around the world, more than 5000 ones are used for medicinal purposes. Among these herbs can point to fennel (*Foeniculum vulgare* Mill) which is of great importance and is used in the pharmaceutical, food, cosmetic and healthcare industries (10). Fennel is one of the oldest spice plants which widely grows in arid and semi-arid and due to its economic

***Corresponding author**: Majid Asadi-Samani, Medical Plants Research Center, Shahrekord University of Medical Sciences, Shahrekord, Iran. Email: biology_2011@yahoo.com importance and pharmaceutical industry usage, it is one of the world's most dimension medicinal herb (11). This plant has anti-inflammatory, antispasmodic, antiseptic, carminative, diuretic and analgesic effect and is effective in gastrointestinal disorder treatment. Also with its anti-ulcer and anti-oxidant properties it is used to treat neurological disorders (12,13). According to importance of fennel as a medicinal herb, the aim of the present study was to evaluate the phytochemical characteristics, and therapeutic properties of this medicinal plant.

Methods

In order to gather the information the keywords Fennel and *Foeniculum vulgare* mill, therapeutic, and pharmacology have been searched until January 1, 2015 from journals accessible in databases such as ScienceDirect, Scopus, EBSCO, Medline, PubMed, Embase, SID and Iran Medex.

Results

Phytology

Foeniculum vulgare Mill with English name of Fennel, Fenouil in French, Shmr (Razianaj) in Arabic and Razianeh in Persian belongs to Apiaceae family. It is an herbaceous and aromatic plant, with a height of 1 to 2 meters, grows in many parts of Europe, the Mediterranean, and Asia. Fennel is a perennial herb with stems grooved, intermittent leaves, often combined with dark green, fluffy with a blade divided into thin pieces, petiole with sheath, flowers are usually bisexual, regular or irregular, with yellow umbrella in the form of oval beads (14,15). On radiating branches linear lines can be diagnosed. Fennel has small seed with a length of about 8 mm and a width of 3 mm with an aromatic odor and sweet taste. Fennel seeds are narrow, long, cylindrical appearance and dimensions vary depending on plant growth. The crack groove light green surface (16).

Phytochemical composition of fennel

All parts of fennel such as roots, leaves, fruit and especially the seeds are used (17). Fennel seed contains 6.3% water, 9.5% protein, 10% fat, 13.4% minerals, 18.5% fibers and 42.3% carbohydrates (18). Its leaves contain vitamins and minerals such as calcium, potassium, sodium, iron, phosphorus, thiamine, riboflavin, niacin and vitamin C (19). Fruits consist 10 to 12 % of oil that is stored in the cotyledons of seeds. Oil obtained from the fennel fruit has 4% palmitic acid, 22% oleic acid, 14% linoleic acid and 6% petrocylic acid. The fruit has value of 4 to 6% essence which its essence and combine ingredients vary according to the location of plant growth (16). The aromatic property of fennel is because of the essence. There are more than 30 types of terpene compounds in the essential oil of fennel, the most important of them are 50 to 80% trans-anethole, 8% fenshon and limonene 5% (20). This herb also contains phenolic compounds such as flavonoids, phenolic acids, hydroxycinnamic acids, coumarin and tannin (21). Phenolic acids include 3-O-Caffeoylquinic acid, 4-O-caffeoylquinic acid, 5-O-caffeoylquinic acid, 1, 3-O-di-caffeoylquinic acid, 1, 4-O-di-caffeoylquinic acid and 1, 5-O-di-caffeoylquinicacid. Its flavonoid contains eriodictyol-7-rutinoside, quercetin-3-rutinoside and rosmarinic acid (22). Also aqueous extract of fennel fruit include quercetin-3-O-galactoside, kaempferol-3-O-rutinoside, kaempferol-3-O-glucoside, quercetin-3-O-glucuronide, kampferol-3-O-glucuronide, isoquercetin, and isorhamnetin-3-O-glucoside (23).

Use of fennel in traditional medicine

Fennel has been used in traditional medicine to treat various diseases for thousands of years in the East Asian countries, India and China (16). People have long been familiar with fennel plant. In the middle ages people believed that chewing the seeds is important to eliminate abdomen noise (24). In the fifth century it was believed that fennel had sedative effect and in 9th to 14th centuries numerous therapeutic properties were attributed to it (25). The Romans believed that fennel seed could help supercharge the vision. The English believed that the plant could offer relief from bloating stomach and facilitate digestion. The fennel therapeutic use has been serious since the 18th century, and many studies have been taken (26). Nowadays, the different parts of the plant are used in treatment of many diseases, particularly pain in the digestive system. Also it is very useful in the treatment of diabetes, bronchitis, chronic cough and kidney stones (27). Fennel seeds are used as a flavoring in cooking meat and fish, prepare ice cream and cream. Due to its diuretic effect the plant is used to treat kidney and bladder diseases. It is also used to relieve nausea and remove vomiting. The herbs is helpful for chronic fever and removing the obstruction in the internal organs, especially the liver, gut, respiratory and urinary tract and also it is used to improve eye diseases such as cataract as well as diseases of the stomach, chronic diarrhea and relieve children colic (28,29).

Pharmacological effects

The pharmacological activities of fennel include following items (30).

Anti-bacterial activity

Fennel is used to treat many bacterial, fungal, viral, and mycobacterial infectious diseases (31). Fennel has antibacterial activity due to compounds such as, linoleic acid, undecanal, 1, 3-benzenediol, oleic acid and 2,4-undecadienal. Fennel has 5-hydroxy-furanocoumarin which has important role antibacterial activity of this plant (32). Aqueous extract of fennel shows bactericidal activity against Enterococcus faecalis, Staphylococcus aureus, Escherichia coli, Pseudomonas aeruginosa, Salmonella typhi, Salmonella typhimurium, and Shigella flexneri (33). During a study it was found that this plant extract has a significant antibacterial effect against a lot of bacteria except Klebsiella pneumoniae and one strain of Pseudomonas aeruginosa. Also this report determined MIC for aqueous and alcoholic extracts of fennel seed which was in the range of 20-80 mg/ml and 5-15 mg/ml and statistical analysis showed better effect of the plant extract compared to standard antibiotics (34). The essence of plant showed very strong antibacterial activity against pathogens in food such as Escherichia coli, Listeria, monocytogenes, Salmonella typhimurium, Staphylococcus aureus, as well as having enormous activity against Helicobacter pylori and Campylobacter jejuni (35,36).

Jazani *et al.* studied the antibacterial activity of fennel extract on Acinetobacter baumannii strains which cause nosocomial infection. The results showed that fennel extract has antibacterial effect on all bacteria strains so its' extract can be used to control multiple-antibiotic resistant bacteria (37).

Anti-fungal activity

Fennel extract has antifungal activity against various fungal species such as Candida albicans, species of Aspergillus, and dermatophytes (21). Also a study on the herb antifungal effect showed significant antifungal activity against fungi in food waste such as Aspergillus niger and Fusarium oxysporum. The MIC of fennel extract for these molds respectively was 750 and 250 micrograms per ml (27).

Another study showed that dillapional the derivative of fennel stalk phenyl propanoid has antimicrobial properties against Aspergillus niger, Bacillus subtilis and Cladosporium cladosporioides. Also derivates of coumarin named scopoletin had antimicrobial properties against above micro-organisms but was less important than dillapional (38).

Antifungal activity of fennel essence on Sclerotinia sclerotiorum was investigated. The antifungal effect of this plant against Sclerotinia sclerotiorum observed based on survival of the microorganisms (39).

A study demonstrated that nitric oxide production in peritoneal macrophages which were treated with fennel extract at a concentration of 10 mg/ml significantly increased. Also the production of reactive oxygen species compared to the control group increased. Lethality study also showed that treated macrophages with concentrations of 10 and 20 mg ml had anti-candidate effects more than control group. Among chemical compositions of the plant extract anethole had the strongest antifungal activity (40).

Antioxidant activity

Fennel is known as an excellent source of natural antioxidants. This plant can inhibit free radicals due to the high content of polyphenols and flavonoids. Phenolic compounds in this herb such as caffeoylquinic acid, rosmarinic acid, eriodictyol-7-orutinoside, quercetin-3-O-galactoside, kaempferol-3-O-glucoside showed antioxidant activity. Fennel volatile oil has strong antioxidant activity, too. Plant ethanolic and aqueous extracts in comparison to its essence has less antioxidant activity (33,41-43).

In a research aqueous and methanolic extracts of fennel seed for Total Antioxidant Capacity (TAC) and determination of total phenolic compounds were studied. TAC was measured using the DPPH, H2O2, and FRAP and phenolic compounds using the Folin-ciocalteu reagent. This study showed that fennel extracts could inhibit free radicals and act as primary antioxidant (41). In another study, the antioxidant activity of aqueous and ethanol extracts of fennel seeds was evaluated by using a variety of antioxidant methods such as total antioxidant, free radical scavenging, superoxide anion radical scavenging, hydrogen peroxide scavenging, metal chelating activity. These antioxidant activities were compared to standard antioxidant such as butylated hydroxyanisole (BHA), and butylated hydroxytoluene (BHT), and a-tocopherol. The results obtained in this study showed that fennel seed was a potential source of natural antioxidants (44). Also antioxidant activity of the ethanol and aqueous extracts of fennel showed that 100 mg of ethanol and watery extracts respectively had the 99.1% and 77.5% of antioxidant activity which was greater than the alpha-tocopherol (36.1%) antioxidant properties with the same dose (45).

Anti-inflammatory activity

Of the pharmacological effects of fennel plant, anti-inflammatory activity can be noted. Research has shown that the methanol extract of fennel has anti-inflammatory effects. Oral administration of 200 mg per kg of methanol extract of fennel fruit shows inhibitory effects on acute and subacute inflammatory diseases and type 4 allergic reactions. In addition, it decreased the activities of superoxide dismutase (SOD) and catalase (CAT). It also significantly increased plasma levels of HDL cholesterol. In contrast, it significantly reduced the level of malondialdehyde (MDA) as a measure of lipid peroxidation. These results indicate that the methanol extract of fennel fruit is effective in reducing inflammation (46). Kataoka et al. studied anti-inflammatory effects of fennel. The results showed that the methanol extract of fennel seeds inhibits inflammation through cyclooxygenase and through lipoxygenase pathways (47,48). Also Choi et al. evaluated fennel methanol extract anti-inflammatory effects. The results showed that the fennel methanol extract had anti-inflammatory activity dependent on the central and peripheral mechanisms (46).

Anti-anxiety activity

Anxiolytic activity of the crude extract of fennel has been reported. Fennel due to phytoestrogens extensively has therapeutic use in the treatment of estrogen deficiency abnormalities. Estrogens are hormones that are involved in the phenomenon of anxiety which appear to act via the GABA A receptors. The results of a study showed that the plant with increase in time spent in the open arm established significant anxiolytic effect. Picrotoxin (GABA receptor antagonist) and Tamoxifen prevented anxiolytic effect. Therefore, fennel probably is an herbal remedy that has anxiolytic effects mediated by GABA-ergic system and estrogen receptors (14).

Mesfin *et al.* studied the anxiolytic activity of fennel on adult mice. It was demonstrated that stress levels in treated group with fennel essence compared to control group significantly decreased. Thus, it can be concluded that this plant can hold promising effects in the treatment of anxiety and stress (49).

Koppula *et al.* investigated the properties of fennel extract in stress reduction and memory enhancement in rats. This study showed that this herb with several functions such as anti-stress proceeding, increase in memory and antioxidant effects may reduce stress and stress-related disorders (50).

Gastro-protective activity

It has been shown that fennel plant has significant protective effect on gastrointestinal disorders. It was shown that the use of fennel oil emulsions eliminated colic in 65% of treated infants which was considerably better than the control group (51,52). In a study Al-Mofleh *et al.* investigated the effect of fennel plant on gastric ulcer. The findings showed that the plant had a protective effect on gastric ulcer. In addition, the herb reduced mucosal lining of the stomach. These functions were attributed to its antioxidant capacity (53).

Estrogenic activity

Fennel has been used for thousands of years as an estrogenic agent. Due to this property, fennel increases milk secretion, reduces menstrual pain, facilitates birth and increases sexual desire. Anatole is the main part of fennel plant that operates estrogenic properties. Researches have shown that active pharmaceutical agents such as dianthole and photoanatole are polymers of anthole (48).

The fennel essence showed fewer side effects in the treatment of primary dysmenorrhea. Administration of different doses of fennel extract significantly decreased contractions intensity induced by oxytocin and prostaglandins (54). Moderate doses increased mammary gland weight and higher doses increased the weight of oviduct, endometrium, myometrium and cervix (55). Myrseyed *et al.* investigated the effect of fennel seed ethanol extract on gonadotropin changes in adult male rats. Testosterone, FSH, LH levels in treatment groups were significantly reduced in comparison to the control group. Significant reduction in the amount of sperm resulting in epididymis weight loss and hormone levels indicates the fennel seed decreases in male reproductive activity (56).

Fennel herb has estrogenic effects and has been traditionally used to treat infertile women. It was shown that the extract of fennel increased serum concentrations of follicle-stimulating hormone and decreased the yolk hormones and testosterone in treatment groups (57). In another study Devi *et al.* investigated fennel fruit acetone extract effect on mammary gland and oviduct. The results of this study confirmed the effects of natural estrogen for this plant seed extract (58).

Cardiovascular and lipid activity

The study of the anti- cholesterol and anti-atherogenic effect of fennel methanol extract showed that treatment with the extract significantly reduced plasma lipid levels. Also the plant had important anti-atherogenic effects. It reduced triglycerides in fatty liver and facilitated blood flow in the coronary arteries by preventing the buildup of fatty deposit in arteries through reduction of plasma and liver fats. As a result because of hypolipidemic and anti-atherogenic activities, this herb could be used for controlling cardiovascular disorders (59,60). Also intravenous injection of the extract significantly reduced blood pressure, without affecting the heart rate and respiration. It seems that fennel extract effect on blood pressure was not mediated by adrenergic, muscarinic, ganglion, serotonergic receptors (61). In other study, oral administration of the extract reduced systolic blood pressure. The fennel extract acts as a diuretic and natriuretic, too (62).

Anti-diabetic activity

A study investigated the effect of aqueous extract Apiaceae family plant such as fennel in lowering blood sugar and anti-diabetic activities. The findings exhibited that the extract could be useful for the control of blood glucose in diabetic patients and in addition, their daily use could be effective in reducing chronic complications associated with diabetes (63).

To evaluate the effect of fennel on blood sugar reduction, a study was conducted on streptozotocin-diabetic rats. The results showed that fennel extract improves hyperglycemia in diabetic rats which part of this related to herb effect on oxidation/restored system. Therefore, this plant can be used in the pharmaceutical industry for the manufacture of anti-diabetic drugs (64). Also methanol extract of fennel fruit reduced blood glucose and triglycerides and led to higher levels of liver and muscle glycogen (65).

Anti-cancer activity

It was shown that TNF-α -dependent responses are involved in inflammation and cancer. It was found that anethole in fennel seed has inhibitory effect on activating TNF-α by transcription factor NF-KB. The results showed that anethole inhibited cellular responses induced by these cytokines which might explain its role in suppressing cancer. It also specified that the fennel with its antiangiogenic mechanisms inhibits prostate tumor xenograft (66).

Bogucka-Kocka *et al.* evaluated apoptotic activity of ethanol extracts of fennel against leukemia. The findings showed that the extract had considerable apoptotic effects on cancer cells (67). In other study, fennel methanol extract effects on antitumor and cytotoxic activities in mice with cancer were investigated. Data of this study showed that the methanol extract of fennel considerably increased MDA levels and significantly reduced CAT activity and glutathione content in the liver and tumor tissue of mice with cancer. In contrast, the total protein content in the ascites fluid decreased. The results demonstrated that the methanol extract of fennel had significant anticancer activity against breast cancer cells (MCF-7) and liver cancer (Hepg) through modulating lipid peroxidation and increasing antioxidant defense system and inhibitory effect on free radicals (68).

Hepato-protective activity

The studies demonstrated that the fennel plant has protective effect on liver. Qiang *et al.* studied the effect of fennel extract in carbon tetrachloride -induced liver injury rats. Data from this study showed that this extract reduced the levels of AST (aspartate aminotransferase), ALT (alanine amino transferase), ALP (alkaline phosphatase) and serum bilirubin (69). Also the effect of fennel on lipid peroxidation in rats with hepatic fibrosis was investigated. After fennel consumption ALT, AST level and MDA content significantly decreased and the TP, ALB and SOD, CAT, GSH-PX activities increased. According to results it might be concluded that fennel probably through effect on regulation of lipid peroxidation might inhibit hepatic fibrosis (70).

Wang *et al.* studied fennel effect on cytokines in rats with hepatic fibrosis. The results demonstrated that degradation of lipids and inflammation was reduced in the fennel treated group. Based on the data obtained from this study can be deduced that fennel might reduce inflammation in the liver and also considerably protect hepatocytes against liver damage (71). In other study, the effect of fennel on hepatic fibrosis and the amount of potassium supplements examined. Patient group with fibrosis, liver tissue inflammation and excessive fat degradation after fennel treatment significantly improved. After treatment with fennel of ascites level and HAase content decreased and potassium levels went up. According to these findings it can be derived that fennel might inhibit hepatic fibrosis (72). Also, the effect of fennel on TNF-α cytokine in liver fibrosis model was examined. In the treated group inflammation was reduced and the amount of TNF-α secretion was reduced by PBMCS (73). Based on these findings, we can conclude that fennel might reduce TNF-α secretion by single –core cells, inhibit inflammation and improve liver fibrosis.

Memory-protective activity

It is believed that some plants including fennel herbs are used to enhance memory and intelligence. Therefore, the effect of fennel extract on memory in amnesiac rats was examined. The results showed that this extract had memory enhancement property (27). In Joshi *et al.* study the effect of fennel extract as a neurotropic factor and anti-acetylcholinesterase in mice were investigated. The findings of this study showed that fennel extract significantly inhibited acetylcholinesterase. According to this study it can be deduced that fennel might be used in treatment of cognitive disorders such as dementia and Alzheimer (74).

Potential mechanisms

According to the literature, some potential mechanisms of the plant's effects have been shown in Table 1.

Side effects

In general, for preparing herbal products minimal toxicity and minimal side effects are very important. Estragole is one of the most important fennel extract compounds. It is reported that this compound led to the development of malignant tumors in rodents, so use of this agent is restricted (18). The Estragole causes tumors in rodents but carcinogenicity in humans has not been established. The total amount of anethole in fennel is 2090 mg/kg. It has been reported that repeated administration of 695 mg/

Table 1. The potential mechanisms of efficacy of some pharmacologic properties of *Foeniculum vulgare* Mill

Pharmacological effects	Possible mechanisms of efficacy
Anti-microbial activity	Presence of active compounds with anti- microbial activity such as oleic acid and coumarin in aqueous and alcoholic extract.
Antioxidant activity	Presence of antioxidant compounds such as flavonoid and phenols in aqueous and ethanolic extract.
Anti-inflammatory activity	The Preventive effects of methanol extract against acute and subacute illness, type 4 allergic reactions through cyclooxygenase and lipoxygenase inhibition.
Anti-anxiety activity	Anxiolytic effects mediated by GABAergic and estrogen receptors
Gastro-protective activity	Regulation of intestinal muscle movement, treatment of gastrointestinal spasm and chronic colitis, protective effect on gastric ulcer, reduce the mucosal lining of the stomach.
Estrogenic activity	Presence of compounds such as anatole effect on increasing milk secretion reduce menstrual pain, facilitate birth, primary dysmenorrhea, and infertility.
Anti- lipid activity	Hypolipidemic effects by reducing plasma triglyceride, total cholesterol, lowering LDL, decreased apolipoprotein B, increased HDL, and increased apolipoprotein A-1.
Cardiovascular activity	Systolic blood pressure reduction, decreased excretion of sodium, potassium and water.
Anti-diabetic activity	The hypoglycemia effect by lowering blood glucose, increasing glutamine peroxide activity, increased levels of liver and muscle glycogen.
Anti-cancer activity	Presence of active compounds such as anethole, inhibitory effect on the activation of TNF-α, antiangiogenic effects, and apoptotic and antitumor effects.
Hepato-protective activity	Decreased levels of AST, ALT, ALP and Bilirubin, reduction of proinflammatory cytokines such as TNF- α and CTGF in fibrosis.
Memory-protective activity	Inhibitory effect on the acetylcholinesterase enzyme.

kg caused a mild lesions in the rat liver. Thus, it was found that normal therapeutic doses of anatole cause mild liver toxicity (75).

It is reported that the use of fennel extract for control and treatment of primary dysmenorrhea causes concern about the teratogenicity potential of it, due to its estrogen-like activity. Investigating the herb extract effect showed teratogenic property that may have toxic effects on the cells of the embryo but no evidence of teratogenicity to concentration of 9.3 mg/ml (76).

Conclusion

Available researches have shown that extracts of fennel possess different pharmacological properties such as anti-allergic, analgesic, anti-inflammatory, antioxidant, antibacterial, anti-cancer, anti-stress and cytotoxicity activity. Medicinal properties of the plant are due to its different chemical compounds. Among the various compounds found in fennel plant essence and phenolic compounds are considered as the most important and most active compounds of it. The fennel bioactive molecules can be used for different drug production and play an important role in human health. The most prominent and best studies have been conducted on the antioxidant, antimicrobial and fennel estrogenic effects in various experimental models. Few studies have been performed on the anticancer effect of this plant, while a high percentage of worldwide deaths occur as various cancer effects. Therefore, it is recommended that future researches be investigate on the effect of this plant on cancer cell lines.

Authors' contributions

All the authors wrote the manuscript equally.

Conflict of interests

The authors declared no competing interests.

Ethical considerations

Ethical issues (including plagiarism, misconduct, data fabrication, falsification, double publication or submission, redundancy) have been completely observed by the authors.

Funding/Support

None.

Reference

1. Tang SY, Halliwell B. Medicinal plants and antioxidants: what do we learn from cell culture and Caenorhabditis elegans studies? Biochem Biophys Res Commun 2010; 394(1): 1-5.
2. Ghasemi Pirbalouti A. Iranian medicinal and aromatic plants. Shahrekord: Islamic Azad University; 2009.
3. Kooti W, Ghasemiboroon M, Asadi-Samani M, Ahangarpoor A, Zamani M, Amirzargar A, *et al.* The effect of hydroalcoholic extract of celery leaves on the delivery rate (fertilization and stillbirths), the number, weight and sex ratio of rat off spring. Adv Environ Biol 2014; 8(10): 824-30.
4. Beyrami-Miavagi A, Farokhi F, Asadi-Samani M. A study of the effect of prostodin and hydroalcoholic extract of Malva neglecta on kidney histopathology and renal factors in female rats. Adv Environ Biol 2014; 8(9): 942-7.
5. Kooti W, Mansouri E, Ghasemiboroon M, Harizi M, Ashtary-Larky D, Afrisham R. The Effects of hydroalcoholic extract of apium graveolens leaf on the number of sexual cells and testicular structure in rat. Jundishapur J Nat Pharm Prod 2014; 9(4): e17532.
6. Asadi-Samani M, Rafieian-Kopaei M, Azimi N. Gundelia: a systematic review of medicinal and molecular perspective. Pak J Biol Sci 2013; 16: 1238-47.
7. Kooti W, Ghasemiboroon M, Asadi-Samani M, Ahangarpoor A, Abadi A, Noori M, *et al.* The effects of hydro-alcoholic extract of celery on lipid profile of rats fed a high fat diet. Adv Environ Biol 2014; 8(9): 325-30.
8. Asadi-Samani M, Kafash-Farkhad N, Azimi N, Fasihi A, Alinia-Ahandani E, Rafieian-Kopaei M. Medicinal plants with hepatoprotective activity in Iranian folk medicine. Asian Pac J Trop Biomed 2015; 5(2): 146-57.
9. Kooti W, Mansori E, Ghasemiboroon M, Harizi M, Amirzarga A. Protective effects of celery (Apium Graveolens) on testis and cauda epididymal spermatozoa in rat. Iran J Reprod Med 2014; 12(5): 365-6.
10. Abe R, Ohtani K. An ethnobotanical study of medicinal plants and traditional therapies on Batan Island, the Philippines. J Ethnopharmacol 2013; 145(2): 554-65.
11. Jamshidi E, Ghalavand A, Sefidkon F, Goltaph E. Effects of different nutrition systems (organic and chemical) on quantitative and qualitative characteristics of Fennel (Foeniculum valgare Mill.) under water deficit stress. Iran J Med Aromat Plants 2012; 28(2): 309-23.
12. Birdane FM, Cemek M, Birdane YO, Gulcin I, Buyukokuroglu ME. Beneficial effects of Foeniculum vulgare on ethanol-induced acute gastric mucosal injury in rats. World J Gastroenterol 2007; 13(4): 607.
13. Delaram M, Kheiri S, Hodjati MR. Comparing the effects of echinop hora-platyloba, fennel and placebo on pre-menstrual syndrome. J Reprod Infertil 2011; 12(3): 221-6
14. Pourabbas S, Kesmati M, Rasekh A. Study of the the anxiolytic effects of fennel and possible roles of both gabaergic system and estrogen receptors in these effects in adult female rat. Physiol Pharmacol 2011; 15(1): 134-43.
15. Bernath J, Nemeth E, Kattaa A, Hethelyi E. Morphological and chemical evaluation of fennel (Foeniculum vulgare Mill.) populations of different origin. J Essent Oil Res 1996; 8(3): 247-53.

16. Ahmadi A, Nasiri Nejad, F, Parivar K. Effect of aqueous extract of the aerial part of the Ruta graveolens on the spermatogenesis of immature Balb/C mice. Razi J Med Sci 2007; 14(56): 13-20
17. Meireles MA. Supercritical fluid extraction from fennel (Foeniculum vulgare): global yield, composition and kinetic data. J Supercrit Fluids 2005; 35(3): 212-9.
18. Rather MA, Dar BA, Sofi SN, Bhat BA, Qurishi MA. Foeniculum vulgare: A comprehensive review of its traditional use, phytochemistry, pharmacology, and safety. Arab J Chem 2012. doi: 10.1016/j.arabjc.2012.04.011
19. Miguel MG, Cruz C, Faleiro L, Simões M, Figueiredo AC, Barroso JG, *et al.* Foeniculum vulgare essential oils: chemical composition, antioxidant and antimicrobial activities. Nat Prod Commun 2010; 5(2): 319-28.
20. Salehi Surmaghi H. Medicinal plants and phytotherapy. Donyaee Taghazie, Tehran, Iran. 2006:59-63.
21. Rahimi R, Ardekani MRS. Medicinal properties of Foeniculum vulgare Mill. in traditional Iranian medicine and modern phytotherapy. Chin J Integr Med 2013; 19(1): 73-9.
22. Faudale M, Viladomat F, Bastida J, Poli F, Codina C. Antioxidant activity and phenolic composition of wild, edible, and medicinal fennel from different Mediterranean countries. J Agric Food Chem 2008; 56(6): 1912-20.
23. Parejo I, Viladomat F, Bastida J, Schmeda-Hirschmann G, Burillo J, Codina C. Bioguided isolation and identification of the nonvolatile antioxidant compounds from fennel (Foeniculum vulgare Mill.) waste. J Agric Food Chem 2004; 52(7): 1890-7.
24. Siyahi M, Shiravi A, Heydari NM. Effect of hydro extract of fennel on prolactine and lactation in female Rat (wistar). J Anim Sci 2009; 1(3): 55-63.
25. Taherian A, Dehghanina M, Vafaei AA, Sadeghi H, Miladi Gorgi H. Effects of aqueous extract of fruit of Foeniculum vulgar on neurogenic and inflamatory pain in mice. Sci J Kurdistan Univ Med Sci 2007; 12(2): 29-36.
26. Ranjbarian P, Sadeghian S, Shirazi MH, Saraf Nejad AF, Fazeli MR, Amin GR. Survey of anti-bacterial effect of plant extracts (Fennel-dill-caraway-cinnamon) by flowcytometry and disk diffusion . Sci J Hamadan Univ Med Sci Health Serv 2004; 11(33): 42-7.
27. Badgujar SB, Patel VV, Bandivdekar AH. Foeniculum vulgare Mill: A Review of its botany, phytochemistry, pharmacology, contemporary application, and toxicology. BioMed Res Int 2014; 2014.
28. Razi M. Content in medicine. Beirut, Lebanon: Dar Al Kotob Al-ilmiyah; 2000.
29. Ibn Sina. Canon in medicine. Translated from Arabic to Persian by AR Sharafkandi. Tehran, Iran: Soroush Publication; 2005.
30. Tonkaboni MM. Gift of believers. Tehran, Iran: Shahid Beheshti University of Medical Sciences Publication; 2007.
31. Duško BL, Comiæ L, Sukdolak S. Antibacterial activity of some plants from family Apiaceae in relation to selected phytopathogenic bacteria. Kragujevac J Sci 2006; 28: 65-72.
32. Esquivel-Ferriño PC, Favela-Hernández JMJ, Garza-González E, Waksman N, Ríos MY, Camacho-Corona MdR. Antimycobacterial activity of constituents from Foeniculum vulgare var. dulce grown in Mexico. Molecules 2012; 17(7): 8471-82.
33. Parejo I, Jauregui O, Sánchez-Rabaneda F, Viladomat F, Bastida J, Codina C. Separation and characterization of phenolic compounds in fennel (Foeniculum vulgare) using liquid chromatography-negative electrospray ionization tandem mass spectrometry. J Agric Food Chem 2004; 52(12): 3679-87.
34. Kaur GJ, Arora DS. Antibacterial and phytochemical screening of Anethum graveolens, Foeniculum vulgare and Trachyspermum ammi. BMC Complement Altern Med 2009; 9(1): 30.
35. Mahady GB, Pendland SL, Stoia A, Hamill FA, Fabricant D, Dietz BM, *et al.* In vitro susceptibility of Helicobacter pylori to botanical extracts used traditionally for the treatment of gastrointestinal disorders. Phytother Res 2005; 19(11): 988-91.
36. Cwikla C, Schmidt K, Matthias A, Bone K, Lehmann R, Tiralongo E. Investigations into the antibacterial activities of phytotherapeutics against Helicobacter pylori and Campylobacter jejuni. Phytother Res 2010; 24(5): 649-56.
37. Jazani N, Zartoshti M, Babazadeh H, Ali-Daiee N, Zarrin S, Hosseini S. Antibacterial effects of Iranian fennel essential oil on isolates of Acinetobacter baumannii. Pak J Biol Sci 2009; 12(9): 738.
38. Kwon YS, Choi WG, Kim WJ, Kyung cKim W, Kim MJ, Kang WH, *et al.* Antimicrobial constituents of Foeniculum vulgare. Arch Pharm Res 2002; 25(2): 154-7.
39. Soylu S, Yigitbas H, Soylu E, Kurt Ş. Antifungal effects of essential oils from oregano and fennel on Sclerotinia sclerotiorum. J Appl Microbiol 2007; 103(4): 1021-30.
40. Naeini A, Naseri M, Kamalinejad M, Khoshzaban F, Rajabian T, Nami H, *et al.* Study on anti-candida effects of essential oil and extracts of Iranian medicinal plants, in vitro. J Med Plant 2011; 2 (38): 163-72.
41. Scalbert A, Manach C, Morand C, Rémésy C, Jiménez L. Dietary polyphenols and the prevention of diseases. Crit Rev Food Sci Nutr 2005; 45(4): 287-306.
42. Chatterjee S, Goswami N, Bhatnagar P. Estimation of phenolic components and in vitro antioxidant activity of fennel (Foeniculum vulgare) and ajwain (Trachyspermum ammi) seeds. Adv Biores 2012; 3(2): 109-18.
43. Díaz-Maroto MC, Díaz-Maroto Hidalgo IJ, Sánchez-

Palomo E, Perez-Coello MS. Volatile components and key odorants of fennel (Foeniculum vulgare Mill.) and thyme (Thymus vulgaris L.) oil extracts obtained by simultaneous distillation-extraction and supercritical fluid extraction. J Agric Food Chem 2005; 53(13): 5385-9.
44. Oktay M, Gülçin İ, Küfrevioğlu Öİ. Determination of in vitro antioxidant activity of fennel (Foeniculum vulgare) seed extracts. LWT-Food Sci Technol 2003; 36(2): 263-71.
45. Shahat AA, Ibrahim AY, Hendawy SF, Omer EA, Hammouda FM, Abdel-Rahman FH, *et al.* Chemical composition, antimicrobial and antioxidant activities of essential oils from organically cultivated fennel cultivars. Molecules 2011; 16(2): 1366-77.
46. Choi EM, Hwang JK. Antiinflammatory, analgesic and antioxidant activities of the fruit of Foeniculum vulgare. Fitoterapia 2004; 75(6): 557-65.
47. Kataoka H, Horiyama S, Yamaki M, Oku H, Ishiguro K, Katagi T, *et al.* Anti-inflammatory and anti-allergic activities of hydroxylamine and related compounds. Biol Pharm Bull 2002; 25(11): 1436-41.
48. Albert-Puleo M. Fennel and anise as estrogenic agents. J Ethnopharmacol 1980; 2(4): 337-44.
49. Mesfin M, Asres K, Shibeshi W. Evaluation of anxiolytic activity of the essential oil of the aerial part of Foeniculum vulgare Miller in mice. BMC Complement Altern Med 2014; 14(1): 310.
50. Koppula S, Kumar H. Foeniculum vulgare Mill (Umbelliferae) attenuates stress and improves memory in wister rats . Trop J Pharm Res 2013; 12(4): 553-8.
51. Chakŭrski I, Matev M, Koĭchev A, Angelova I, Stefanov G. Treatment of chronic colitis with an herbal combination of Taraxacum officinale, Hipericum perforatum, Melissa officinaliss, Calendula officinalis and Foeniculum vulgare. Vutr Boles 1980; 20(6): 51-4.
52. Alexandrovich I, Rakovitskaya O, Kolmo E, Sidorova T, Shushunov S. The effect of fennel (Foeniculum vulgare) seed oil emulsion in infantile colic: a randomized, placebo-controlled study. Altern Ther Health Med 2003; 9(4): 58-61.
53. Al-Mofleh I, Al-Sobaihani M, Alqasoumi S, Al-Said M, Al-Dosari M, Al-Yahya M, *et al.* Fennel" Foeniculum vulgare" treatment protects the gastric mucosa of rats against chemically-induced histological lesions. Int J Pharm 2013; 9(3): 182.
54. Ostad S, Soodi M, Shariffzadeh M, Khorshidi N, Marzban H. The effect of fennel essential oil on uterine contraction as a model for dysmenorrhea, pharmacology and toxicology study. J Ethnopharmacol 2001; 76(3): 299-304.
55. Malini T, Vanithakumari G, Devil Nmsak, Fiango V. Effect of Foeniculum vulgare Mill. seed extract on the genital organs of male and female rats. Indian J Physiol Pharmacol 1985; 29(1): 21-26
56. Myrseyed F, Shiravi A, Nasr-Abadi M. The effect of intraperitoneal injection of alcoholic extract Foeniculum vulgare seed on gonadotropic and testosterone hormones in male wistar rats. J Anim Sci 2088; 1(1): 49-56.
57. Mirabolghasemi G, Alizadeh F. The Effect of hydroalcoholic extract of Fennel (Foeniculum vulgare) seed on serum levels of sexual hormones in female Wistar rats with Polycystic Ovarian Syndrome (PCOS). Arak Med Univ J 2014; 17(5): 70-8.
58. Devi K, Vanithakumari G, Anusya S, Mekala N, Malini T, Elango V. Effect of Foeniculum vulgare seed extract on mammary glands and oviducts of ovariectomised rats. Anc Sci Life 1985; 5(2): 129.
59. Oulmouden F, Ghalim N, El Morhit M, Benomar H, Daoudi EM, Amrani S. Hypolipidemic and Anti-Atherogenic effect of methanol extract of Fennel (Foeniculum Vulgare) in hypercholesterolemic mice. Int J Sci Knowl 2014; 3(1): 42-52.
60. Oulmouden F, Saïle R, Gnaoui N, Benomar H, Lkhider M, Amrani S, *et al.* Hypolipidemic and anti-atherogenic effect of aqueous extract of fennel (Foeniculum Vulgare) extract in an experimental model of atherosclerosis induced by triton WR-1339. Eur J Sci Res 2011; 52(1): 91-9.
61. Abdul-Ghani AS, Amin R. The vascular action of aqueous extracts of Foeniculum vulgare leaves. J Ethnopharmacol 1988; 24(2): 213-8.
62. Bardai SE, Lyoussi B, Wibo M, Morel N. Pharmacological evidence of hypotensive activity of Marrubium vulgare and Foeniculum vulgare in spontaneously hypertensive rat. Clin Exp Hypertens 2001; 23(4): 329-43.
63. Sushruta K, Satyanarayana S, Srinivas S, Sekhar JR. Evaluation of the blood-glucose reducing effects of aqueous extracts of the selected umbelliferous fruits used in culinary practices. Trop J Pharm Res 2007; 5(2): 613-7.
64. El-Soud N, El-Laithy N, El-Saeed G, Wahby M, Khalil M, Morsy F, et al. Antidiabetic activities of Foeniculum vulgare Mill. essential oil in streptozotocin-induced diabetic rats. Maced J Med Sci 2011; 4(2): 139-46.
65. Dongare V, Arvindekar A, Magadum C. Hypoglycemic effect of Foeniculum vulgare Mill. fruit on dexamethasone induced insulin resistance rats. Res J Pharmacogn Phytochem 2010; 2(2): 163-5.
66. Garga C, Khan S, Ansari S, Suman A, Garg M. Chemical composition, therapeutic potential and perspectives of Foeniculum vulgare. Pharmacogn Rev 2009; 3(6): 346-352
67. Bogucka-Kocka A, Smolarz H, Kocki J. Apoptotic activities of ethanol extracts from some Apiaceae on human leukaemia cell lines. Fitoterapia 2008; 79(7): 487-97.
68. Mohamad RH, El-Bastawesy AM, Abdel-Monem MG, Noor AM, Al-Mehdar HA, Sharawy SM, et al. Antioxidant and anticarcinogenic effects of methanolic extract and volatile oil of fennel seeds (Foeniculum vulgare). J Med Food 2011;

14(9):986-1001.
69. Ozbek H, Ugras S, Bayram I, Uygan I, Erdogan E, Ozturk A, *et al.* Hepatoprotective effect of Foeniculum vulgare essential oil: A carbon-tetrachloride induced liver fibrosis model in rats. Scand J Lab Anim Sci 2004; 31(1): 9-17.
70. Qiang F, Yiming A, Shui-quan W, Zi-ming G. Effects of foeniculum vulgare Mill on lipid peroxidation in rats with liver hepatic fibrosis. Prog Mod Biomed 2011; 21: 13.
71. Liu YP, Xu Y, Gan ZM. The influence of the Foeniculum vulgare Mill on cytokine in hepatic fibrosis rats. J Xinjiang Med Univ 2009; 6: 8.
72. Wang L, Zhang T, Zhang JL, YU Y, Gan ZM. Experimental study of Chinese herb Foeniculum vulgare Mill on liver hepatic fibrosis and potassium supplement in rats. J Xinjiang Med Univ 2012; 9: 12.
73. Liu YP, Xu Y, Gan ZM. The effect on the TNF-αin CCL4-induced liver fibrosis rat by the Foeniculum vulgare Mill [J]. J Xinjiang Med Univ 2008; 4: 21.
74. Joshi H, Parle M. Cholinergic basis of memory-strengthening effect of Foeniculum vulgare Linn. J Med Food 2006; 9(3): 413-7.
75. Taylor JM, Jenner PM, Jones WI. A comparison of the toxicity of some allyl, propenyl, and propyl compounds in the rat. Toxicol Appl Pharmacol 1964; 6(4): 378-87.
76. Ostad S, Khakinegad B, Sabzevari O. Evaluation of the teratogenicity of fennel essential oil (FEO) on the rat embryo limb buds culture. Toxicol Iin Vitro 2004; 18(5): 623-7.

10

A study on anti-diabetic and anti-hypertension herbs used in Lorestan province, Iran

Bahram Delfan[1], Kourosh Saki[2], Mahmoud Bahmani[1*], Nader Rangsaz[3], Mohammad Delfan[4], Nima Mohseni[5], Hedayatollah Shirzad[6], Zahra Babaeian[7]

[1]Razi Herbal Medicines Research Center, Lorestan University of Medical Sciences, Khorramabad, Iran
[2]Shahid Beheshti University of Medical Sciences, Tehran, Iran
[3]Faculty of Veterinary Medicine, Islamic Azad University, Shahrekord Branch, Shahrekord, Iran
[4]Deputy for Food and Drug, Lorestan University of Medical Sciences, Khorramabad, Iran
[5]Faculty of Veterinary Medicine, Islamic Azad University, Karaj Branch, Karaj, Iran
[6]Medical Plants Research Center, Shahrekord University of Medical Sciences, Shahrekord, Iran
[7]Deputy of Research and Technology, Ministry of Health and Medical Education, Tehran, Iran

ARTICLE INFO

Keywords:
Lorestan province
Herbs
Traditional medicine
Diabetes
High blood pressure
Iran

ABSTRACT

Introduction: Diabetes and hypertension are amongst the most prevalent diseases in the world, while they can be controlled and prevented, create many problems and complications for affected patients. This study was aimed to identify and report the most important and effective herbs for diabetes and high blood pressure treatment in Lorestan province (West of Iran).
Methods: By gathering and integrating indigenous data from local inhabitants of Lorestan, Iran, the goal of this study was accomplished. Data were gathered by cooperation of the agents of public health services network all over the towns of Dorud, Boroujerd, Khorramabad, Aleshtar, Poledokhtar, Aligoodarz, Nurabad and Kouhdasht.
Results: Results of this study showed that there were overall 17 medicinal plants which were used for treatment and controlling of diabetes and high blood pressure.
Conclusion: Medicinal plants reported in this study are indigenous to the Lorestan province. Some of the foresaid herbs seem to have some unknown therapeutic effects which are reported in this study for the first time, and some others have various known therapeutic effects mentioned in other similar studies. It is essential for researchers to find out the actuality of clinical effectiveness of the herbs and their active substances. Once the positive effects of these herbs proved, it would be possible to produce drugs which are useful in curing and controlling diabetes and hypertension.

Implication for health policy/practice/research/medical education:
Medicinal plants reported in this study are indigenous to the Lorestan province. If their effects are confirmed by researchers, it would be possible to produce drugs useful in curing and controlling diabetes and hypertension.

Introduction

Diabetes is one of the most common chronic diseases in the world which is becoming increasingly prevalent. It is also the third leading cause of death in the most developed countries (1). Diabetes mellitus is a complex disorder with metabolic and vascular complications. This chronic disease causes hyperglycemia then it affects different body systems, including the kidneys, eyes and mucous membrane. 9.5% of U.S population is diagnosed to have diabetes (2).

Diabetes is the most common carbohydrate metabolism disorder in which blood glucose level rises due to a deficiency of Insulin secretion or its abnormal activity. Long-term complications of diabetes include heart disease, stroke, kidney failure, blindness, nerve damage and neuropathy, atherosclerosis, chronic infections, immune deficiency and peripheral vascular disease that may lead to ulcers, gangrene and amputation (3-5).

*Corresponding author: Dr. Mahmoud Bahmani; Razi Herbal Medicines Research Center, Lorestan University of Medical Sciences, Khorramabad, Iran; Email: mahmood.bahmani@gmail.com

In 2011, approximately 7% of world population was diagnosed with diabetes, while 80% of these people were living in developing countries (6). Studies conducted in Iran show a prevalence of approximately 4.2% to 15.9% (7). Hypertension is defined as a blood pressure more than 90/140 mmHg. In 95% of cases, the cause of hypertension is unknown, which is called primary hypertension. Some main causes of hypertension include oral contraceptive drugs, hyperaldosteronism, cushing's syndrome, renal artery stenosis and renal failure. Other possible causes of hypertension include genetic-related disorders of renal sodium secretion, genetic-related disorders of Na/Ca exchange in smooth muscles of arteries, changes in the genes coding angiotensin, other proteins of renin-angiotensin system, and hormonal-neurogenic vasoconstriction (8-17). Almost a quarter of deaths in elderly patients are resulted from hypertension and its complications (18).

Blood pressure is a common asymptomatic, identifiable and usually treatable disease but if left untreated the consequences of that could be fatal for the patient. Hypertension is the most common risk factor for acute myocardial infarction, stroke, peripheral vascular disease, and is the major known factor for cardiovascular disease and its mortality (19-21).

Regarding the importance of producing therapeutic agents and drugs from medicinal plants and preparing documentations about valuable indigenous information in the field of traditional medicine and finding cheap, safe and effective ways of preventing diabetes and hypertension, this ethnobotanical study was performed to collect the information about traditional medicine in Lorestan region and to identify medicinal plants claimed to be effective in treating diabetes and hypertension.

Materials and Methods

The study setting

Lorestan is a province of western Iran, located latitude and longitude of 33.4871° N, 48.3538°. Lorestan has four different climates (semi-dry, semi-moist temperate, semi-moist cold and altitude climate). Its area is approximately 28,300 square acres of land. Minimum height above sea level is 330 m in Pole-Zal and maximum height above sea level is 4050 m in Oshtoran-kooh.

This province has a varied climate and this variability is quite evident from the northeast to the southwest. Lorestan is a neighbor of Hamedan and Markazi provinces in north, Isfahan in east, Khuzestan in south and Ilam and Kermanshah in west.

Method of identifying and collecting the plants

Data of traditional medications were provided through interviews and questionnaires, with assistance of Management and Planning Organization of Lorestan province and Lorestan University of Medical Sciences. Local inhabitants data were also collected through cooperation with Health Networks of Dorud, Burujird, Khorramabad, Aleshtar Poldokhtar, Aligoodarz, Nurabad and Kouhdasht.

Results

After collecting and classifying the data, a total number of 17 medicinal plants effective for controlling and treating of diabetes and hypertension were identified, which were marked in Table 1.

Discussion

Despite the presence of anti-diabetic drugs in pharmacies, diabetes and its complications are still a major medical problem. So, many studies and efforts have been done to manage clinical treatment of diabetes by applying medicinal plants. Hence, ethnobotanical studies are necessary for identifying anti-diabetic herbs and providing information for researchers. The World Health Organization (WHO) has declared about the use of herbal agents in controlling diabetes and conducting researches in this direction as a necessity (27).

In traditional medicine, berries are used as antidiabetic agents in lowering blood glucose, diuretic, laxative, effective in smallpox and typhoid, fattening agent, aphrodisiac, relieve coughing, asthma, effective in rheumatism, mucokinetic, anti-phlegmatic, treatment of hypotension and bactericidal and virucidal effects (28-32). Berry is introduced as one of the anti-diabetic plants in Lorestan province in traditional medicine which is effective in reducing blood sugar.

Berries are important sources of antioxidant and phenolic compounds. Flavones, hydroxycinamic acid and cyanidin 3-glucoside are other compounds found in the berries (33-35). Berry lowers blood glucose and increases glucose uptake by the cells (36). Given the known mechanisms of berry in treatment and prevention of diabetes and hyperglycemia and its complications, it can be used as an alternative to sugar to sweeten tea in diabetic persons.

Barberries are used in treating infectious fevers, typhus and diarrhea. Experimental studies performed on animals reportedly show anti-inflammatory effects of barberry (37,38). Flavonoids aglycones inhibit facilitated diffusion of glucose and flavonoids glycosides inhibit glucose uptake through active transport. In addition, certain polyphenols such as catechin and gallic acid have no effect on insulin-mediated glucose uptake, whereas quercetin, myristin and catechin gallate inhibit glucose uptake in a dose-dependent manner (39,40). Another study proved that barberry has a depressing effect on blood pressure (41). Other studies have also shown the arterial blood pressure lowering effects of barberry. Barberry fruits contain bioactive substances such as malic acid, pectic substances, glycoside substances and berberine. Most properties of Barberries can be attributed to berberine (42-44).

Citrullus colocynthis has been mentioned as a healing drug of diabetes in traditional medicine (45). Acute

Table 1. Complete information of ethnobotany, route of use and therapeutic effects of herbs effective in diabetes and high blood pressure in Lorestan province.

Scientific name	Family	Local Name	Persian Name	Usable Part	Method of application	Gathering Season	Traditional Therapeutic Effect
Morus alba	Moraceae	Ti	Toot	Fruit	Raw berry or dried berry is eaten as sugar	Spring	Lowers blood pressure
Berberis integrima	Berberidaceae	Zereshk	zereshk	Leaf and stem	Cooked and sodden	Spring	Diabetes treatment
Pistacia atlantica	Anacardiaceae	Zhevi	baneh (peste koohi)	Juice	After softened by drenching, it is applied on the ulcer and covered with fabric ,to be replaced each day	Spring, Summer	Diabetic ulcers and hyperglycemia
Capparis spinosa	Capparaceae	Shomi-sheytoni	Hendevaneh aboujahl	Fruit and leaf	Raw fruit or dry leaf distillate is eaten	Spring, Summer	Lowers blood glucose
Urtica dioica	Urticaceae	gezgezo	gazaneh	Twig	The leaf is tied on muscles, sodden stems is eaten with soup	Spring, Summer, Autumn	Lowers blood glucose
Valeriana officinalis L	Valerianaceae	Midareh	sonbol-el-tib	Fruit	Ripe fruit is eaten raw, unripe fruit is used to provide distillate	Spring	Lowers blood glucose
Melilotus officinalis	Leguminosae	Yonje	yonje	Flower, leaf, stem	Distillate or infusion is drunk after eating food. Raw leaves and stem is used	Any season	Lowers blood glucose
Nectaroscordeum tripedale Nectaroscordeum coelzi	Amaryllidaceae	Aneshk	Piaz tabestani lorestan	Twig	Raw or through sauces, with beverages like dough, infusions is eaten	Spring	Lowers blood glucose
Falcaria vulgaris	Apiaceae	Paghazou	ghaziaghi	Flower, leaf, stem	Leaves are cooked and eaten with food, a glass of infusion once a day	Spring and Winter	Lowers blood pressure
Smyrnium cordifolium	Umbelliferae	Pinomeh	andool	Seed	Squeezed seeds	Spring	Lowers blood pressure
Crocus hasskenechtii	Iridaceae	Pishok	soffron	Root	Raw and cooked	Spring	Lowers blood pressure
Berberis integrima	Berberidaceae	Zereshk	zereshk	Leaf and stem	Cooked or sodden	Spring	Lowers blood pressure
Ziziphus spina-christi Ziziphus nummularia	Rhamnaceae	Konar	sedr	Flower, leaf, fruit	Sodden leaves and flower	Spring, midsummer	Lowers blood pressure
Allium ursinum	Liliaceae	Sir kohi	Sir	Scallion	Raw or with food	Spring	Lowers blood pressure
Tragapogon caricifolius	Compositae	Sheng	shang	Whole parts	Raw, dried or infusion	Spring	Lowers blood pressure
Anethum graveolens	Umbelliferae	shevit	shevid	Whole parts	Dried or fresh with food	Summer	Lowers blood pressure
Amygdalus scoparia	Rosaceae	Badam	badam	Fruit	Sodden peel	Spring	Lowers blood pressure

hypoglycaemic and anti-hyperglycaemic effects of various root extracts of this plant have been shown in vivo models of normal and diabetic rabbits (46). Another study has shown the mechanism of action of the fruit of Citrullus colocynthis. This means that the fruit extract immediately and in a stable way stimulates secretion of insulin from pancreatic beta cells of rats (47). It also contains colocynthin, colocynthilin, citrulline, citronellol, resinous substances, pectin and various salts (48).

Valerian has blood pressure lowering effects in animals (49). Garlic has anti-parasitic, anti-viral, anti-fungal and anti-oxidant effects, improves peripheral blood flow and reduces blood lipids. These effects are attributed to its antioxidant activity (50-53).

Tragopogon dubius treats dysentery and bile flows. Its extract is used for healing gastric ulcer and known to be beneficial as stomach tonic. Its sodden is effective in liver disorders, gastric burning pains and regurgitation. Zakaryia al-Razi has recommended the use of sheng for excreting toxins (54). Sheng has been used for reducing blood lipids, increasing appetite, stomach and liver tonic in traditional medicine and is known to be beneficial in liver disorders and kidney stones (55,56). Sheng is one of the main sources of inulin (57). It seems that inulin is the main ingredient of sheng to have hypotensive effects.

Dill in traditional medicine is used to treat flatulence, indigestion and gastric ulcers. Dill has a strong antibacterial effect (58-60). Dill extract is used as cholestero-lowering drug in Iran. Furocoumarins can reduce total triglyceride and total cholesterol in hyperlipidemic rats (61). Dill seed contains D-carvone, D-limonene, α-phellandrene and dihydrocarvone (62). Dill Lowers blood glucose and reduces the blood lipids and cholesterol (63,64). Bioactive substances of dill may be a source of herbal medicines effective against hypertension and diabetes. Almonds play an important role in reducing the risk of heart disease in diabetic patients (65).

Besides predicating traditionally believed effects of

these herbs, it is essential for researchers to find out the actuality of clinical effectiveness of the herbs and their active substances. Once the positive effects of these herbs proved, it is possible to produce drugs which are useful in curing and controlling diabetes and hypertension (66-70). Moreover, it has a great significance to make documented records of traditional medical information to prevent them from shrinking.

Acknowledgments
This study was carried out with the collaboration of the Management and Planning Organization of Lorestan, Lorestan University of Medical Sciences, Deputy of Research & Technology. Authors require to acknowledge the efforts done by Mrs. M. Rashidi-pour, Dr. Abbasi, Dr. Salarvand, Dr. Jamshidi, Dr. Maknly, Dr. Hejazi, Dr. Refahi, Dr. Veysi, Dr. Roshani, Dr. Rezaei, Dr. Mosadegh, gentlemen, Mr. Vali Khorramabadi, Hassan Niknam, Salar Alizadeh, Bahman Hassanzadeh. They also appreciate the assistance and coopration of Dorud health and treatment organization, Borojerd, Khorramabad, Aleshtar Poldokhtar, Aligoodarz, Nurabad and Kouhdasht.

Authors' contributions
All the authors wrote the manuscript equally.

Conflict of interests
The authors declared no competing interests.

Ethical considerations
Ethical issues (including plagiarism, misconduct, data fabrication, falsification, double publication or submission, redundancy) have been completely observed by the authors.

Funding/Support
None.

References

1. Little J, Falace D. Dental management of the medically compromised patient. 7th ed. St Louis: Mosby; 2008. p. 145-50.
2. Greenberg MS, Glick M. Burket's oral medicine diagnosis & treatment, 11th ed. Hamilton: BC Becker Co; 2008. p. 63-5.
3. Hunt JV, Smith CC, Wolff SP. Autoxidative glycosylation and possible involvement of peroxides and free radicals in LDL modification by glucose. Diabetes 1990; 39(11):1420-4.
4. Koya D, Hayashi K, Kitada M, Kashiwagi A, Kikkawa R, Haneda M. Effects of antioxidants in diabetes-induced oxidative stress in the glomeruli of diabetic rats. J Am Soc Nephrol 2003; 14(8 Suppl 3): 250-3.
5. Engelgau M, Geiss L, Saaddine J, Boyle J, Benjamin S, Gregg E, *et al.* The evolving diabetes burden in the United States. Annals of Internal Medicine 2004;140(11):945-50.
6. Boulton AJ, Vileikyte L, Ragnarson-Tennvall G, Apelqvist J. The global burden of diabetic foot disease. Lancet 2005; 366(9498):1719-24.
7. Baghianimoghadam MH , Afkhami Ardekani M. The effect of educational intervention on quality of life of diabetic patients type 2, referee to diabetic research centre of Yazd. Horizon Med Sci 2008; 13(4):21-8.
8. Carretero OA, Oparil S. Essential hypertension. Part I: definition and etiology. Circulation 2000;101(3):329-35.
9. Palmer BF. Renal dysfunction complicating the treatment of hypertension. N Engl J Med 2002;347(16):1256-61.
10. Pickering TG, Herman L, Devereux RB, Sotelo JE, James GD, Sos TA, *et al.* Recurrent pulmonary oedema in hypertension due to bilateral renal artery stenosis: treatment by angioplasty or surgical revascularisation. Lancet 1988;2(8610):551-2.
11. Hanenson IB, Taussky HH, Polasky N, Ransohoff W, Miller BF. Renal excretion of sodium in arterial hypertension. Circulation 1959;20:498-510.
12. Zhang Y, Jose PA, Zeng C. Regulation of sodium transport in the proximal tubule by endothelin. Contrib Nephrol 2011;172:63-75.
13. Patel SK, Wai B, Ord M, MacIsaac RJ, Grant S, Velkoska E, *et al.* Association of ACE2 genetic variants with blood pressure, left ventricular mass, and cardiac function in Caucasians with type 2 diabetes. Am J Hypertens 2012;25(2):216-22.
14. Edvardsson B, Persson S. Reversible cerebral vasoconstriction syndrome associated with autonomic dysreflexia. J Headache Pain 2010;11(3):277-80.
15. Magiakou MA, Smyrnaki P, Chrousos GP. Hypertension in Cushing's syndrome. Best Pract Res Clin Endocrinol Metab 2006;20(3):467-82.
16. Douma S, Petidis K, Doumas M, Papaefthimiou P, Triantafyllou A, Kartali N, *et al.* Prevalence of primary hyperaldosteronism in resistant hypertension: a retrospective observational study. Lancet 2008;371(9628):1921-6.
17. Oparil S. Hypertension and oral contraceptives. J Cardiovasc Med 1981; 6(4):381,384-7.
18. Black JM, Matassarin-Jacobs E, editors. Luckmann and Sorensen's Medical-Surgical Nursing: A Psychophysiologic Approach. 4th ed. Philadelphia: W.B. Saunders; 1993.
19. Harison. Harrison Principles of Internal Medicine: Cardiovascular Disease. Tarbiat Translation. Tehran: Publication of Noore Danesh; 1385. p. 403.
20. Vasan RS, Beiser A, Seshadri S, Larson MG, Kannel WB.. Residual lifetime risk for developing hypertension in middle-aged women and men: the Framingham Heart Study. JAMA 2002; 287:1003–10.
21. Stamler J, Stamler R, Neaton JD. Blood pressure, systolic and diastolic, and cardiovascular risks: US

population data. Arch Intern Med 1993; 153:598–615.
22. Choi CW, Kim SC, Hwang SS, Choi BK, Ahn HJ, Lee MY, *et al.* Antioxidant activity and free radical scavenging capacity between Korean medicinal plants and flavonoids by assay-guided comparison. Plant Sci 2002; 163:1161-8.
23. Bhattaram VA, Ceraefe M, Kohlest C, Vest M, Deundorf H. Pharmacokinetics and bioavailability of herbal medicinal products. Phytomed 2002; 9:1-36.
24. Frenz MJ. Medical nutrition therapy for diabetes mellitus and hypoglycemia of nondiabetic origion. In: Mahan LK, Escott-stumps S, Editors. Krause's Food, Nutrition and Diet therapy. 11th ed. Philadelphia: Sunders press; 2004. p. 792-837.
25. Gleckman R, Mory J. Diabeted-related foot infection. J Contemporary Inter Med 1994; 6:57-62.
26. Mitra SK, Gopumadhavan S, Muralidhar TS, Anturlikar SD, Sujatha MB. Effect of a herbomineral preparation D-400 in streptozotocininduced diabetic rats. J Ethnopharmacol 1996; 54:41-6.
27. Rai MK. A review on some antidiabetic plants of India. Ancient Sci Life 1995; 14:42-54.
28. Loew D, Kaszkin M. Approaching the problem of bioequivalence of herbal medicinal products. Phytother Res 2002; 16:705-11.
29. Chen MD, Song YM, Lin PY, Zin C. Effects on hyperglycemia and hypoleptinemia in sterptozotosin-induced diabetic mice. Horm Metab Res 2000;32: 107-9.
30. Chu Q, Lin M, Tian X, Ye J. Study on capillary electrophoresis amperometric detection profiles of different parts of Morus alba L. J Chromatogr 2006; 16(1-2):286-90.
31. Kim H, Jang MH, Shin MC, Chang HK, Lee TH, Lim BV, *et al.* Folium mori increases cell proliferation and neuropeptide Y expression in dentate gyrus of streptozotocin induced diabetic rats. Biol Pharm Bull 2003; 26:434-7.
32. Nomura T. Phenolic compounds of the mulberry tree and related plants. In: Herz W, Grisebach H, Kirby GW, Tamm C, Editors. Progress in the Chemistry of Organic Natural Products, vol. 53. Vienna: Springer;1988. p. 87–201.
33. Mazza G, Miniati E. Small Fruits. In: Boca Raton FL, editor. Anthocyanins in Fruits, Vegetables, and Grains. Boca Raton, FL:CRC Press:1993.
34. Heinonen IM, Meyer AS, Frankel EN. Antioxidant activity of berry phenolics on human low-density lipoprotein and liposome oxidation. Journal of Agricultural Food Chemistry 1996; 44:4107-12.
35. Fukumoto LR, Mazza G. Assessing antioxidant and prooxidant activity of phenolic compounds. Journal of Agriculteral Food Chemistry 2000; 48:3597-604.
36. Arzi A, Zahedi S, Ghanavati J. Effect of Morus alba leaf extract on streptozocininduced diabetes in mice. Ahvaz Journal of Medical Sciences 2001; 30:20.
37. Fatehi M, Saleh TM, Fatehi-Hassanabad Z, Farrokhfal K, Jafarzadeh M, Davodi S. A pharmacological study on Berberis Vulgaris fruit extract. J Ethnopharmcol 2005; 102: 46-52.
38. Zargari A, editor. Medicinal Plants. 7th ed. Tehran: Tehran University Press; 1993. p. 72-9.
39. Johnston K, Sharp P, Clifford M, Morgan L. Dietary polyphenols decrease glucose uptake by human intestinal Caco-2 cells. FEBS Lett 2005; 579:1653-7.
40. Strobel P, Allard C, Perez-Acle T, Calderon R, Aldunate R, Leighton F. Myricetin, quercetin and catechin-gallate inhibit glucose uptake in isolated rat adipocytes. Biochem J 2005; 386:471-8.
41. Shamsa F, Ahmadiani A, Khosrokhavar R. Antihistaminic and anticholinergic activity of barberry fruit (Berberis vulgaris) in the guineapig ileum. J Ethnopharmacol 1999; 64(2):161-6.
42. Baytop T. Phytotherapy in Turkey: past and present. Nobl Pub l, Stanbul, Turkey, 1999
43. Blumenthal Busse WR, Goldbert A, Grenwald J, Hall T, Klein S, Riggins CW, *et al.* The complete German E Monographs - therapeutic guide to herbal medicines. Austin, TX: American butanical council; 1998. p. 310.
44. Gudima SO, Memelova LV, Bordulin VB. Kinetic analysis of interaction of human immunodeficiency virus revers transcriptase with alkaloids. Mol Biol (Mosk) 1991; 28:1308-14.
45. Fallah Hosseini H, Heshmat R, Larijani B, Fakhr Zadeh H, Jafari Azar Z, Darvish Zadeh F, *et al.* The clinical investigation of Citrullus Colocynthis (L.) Schrad. fruit in treatment of type II diabetic patients: A randomized, double-blind, placebo-controlled study. Journal of Medicinal Plants 2006;5:31-5.
46. Nmila R, Gross R, Rchid H, Roye M, Manteghetti M, Petit P, *et al.* Insulinotropic effect of Citrullus colocynthis fruit extracts. Planta Med 2000; 66:418-23.
47. Abdel-Hassan IA. Abdel-Barry JA. Tariq Mohammeda S. The hypoglycaemic and antihyperglycaemic effect of citrullus colocynthis fruit aqueous extract in normal and alloxan diabetic rabbits. J Ethnopharmacol 2000;71:325-30.
48. Zargari A. Pharmaceutical plants. 8th Edition, Tehran: Publication of Tehran University; 1993. p. 90-4.
49. British Pharmacopeia Addendum. London: LLMSOL;1993. p. 2035
50. Ayaz E. Alpsoy HC. Garlic (Allium sativum) and traditional medicine. Acta Parasitol Turcica 2007; 31 (2):145-9.
51. Ebadi A, Rahimielenji A, Taghadosi M, Khorshidi A, Akbri H. Effect of garlic on blood glucose in type 2 diabetic patients. Quarterly Journal of Feiz 2007; 11(1):76-85.
52. Borek C. Antioxidant health effects of aged Garlic extract. Journal of Nutrition 2001; 131(3s):1010-5.

53. Ide N, Lau BH, Ryu K. Antioxidant effects of fructosyl arginine, a Maillard reaction product in aged garlic extract. Journal of Nutrition Biochemistry 1999; 10(6):372-6.
54. Bahmani M, Zargaran A, Rafieian-Kopaei M, Saki M. Ethnobotanical study of medicinal plants used in the management of diabetes mellitus in the Urmia, Northwest Iran. Asian Pac J Trop Med 2014; 7(Suppl 1): 348-54.
55. Zargari A. Medicinal Plants. Sixth Ed. Vol 1. Tehran:Tehran University Press;1990. p. 72-166.
56. Shafizadeh F. Popular Medicinal Plants of Lorestan. Tehran:Hayan Publication; 2002. p. 128.
57. Rastall RA, Maitin V. Prebiotics and synbiotics: towards the next generation. Curr Opin Biotech 2002; 13:490-6.
58. Duke J. Hanbooke of medical herbs. London: CRC Press; 2001.
59. Hosseinzadeh H, Karimi GR, Ameri M. Effects of Anethum graveolens L. seed extracts on experimental gastric irritation models in mice. BMC Pharmacol 2002; 2:21.
60. Delaquis PJ, Stanich K, Girard B, Mazza G. Antimicrobial activity of individual and mixed fractions of dill, cilantro, coriander and eucalyptus essential oils. Int J Food Microbiol 2002; 74(1-2): 1019.
61. Bahramikia S, Yazdanparast R. Efficacy of different fractions of Anethum graveolens leaves on serum lipoproteins and serum and liver oxidative status in experimentally induced hypercholesterolaemic rat models. Am J Chin Med 2009; 37(4): 685-99.
62. Carla CCR, de Carvalho M. Carvone: Why and how should one bother to produce this terpene. Food Chem 2006; 96(3):413-22.
63. Panda S. The effect of Anethum graveolens L. (dill) on corticosteroid induced diabetes mellitus: involvement of thyroid hormones. Phytother Res 2008;22(12):1695-7.
64. Yazdanparast R, Bahramikia S. Evaluation of the effect of Anethum graveolens L. crude extracts on serum lipids and lipoproteins profiles in hypercholesterolemia rats. Daru 2008; 16(2):88-94.
65. Darvish Damavandi R, Shidfar F, Rajab A, Mohammadi V, Hosseini S. The Effects of Cashew Consumption on Serum Glucose, Insulin and Lipoprotein in Type 2 Diabetic Patients. Iranian Journal of Endocrinology and Metabolism 2012; 14(4): 325-334.
66. Bahmani M, Saki K, Rafieian-Kopaei M, Karamati SA, Eftekhari Z, Jelodari M. The most common herbal medicines affecting Sarcomastigophora branches: a review study. Asian Pac J Trop Med 2014; 7(Suppl 1): 14-21.
67. Bahmani M, Rafieian-Kopaei M, Hassanzadazar H, Saki K, Karamati SA, Delfan B. A review on most important herbal and synthetic antihelmintic drugs. Asian Pac J Trop Med 2014; 7(Suppl 1): 29-33.
68. Bahmani M, Rafieian-Kopaei M, Jeloudari M, Eftekhari Z, Delfan B, Zargaran A, *et al.* A review of the health effects and uses of drugs of plant licorice (Glycyrrhiza glabra L.) in Iran. Asian Pac J Trop Dis 2014; 4(Suppl 2): 847-9.
69. Saki K, Bahmani M, Rafieian-Kopaei M. The effect of most important medicinal plants on two important psychiatric disorders (anxiety and depression)-a review. Asian Pac J Trop Med 2014; 7(Suppl 1): 34-42.
70. Asadbeigi M, Mohammadi T, Rafieian-Kopaei M, Saki K, Bahmani M, Delfan B. Traditional effects of medicinal plants in the treatment of respiratory diseases and disorders: an ethnobotanical study in the Urmia. Asian Pac J Trop Med 2014; 7(Suppl 1): S364-8.

Antifungal effects of *Allium ascalonicum, Marticaria chamomilla* and *Stachys lavandulifolia* extracts on *Candida albicans*

Hassan Moghim[1,*], Simin Taghipoor[1], Najmeh Shahinfard[1], Soleiman Kheiri[1], Zahra Heydari[1], Samira Rafieian[2]

[1]Medical Plants Research Center, Shahrekord University of Medical Sciences, Shahrekord, Iran
[2]Pharmaceutical Faculty, Isfahan University of Medical Sciences, Isfahan, Iran

ARTICLE INFO

Keywords:
Antifungal activity
Candida albicans
Allium ascalonicum
Marticaria chamomilla
Stachys lavandulifolia

ABSTRACT

Introduction: Due to increased risk for opportunistic fungal infections and increasing prevalence of hospital infections caused by pathogenic yeasts and fungus resistance to antifungal drugs, discovery of antifungal compounds with high efficiency is necessary. This study was aimed to evaluate and compare the antifungal activities of *Allium ascalonicum*, *Marticaria chamomilla* and *Stachys lavandulifolia* on *Candida albians*.
Methods: In this study the plants extracts were prepared with macerated method using ethanol 70%. Antifungal activities of the extracts were performed according to microbroth dilution method in 96 well microdilution plates. The amount of Minimum Inhibitory Concentration (MIC) and Minimum Fungicidal Concentration (MFC) based on counting the number of fungal colonies (CFU) were evaluated for each of *Allium ascalonicum*, Chamomile and *Stachys lavandulifolia* extracts compared with the control group.
Results: MIC of *Allium ascalonicum*, *Marticaria chamomilla* and *Stachys lavandulifolia* were respectively 0.31, 3.75 and 15.13 mg/ml and also MIC50% of *Allium ascalonicum*, *Marticaria chamomilla* and *Stachys lavandulifolia* were respectively 0.93, 10.59 and 41.32 mg/ml and MIC 90% of them were respectively 8.65, 16.88 and 60.55 mg/ml and their MFC were respectively 20, 20 and 65 mg/ml.
Conclusion: The results indicate that all three extracts are effective, but *Allium ascalonicum* possesses the highest antifungal activity on *Candida albicans*. If clinical trials approve these findings, this plant may represent a new source of antifungal agent for control of *Candida albicans*.

Implication for health policy/practice/research/medical education:
The results indicate that *Allium ascalonicum* possesses high antifungal activity on *Candida albicans*. If clinical trials approve these findings, this plant may represent a new source of antifungal agent for control of *Candida albicans*.

Introduction

Candidiasis is one of the most important and most common opportunistic fungal diseases in humans (1,2). *Candida albicans* is the most important agent in causing *Candidiasis*. Infection can be seen as acute, subacute or chronic in skin, nails, vaginal mucosa, bronchus, lung and gastrointestinal tract. Host response against infection is usually mild irritation and inflammation, then chronic form and acute purulent or granulomatous changes (3). Pravin in 2006 reported that 70% of human population always or occasionally use herbal medicines. WHO estimated that 80% of the population at risk of some diseases, use herbal medicines as first line treatment (4). Due to increased risk for opportunistic fungal infections and the increasing prevalence of hospital infections caused by pathogenic yeasts and fungus resistance to antifungal drugs, discovery of antifungal compounds with high efficiency and low toxicity is necessary. Plants present a

***Corresponding author**: Hassan Moghim,
E-mail: hassan.moghim@yahoo.com

great variety of compounds with therapeutic properties and might be considered as suitable alternative (4).
Synthetic drugs and chemicals used in fungal infections, especially in patients with underlying disease have many side effects (5). Researches on medicinal plants have shown promising results on different diseases (6-9). Some herbs have strong anti-oxidant activities and are rich in anti-microbial components that can be used to treat fungal infections and bacteria (10,11).
Allium genus have been shown to have antifungal activity which basically depends on the presence of sulfur compounds (12). The main compounds of scallion are composed of disulfide compounds, trisulfide, flavonoids (quercetin), saponins and sapogenine (13,14). The amount of flavonoids present in one ml of ethyl acetate extract of scallion is 156.87±5 µg or 38% of its extract (15).
Marticaria chamomilla is from Asteraceae family (16). The main components of *Marticaria chamomilla* are Chamazulen and α-Bisabolol with high antimicrobial properties against gram positive and gram negative bacteria (17).
Marticaria chamomilla and some components of this plant such as α- bisabolol, apigenin and luteolin have been shown to have antibacterial and antifungal activities (18).
Stachys lavandulifolia has antioxidant activity and destroys free radicals (19).
This study was aimed to evaluate and compare the antifungal activities of *Allium ascalonicum*, *Marticaria chamomilla* and *Stachys lavandulifolia* on *Candida albians*.

Material and Methods

Extraction method

To prepare extracts, the plants, *Allium ascalonicum*, *Marticaria chamomilla* or *Stachys lavandulifolia* were purchased from a reputable grocery and after separation of brushwood with an electric mill, they were powdered. The resulting powder after passing through sieve No. 10 was poured in the flasks and mixed with 300 cc ethanol 70%. The solution was kept for 72 hours in a dry environment. After the solution was passed through the filter paper, it was transferred for extracting to percolation system. While the temperature was 38 °C on the system, the extract was transferred to the incubator and the alcohol was completely removed (20,21). When needed different concentrations of the extracts were prepared using distilled water and 0.5 ml of DMSO (Dimethyl Sulfoxide).

Preparation of Candida albicans suspensions

The standard fungal strain with PTCC5027 code used in this project was provided from Scientific Research Center of Iran. *Canida albicans* was cultured on dextrose agar medium at 35 °C. After 24 hours, some colonies were transferred to one ml of normal saline to prepared a solution with concentration of 0.5 McFarland 1.5×10^6 cfu/ml (neobar slides were used for colony counting). Then, the resulting solution was diluted to a ratio of 1:1000 and suspensions with concentrations of 0.5-2.5×10^3 cfu/ml was provided (22).
Different dilutions were prepared from *Allium ascalonicum*, *Marticaria chamomilla* and *Stachys lavandulifolia* extracts using Microbroth dilution method, and according to the method proposed by the National Committee for Clinical Laboratory Standards for yeasts (NCCLSM27-A). Thus, to the first well of Ninety-six well plates, two-fold dilution of the extract was poured, and subsequent dilutions were prepared with serial dilution (22).
Different Concentrations of the extracts were prepared as follows:
Allium ascalonicum: 0.31, 0.625, 0.93, 1.25, 1.87, 2.5, 3.75, 5, 7.5, 10, 12, 15 and 20 mg/ml,
Marticaria chamomilla: 2.5, 3.75, 5, 7.5, 10, 12,15 and 20 mg/ml,
Stachys lavandulifolia: 15, 20, 25, 30, 35, 40, 45, 50, 55, 60 and 65 mg/ml.
100 microliters of each dilution of the extract was added separately to the socket of ninety-six well plates that contained 100 ml of Sabouraud broth liquid medium (Sabouraud broth). Then 100 ml of yeast cell suspension in volumes equivalent to 2500 cells per ml were inoculated into the all sockets, except the control plates. The plates were kept at 35 °C for 48 h in the incubator on the Shaker. After incubation time, 10 micro liters of the contents of each socket was cultured on Sabouraud dextrose agar medium and were placed for 48 hours at 35 °C. After this period, the amount of Minimum Inhibitory Concentration (MIC) and Minimum Fungicidal Concentration (MFC) based on counting the number of fungal colonies (CFU) were evaluated for each of *Allium ascalonicum*, Chamomile and *Stachys lavandulifolia* extracts compared with the control group (23).

Results

Results of Allium ascalonicum extract

As can be seen in Figure 1, the extract has antifungal activity on *Candida albicans* and the effect is dose dependent.

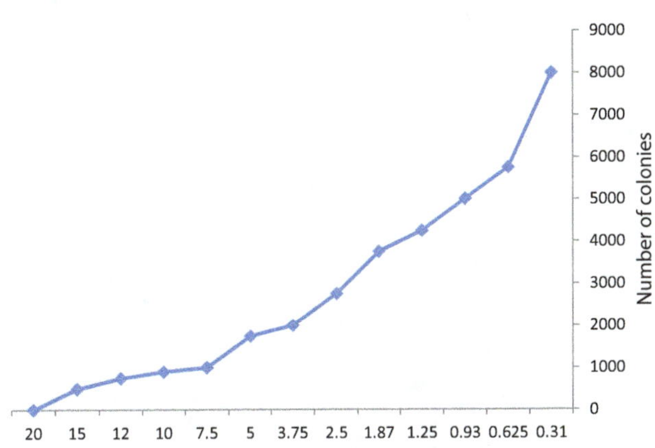

Figure 1. The number of colonies grown in culture medium, in different concentrations of *Allium ascalonicum* extract

MIC, MIC 50%, MIC 90% and MFC of *Allium ascalonicum* extract on *Candida albicans* were respectively 0.31, 0.93, 8.65 and 20 mg/ml (Figure 2).

Results of *Marticaria chamomilla* extract

The effect of the extract against *Candida albicans* was dependent on the dose of the extract. Hence, with increasing concentrations of *Marticaria chamomilla* extract the number of *Candida albicans* colonies reduced. In the concentration of 20 mg/ml, no colony was grown (Figure 3).

MIC, MIC 50%, MIC 90% and MFC of *Marticaria chamomilla* were respectively 3.75, 10.59, 16.88 and 20 mg/ml (Figure 4).

Results of *Stachys lavandulifolia* extract

The effect of *Stachys lavandulifolia* extract on the growth of *Candida albicans* was also examined. The extract the same as two other extracts had antifungal activity and in the concentration of 65 mg/ml, no colony could grow (Figure 5).

MIC, MIC 50%, MIC 90% and MFC of *Stachys lavandulifolia* on *Candida albicans* were respectively 15.13, 41.32, 60.55 and 65 mg/ml (Figure 6).

The MIC 50%, MIC 90% and MFC values (mg/ml) of three plants are compared in Table 1.

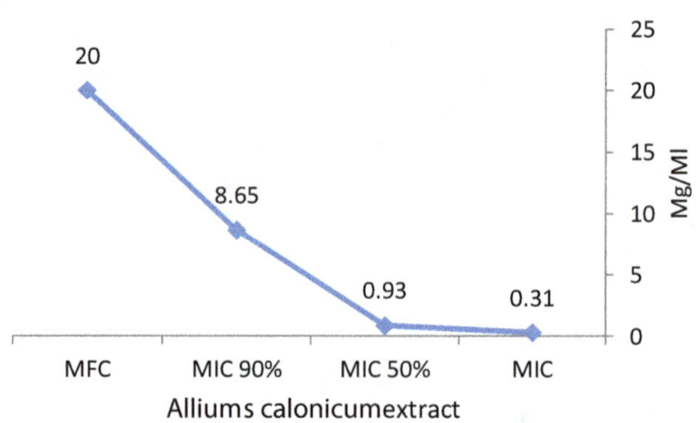

Figure 2. Comparison the MIC and MFC of *Allium scalonicum* extract on *Candida albicans*

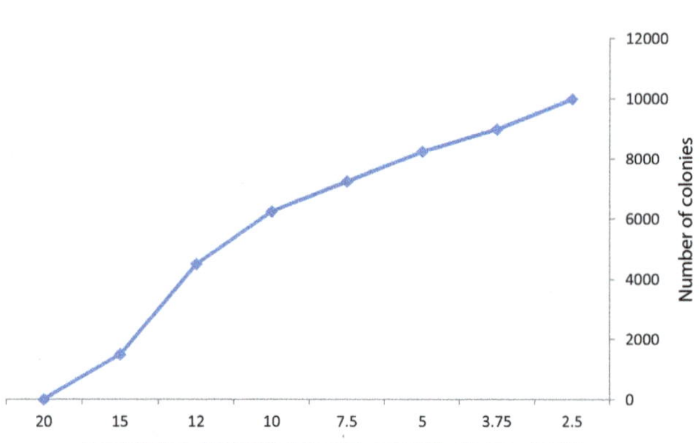

Figure 3. The number of colonies grown in culture medium, in different concentrations of *Marticaria chamomilla* extract

Comparison of inhibitory and fungicidal effects of plant extracts

The logistic regression test showed that there were significant differences between the inhibitory and fungicida effects of each of the plants extracts ($P<0.05$). *Allium ascalonicum* had the greatest inhibitory and fungicidal effects on *Candida albicans* then *Marticaria chamomilla*, and *Stachys lavandulifolia* had the least antifungal effect (Figure 7).

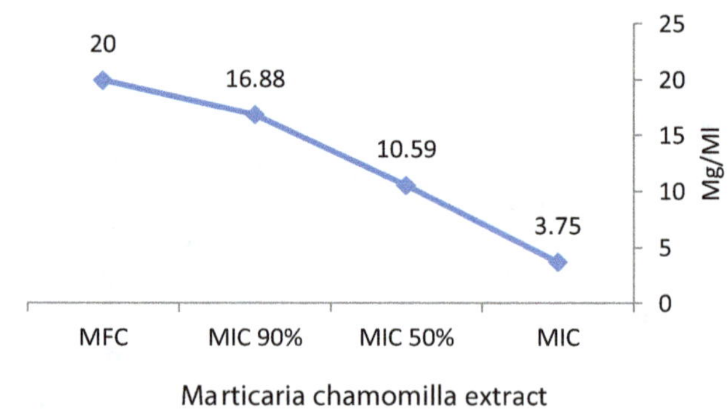

Figure 4. Comparison the MIC and MFC of *Marticaria chamomilla* extract on *Candida Albicans*

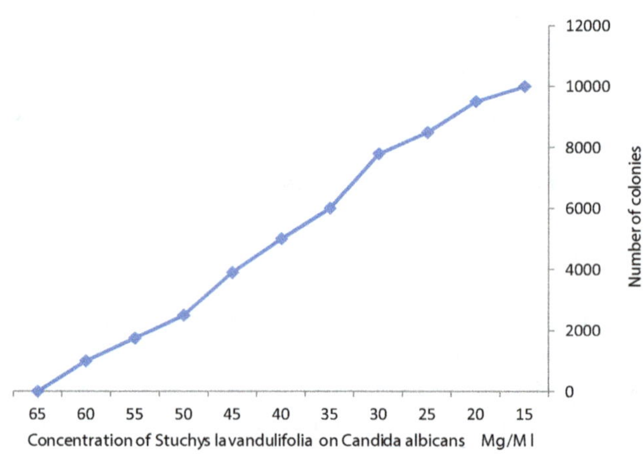

Figure 5. The number of colonies grown in culture medium, in different concentrations of *Stachys lavandulifolia* extract.

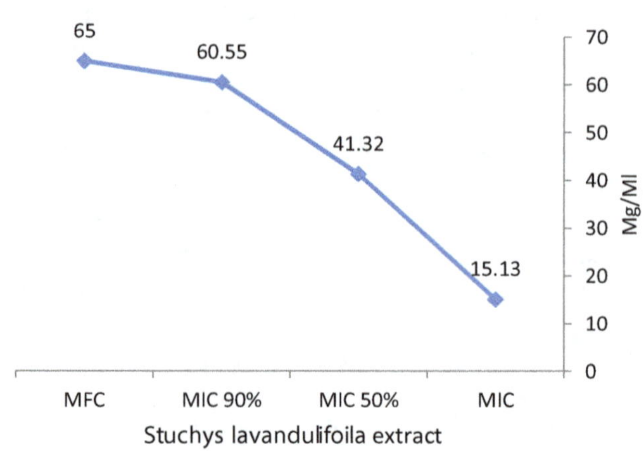

Figure 6. Comparison the MIC and MFC of *Stachys lavandulifolia* extract on *Candida Albicans*

Table 1. MIC 50%, MIC 90% and MFC values of the plants studied (mg/ml) and their 95% Confidence intervals

Plant	MIC 50%		MIC 90%		MFC	
	Value	95% confidence interval	Value	95% Confidence interval	Value	95% Confidence interval
Allium ascalonicum	0.93	0.15-1.92	8.65	7.19-10.31	20	19.5-20.95
Marticaria chamomilla	10.59	10.10-11.11	16.88	16.00-17.97	20	18.9-20.5
Stachys lavandulifolia	41.32	38.91-43.70	60.55	56.83-65.69	65	61.3-66.8

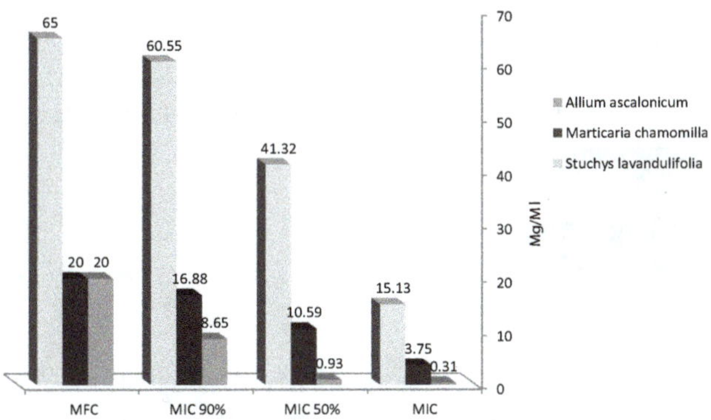

Figure 7. Comparison of MIC 50%, MIC 90%, and MFC *Allium ascalonicom*, *Marticaria chamomilla* and *Stuchys lavanulifolia* extracts on *Candida albicans*

Discussion

In this study the plants showed antifungal activity against *Candida albicans. Candidiasis* is the most common opportunistic fungal infection that can be seen on the skin, mucous membranes, respiratory tract and genitourinary system (3).

The results of this study are partially in agreement with previous ones which have proved the inhibitory effects of Allium genus especially *Allium ascalonicum* against bacteria, fungi, viruses and protozoa (24).

In a study Amin and colleagues evaluated and expressed anti-fungal and anti-bacterial effects of Allium ascalonicum, garlic and onion. Fungal species were more sensitive than bacteria. MIC values of dried *Allium ascalonicum* extracts for *Trichophyton mentagrophytes* was 0.62 mg/ml and for *Aspergillus flavus*, *Aspergillus fumigatus* and *Aspergillus niger* was 20 mg/ml (25).

In another study Yin and colleagues studied the antifungal effects of seven Allium species on three species of *Aspergillus*. In this study, the obtained MIC values of *Allium ascalonicum* extracts for *Aspergillus flavus*, *Aspergillus fumigatus* and *Aspergillus Niger* were respectively 0.474 mg/ml, 0.558 and 0.228 mg/ml (26).

Antifungal effect of aqueous and alcoholic extracts of *Allium hirtifolium* has also been tested. In this study, MIC values of *Allium hirtifolium* extract against the fungal species tested for the alcoholic extract were between 0.058 and 0.8 mg/ml and for aqueous extract between 0.26 and 3.84 mg/ml, and MFC of alcoholic and aqueous extracts were reported respectively between 0.1-12.8 mg/ml and 0.6-68.29 mg/ml (27).

It was shown by Zarei Mahmudabadi that the effect of *Allium ascalonicum* on saprophyte was more than its effect on *Candida albicans* (28).

In a study antifungal effect of onion and garlic on *Candida* albicans was evaluated. The MIC values of onion and garlic were respectively 4.522 mg/ml and 0.569 mg/ml, in which, the MIC values of *ketoconazole* for *Candida albicans* was 23.582 mg/ml (29).

In our study, MIC, MIC 50%, MIC 90% and MFC of *Allium ascalonicum* extract on *Candida albicans* were respectively 0.31, 0.93, 8.65, and 20 mg/ml, which they are consistent with the results of previous studies. These results may indicate that *Allium ascalonicum* has antifungal effect against the *Candida albicans* and may be a good candidate to be used in fungi infections.

Few studies have examined antifungal properties of *Marticaria chamomilla*, especially its effect on *Candida albicans.* Some studies have rejected the antifungal properties of this plant. For example Naiini and colleagues in 2009 evaluated the MIC and MFC of some plant extracts, including, *Marticaria chamomilla* against *Candida albicans.* In this study, the highest rate of used extracts, was 6.4 mg/ml. *Marticaria chamomilla* extract did not show antifungal effect in none of the concentrations (30).

In contrast, some studies have emphasized on antifungal activity of *Marticaria chamomilla.* Magro has mentioned, that dried *Roman chamomile* extract could inhibit the growth of *Aspergillus niger* in 920 mg/ml concentration (31).

In a research, by Abud latif in 2011, has been examined the pure and methanolic extracts of *Marticaria chamomilla* on the growth of *Candida albicans* and *Aspergillus niger.* In this study, MIC values of pure extract and methanol extracts of *Marticaria chamomilla* were obtained 0.002 mg/ml and 0.1 mg/ml, respectively (32).

In our study, MIC, MIC 50% , MIC 90% and MFC of *Marticaria chamomilla* were respectively 3.75, 10.59, 16.88, and 20 mg/ml.

Berry in 1995 has mentioned that α-bisabolol, spirother, camazolen and umbeliferone are some components with antifungal activities which all are present in *Marticaria chamomilla* (33).

The discrepancies in the results of different researchers can be due to differences in the types of used native plants or differences in the types of extracts and compounds and/ or differences in the used methods in the study. It seems that in this regard more studies are needed to evaluate the antifungal effects of *Marticaria chamomilla.*

Studies are also limited on the effects of antimicrobial and especially antifungal of *Stachys lavandulifolia.*

Dulger in Turkey studied the antifungal effects of methanolic extracts of four different types of *Stachys lavandulifolia* on several bacteria and yeasts. In this study the MIC and MFC of yeasts were obtained 0.032 mg/ml. It seems that due to equal amounts of MIC and MFC, *Stachys lavandulifolia* extract is a fungicidal plant (34). In another study by Skaltsa, the antifungal effect of *Stachys lavandulifolia* extract on *Candida albicans* was obtained between 0.3 and 1 mg/ml of extract (35). The results of this study indicate that *Stachys lavandulifolia* has a strong antifungal effect and plants of this family can inhibit fungal growth very well. In our study, MIC, MIC 50%, MIC 90% and MFC of *Stachys lavandulifolia* on *Candida albicans* were respectively 15.13, 41.32, 60.55 and 65 mg/ml.

Saidi *et al.* evaluated the effect of extracts of *S. Lavandulifolia* on *Candida albicans* using microbroth dilution method that the method used, is consistent with our study and results of both studies show that the extract had no effect on *Candida albicans* (17).

Conclusion

In the present study in order to be stopped Candida fungus growth, There were significant differences between the MIC, MIC 50% and MIC 90% three groups of plant extracts (*Allium ascalonicum*, *Marticaria chamomilla* and *Stachys lavandulifolia*). All three plants had the ability to inhibit the growth of *Candida albicans* but *Allium ascalonicum* extract had the greatest impact on controlling fungal. Also *Marticaria chamomilla* extract was in the next position, but the concentration required for *Marticaria chamomilla* extract was much higher than the other two plants.

In this study, the antifungal effect of *Allium ascalonicum, Marticaria chamomilla* and *Stachy lavandulifolia* extracts were determined on *Candida albicans* that as from increasing concentrations of plant extracts, growth of fungi was limited and since the chemical antifungal drugs are too expensive and also have some side effects and Harmful for patients, so if the herbal medicines produce, can be reduced side effects and drug resistance to chemical drugs.

Alliums ascalonicum extract had high effect on *Candida albicans,* so, this plant extract might be used to treat fungal infections. However, to better determine the impact of this plant to treat fungal infections, further researches should be done on clinical samples and directly effect of plant extract should be studied on *Candidiasis* patients.

Acknowledgements

This paper has been derived from MD theses of the Zahra Heydari. The authors gratefully thank the Medical Plants Research Center and Deputy of Shahrekord University of Medical Sciences, Iran, which funded the research (code number of 290-75-01-1389).

Authors' contributions

All the authors wrote the manuscript equally.

Conflict of interests

The authors declared no competing interests.

Ethical considerations

Ethical issues (including plagiarism, misconduct, data fabrication, falsification, double publication or submission, redundancy) have been completely observed by the authors.

Funding/Support

None.

References

1. Moghim H. Detection of CH50 and role of C3, C4 complement in patients with Candidiasis. J Shahrekord Univ Med Sci 2000;2(1):61-5.
2. Moghim H. Role of cellular immunity in prevention of Candidiasis in leukemic and lymphomatic patients using flowcytometry method. J Shahrekord Univ Med Sci 2001; 3(3):42-8.
3. Rippon JW. Candidiasis and the pathogenic yeasts. Medical Mycology. 3nd ed. Philadelphia: W.B. Saunders Company; 1988. p. 532-8.
4. Khajehdehi P. Turmeric: Reemerging of a neglected Asian traditional remedy. J Nephropathol 2012; 1(1):17-22.
5. Bannerman RH, Burton J, Wen C. Traditional Medicine and health care coverage. England. MAC Millan/Spoottis Wood 1983; 9-17,90 and 99-100. Geneva: World Health Organisation; 1993.
6. Asgari S, Setorki M, Rafieian-kopaei M, Heidarian E, Shahinfard N, Ansari R, *et al.* Postprandial hypolipidemic and hypoglycemic effects of Allium hertifolium and Sesamum indicum on hypercholesterolemic rabbits. Afr J Pharm Pharmacol 2012;6(15):1131-5.
7. Asgary S, Rafieian-Kopaei M, Adelnia A, Kazemi S, Shamsi F. Comparing the effects of lovastatin and cornus MAS fruit on fibrinogen level in hypercholesterolemic rabbits. ARYA Atheroscler 2010;6(1):1-5.
8. Asgari S, Rafieian-kopaei M, Pourgheysari B, Ansari-Samani R, Deris F, Shahinfard N, et al. Allium hirtifolium Boiss: Radical scavenging property and the lowering effects on blood fibrinogen and factor VII. Life Sci J 2012;9(3):1793-8
9. Bahmani M, Rafieian-kopaei M, Parsaei P, Mohsenzadegan A. The anti-leech effect of Peganum harmala L. extract and some anti-parasite drugs on

Limnatis Nilotica. Afr J Microbiol Res 2012; 6(10): 2586-90.

10. Shirzad H, Taji F, Rafieian-Kopaei M. Correlation between antioxidant activity of garlic extracts and WEHI-164 fibrosarcoma tumor growth in BALB/c mice. J Med Food 2011; 14(9):969-74.
11. Kung KH. Antimicrobial properties of allium species. Cur Opin Biotechnol 2012; 23(2)142-147.
12. Fujisawa H, Watanabe K, Suma K, Origuchi K, Matsufuji H, Seki T, *et al.* Antibacterial potential of garlic-derived allicin and its cancellation by sulfhydryl compounds. Biosci Biotechnol Biochem 2009;73:1948-1955.
13. Rahbar M, Hosseini Taghavi SA, Diba K, Heidari A. In vitro antibacterial activity of shallot (Allium ascalonicum) crude juice. J Med Plants 2005; 4(13):26-29.
14. Fattorusso E, Lorizzi M, Lanzotti V, Taglialatela-Scafati O. Chemical composition of shallot (Allium ascalonicum Hort). J Agric Food Chem 2002; 50(20):5686-90.
15. Seyfi P, Mostafaie A, Mansouri K, Arshadi D, Mohammadi-Motlagh HR, Kiani A. In vitro and in vivo anti-angiogenesis effect of shallot (Allium ascalonicum): a heat-stable and flavonoid-rich fraction of shallot extract potently inhibits angiogenesis. Toxicol In Vitro 2010; 24(6):1655-61.
16. Tolouee M, Alinezhad S, Saberi R, Eslamifar A, Zad SJ, Jaimand K, *et al.* Effect of Matricaria chamomilla L. flower essential oil on the growth and ultrastructure of Aspergillus niger van Tieghem. Int J Food Microbiol 2010; 139(3):127-33.
17. Saeedi M, Morteza-Semnani K, Mahdavi MR, Rahimi F. Antimicrobial studies on extracts of four spacies of Stuchys. Indian J Pharm Sci 2008; 70(3):403-6.
18. Abdoul-Latif FA, Nabil M, Edou P, Ali AA, Djama SO, Obamé LC, *et al.* Anti microbial and antioxidant activities of essential oil and methanol extract of Marticaria chamomilla L. from Djibuti. *J Med Plants Res* 2011; 5(9):1512-7.
19. Taghikhani M, Nasri H, Asgari A, Afrough H, Namjoo AR, Ansari-Samani R, *et al.* The renal toxicity of hydroalcoholic extract of Stachys lavandulifolia Vahl in Wistar rats. Life Sci J 2012;9(4): 3025-31.
20. Sharafati R, Sherafati F, Rafieian-Kopaei M. Biological characterization of Iranian walnut (Juglans regia) leaves. Turk J Biol 2011; 35:635-9.
21. Namjoo A, Nasri H, Talebi-Juneghani A, Baradaran A, Rafieian-Kopaei M. Safety Profile of Carthamus tinctorius L. in lactation: Brain, Renal and Hepatotoxicity. Pak J Med Sci 2013;29(1):378-383.
22. Willinger B, Apfalter P, Hirschl AM, Makristathis A, Rotter M, Seibold M. Susceptibility testing of Candida species: comparison of NCCLS microdilution method with Fungitest. *Diagn Microbiol Infect Dis* 2000; 38(1):11-15.
23. Razzaghparast A, Shams Ghahfarokhi M, Yadegari MH, Razzaghi Abyaneh M. Antifungal effects of Allium cepa and some azoles in intact forms and in combinations to each other against pathogenic yeasts. Kowsar Med J 2008;13(2):103-13.
24. Asili A, Behravan J, Naghavi MR, Asili J. Genetic diversity of persion shallot (Allium hirtifolium) ecotypes based on morphological traits, allicin content and RAPD markers. J Med Arom Plants 2010; 1(1):1-6.
25. Amin M, Kapadnis BP. Heat stable antimicrobial activity of Allium ascalonicum against bacteria and fungi. Indian J Exp Biol 2005; 43(8):751-4.
26. Yin MC, Tsao SM. Inhibitory Effect of Seven Allium Plants Upon Three Aspergillus Species. Int J Food Microbiol 1999; 49:49-56.
27. Fateh R, Nasiri Kashani MJ, Motevallian M, Falahati M, Yazdanparast A. In vitro Antifungal activity of Allium hirtifolium in comparison with the Miconazole. Med J Islamic Rep Iran 2010; 24(1):17-22.
28. Zarei Mahmudabadi A, Gharib Nasery MK. Antifungal activity of shallot, Allium ascalonicum Linn (Liliaceae), In Vitro J Med Plants Res 2009; 3(5):450-3.
29. Shams-Ghahfarokhi M, Shokoohamiri MR, Amirrajab N, Moghadasi B, Ghajari A, Zeini F, *et al.* In vitro antifungal activities of Allium cepa, Allium sativum and ketoconazole against some pathogenic yeasts and dermatophyts. Fitoterapia 2006;77:321-3.
30. Naeini A, Khosravi AR, Chitsaz M, Shokri H, Kamlnejad. Anti candida albicans activity of some Iranian plants used in traditional medicine. J Mycol Med 2009;19(3):168-72.
31. Magro A, Carolino M, Bastos M, Mexia A. Efficacy of plant extracts against stored-products fungi. Rev Iberoam Micol 2006;23:176-8.
32. Abdoul-Latif FM, Mohamed N, Edou P. Anti microbial and antioxidant activity of essential oil and methanol extract of marticaria chamomilla L. Flower from Djibuti. J Med Plants Res 2011; 5:1512-7.
33. Berry M. Herbal products. Part 6. Chamomiles. Pharm J 1995;245:191-3.
34. Dulger G, Aki C. Antimicrobial activity of the leaves of endemic Stachys pseudopinardii in Turkey. Trop J Pharm Res 2009; 8(4):371-5.
35. Skaltsa HD, Demetzos C, Lazari D, Sokovic M. Essential oil analysis and antimicrobial activity of eight Stachys species from Grecc. Phytochemistry 2003;64(3):743-52.

12

Effect of *Kelussia odoratissima* Mozaff essential oil on promastigot form of *Leishmania major* (*in vitro*)

Khodadad Pirali Kheirabadi[1*], Siavash Saei Dehkordi[2], Parviz Kheibari[3]

[1]Department of pathobiology, Faculty of Veterinary Medicine, Shahrekord University, Shahrekord, Iran
[2]Department of Food Hygiene and Quality Control, Faculty of Veterinary Medicine, Shahrekord University, Shahrekord, Iran
[3]Faculty of Veterinary Medicine, Shahrekord University, Shahrekord, Iran

ARTICLE INFO

Keywords:
Essential oil
In vitro
Kelussia odoratissima
Leishmaniasis
Promastigot form

ABSTRACT

Introduction: Leishmaniasis is a zoonotic disease caused by a protozoan of the genus *Leishmania*. In this study, the effects of *Kelussia odoratissima* Mozaff essential oil on the promastigot form of *Leishmania* major were studied.
Methods: In this study, the effects of *Kelussia odoratissima* Mozaff essential oil on the promastigot form of *Leishmania major* were assessed by calculating the average number of surviving promastigots after exposure to different concentrations of essential oil, relative to the control Glucantime, at different time intervals. To achieve this, various essential oil concentrations (7.5 μl, 15 μl, 25 μl, 35.25 μl, 50 μl) were added to parasites. Different groups in this study were kept in a 26°C incubator under identical conditions. 24, 48 and 72 hours after incubation, living promastigots were counted.
Results: The effect of the essential oil of *Kelussia odoratissima* Mozaff differed from the negative and positive controls and depended on the concentration: higher concentrations (35.25 μl, 50 μl) had a stronger effect on promastigots, causing total mortality.
Conclusion: This study showed that *Kelussia odoratissima* Mozaff essential oil had effects on promastigot form of *Leishmania major.* So it might be possible to use the essential oil of *Kelussia odoratissima* instead of chemical drugs.

Implication for health policy/practice/research/medical education:
It is possible to use the essential oil of *Kelussia odoratissima* instead of chemical drugs. The use of any concentration of essential oil of *Kelussia odoratissima* controlled *L. major* more effectively by increasing in essential oil concentration. Future research would assess the effect of this essential oil on the amastigote form of *L. major.*

Introduction

Medicinal herbs contain physiologically active principles that have been exploited in traditional medicine for the treatment of various ailments due to their anti-microbial properties (1,2). The antifungal and antibacterial activity exhibited by extracts and essential oils of medicinal plants is well proved (3).

Kelussia odoratissima Mozaff. (wild celery; Apiaceae) is a sweet-smelling, glabrous, perennial aromatic herb, which is traditionally consumed in Iran and grows to a height of 120 to 200 cm. The flowers are 1-2 mm in diameter and all are hermaphroditic. *K. odoratissima* is an Iranian endemic plant native to Zagros (central region of Iran) (4).

Kelussia grows in April and its aerial parts are harvested (5,6). Flavonoids have anti-inflammatory (7), anti-allergy (8), anti-diabetes, antihyperlipidemic and anti-hypercholesterolemic effects (9,10) and improves spatial memory (11). Phthalides constitute 70% of the *Kelussia* essence with several effects: liver protection, prostaglandin F2α inhibition, prevention of cancer tumors, treatment of epilepsy and liver disorders and reduction in blood viscosity (5,12,13). Despite this, there are no study related to the antileishmanial effect of the essential oil of *K. odoratissima*, this being the focus of our study.

Leishmaniasis affects more than 12 million people in 88 countries (14). Cutaneous leishmaniasis (CL), with 1 to 1.5 million annual cases, is the most common form of this disease (15). There is no vaccine available against any form of leishmaniasis and chemotherapy is the only currently available treatment (16,17). The standard treatment for

***Corresponding author**: Khodadad Pirali Kheirabadi, Department of Pathobiology, Faculty of Veterinary Medicine, University of Shahrekord, Shahrekord, Iran. Email: khpirali@yahoo.com

CL is antimoniate, which requires long-term injections, and resistance is emerging, which cause high dose usage, resulting side effects (17,18).

The search for new, safe and inexpensive drugs to treat and control CL, especially anthroponotic CL, is needed. Conventional healers are usually cheap and sometimes more effective than chemical drugs (19).

In this study, the effect of the essential oil of *K. odoratissima* on promastigot form of *Leishmania major* was studied. The results obtained from this study help us to find the alternative natural drug instead of chemical ones.

Materials and Methods

Plant material

A wild-growing plant from Kogiluye and Buyer Ahmad province located in the southwest of Iran, was collected in April and May, 2012. The samples, which were identified and confirmed as *K. odoratissima* Mozaff, were deposited in the Herbarium of the Research Institute of Jahade Keshavarzi of Shahrekord, Iran.

Isolation of the volatile oil

20 kg from aerial parts of the plant was dried in an oven equipped with warm air circulation. One hundred grams of the air-dried material was ground and powdered. The powder was subjected to hydro-distillation for 3 hours using a Clevenger-type system. Finally, 30 ml essential oil extracted. The oil was kept at 2°C to 4°C in a sealed brown vial.

Chemical analysis of the oil

Analysis of the essential oil was performed on a Hewlett-Packard Model 6890 GC-MS using a HP-5MS capillary column (30 m×0.25 mm i.d., 0.25 m film thickness). The injector temperature and detector temperature was 250°C. Helium was used as the carrier gas at a flow rate of 1.00 ml/min. The column temperature was programmed from 40°C to 280°C at a rate of 4°C/min. The EI mode was at 70 eV, while the mass spectra were recorded from 30 to 450 m/z. Confirmation of identity was carried out by comparing their retention indices with the Wiley 275 library data of the GC–MS system and with the mass spectra literature data (20).

Preparing the promastigot form of Leishmania major

The promastigot form of *Leishmania major* strain MRHO/IR/ER/75 was prepared from department of Parasitology Research, University of Medical Sciences of Isfahan, Iran. The promastigots were transferred to RPMI 1640 medium and incubated at 26°C for 72 hours.

Preparing the different concentrations and control groups

After the promastigots increased in the medium, they were counted using a Neobar chamber (0.100 mm, Tiefe, Depth, Profondeur, Neubauer Improved, Precicolor, HBG, Germany) in which 10 µl of this medium was mixed with 10 µl of formalin, which was used to kill the promastigots. 150 µl of medium contained 10^6 promastigots. Next, different concentrations of *K. odoratissima* essential oil (15, 30, 50, 75 and 100 mg/ml) were prepared, to achieve this, various essential oil concentrations (7.5 µl, 15 µl, 25 µl, 35.25 µl, 50 µl) were added to parasites. There was a negative control (no essential oil) and a positive control (Glucantime®, Specia, Paris, France) by mixing with sterile RPMI 1640 medium in different tubes. 10^6 promastigots (i.e., 150 µl of medium containing promastigots) were added to each tubes, as presented in Table 1. The total volume of all tubes was 500 µl after mixing.

Counting the number of living promastigots after the mixing

After mixing the promastigots with different concentrations of *K. odoratissima* essential oil, those tubes, as well as the negative and positive controls, were incubated in dark incubator and in 26°C for 72 hours. The number of living promastigots was counted at 24, 48 and 72 hours after incubation.

Statistical analysis

The data were analyzed by one-way analysis of variance (ANOVA) and significant differences ($P<0.05$) between means were assessed by Tukey's test using SPSS software version 19.0.

Results

Composition of essential oil

In the essential oil of *K. odoratissima*, the sesquiterpene hydrocarbons were the most abundant compounds (57.77%). In addition, the least quantitative percentage (2.7%) was belonged to monoterpene hydrocarbons. The major components were *Z*-ligustilide (34.5%), *E*-ligustilide (11.79%), 3-*Z*-butylidenephthalide (8.81%) and Dec-9-en-1-ol (5.86%).

24 and 48 hours after incubation

Effects of essential oil of *Kelussia odoratissima* Mozaff on promastigot form of *Lishmania major* differenced from

Table 1. Volume of materials in each tube prepared for different concentrations of essential oil

Tubes Materials	15 mg/ml	30 mg/ml	50 mg/ml	75 mg/ml	100 mg/ml	Negative control	Positive control (Glucantime)
Promastigots	150 µl	150 µl	150 µl	150 µl	150 µl	150 µl	150 µl
RPMI 1640	342.5 µl	335 µl	325 µl	314.75 µl	300 µl	350 µl	181 µl
Glucantime	-	-	-	-	-	-	169 µl
Essential oil	7.5 µl	15 µl	25 µl	35.25 µl	50 µl	-	-
Total volume	500 µl	500 µl	500 µl	500 µl	500 µl	500 µl	500 µl

Table 2. Mean number of living promastigots ± SEM 24, 48 and 72 hours after incubation

Tube	Mean number of living promastigots ± SEM						
	15 mg/ml	30 mg/ml	50 mg/ml	75 mg/ml	100 mg/ml	Negative Control	Positive Control
24 h	127.25±3.12 a	119.11±4.54 a	116.63±3.96 a	111.76±4.32 a	103.51±3.81 a	125.3±1.96 b	79.47±0.44 c
48 h	124.12±2.68 a	117.63±2.96 a	110.17±4.23 a	104.00±3.69 a	98.99±1.99 a	148.25±2.25 b	74.23±0.97 c
72 h	119.08±1.75 a	102.45±1.85 a	93.27±2.17 a	87.00±4.44 a	73.93±3.12 d	211.63±2.19 b	67.56±0.82 c
Mean of 3 Times	123.48±2.51 a	113.06±3.11 b	106.69±3.45 c	100.92±4.15 d	92.14±2.97 e	161.72±2.13 f	73.75±0.74 g

Different letters within each row (i.e., within each time interval) indicate significant differences (P<0.05) between mean of living promastigots number in each tube according to Tukey's test.

negative control and positive controls. However, there were no significant differences between groups with different concentrations of essential oil (Table 2).

72 hours after incubation

In this time decreasing in living promastigots in different tubes were more than past times. Same as past times, effect of essential oil of *Kelussia odoratissima* Mozaff on promastigot form of *Lishmania major* was differenced from negative control and positive control (Table 2).

Totally the *K. odoratissima* essential oil had a different effect on the promastigot form of *L. major* relative to the negative and positive control, but this depended on the essential oil concentration; higher concentrations (35.25 µl, 50 µl) had a stronger effect on promastigots, causing total mortality (Table 2). In all three-time intervals, the use of any concentration of essential oil of *Kelussia odoratissima* controlled *L. major* more effectively by increasing in essential oil concentration (Table 2).

Discussion

The application of natural plant products for control of bacterial, fungal and parasitic bee and brood diseases has several advantages over conventional means. In the specialized literature resistance of bacteria to essential oils has not yet been documented. In addition, natural substances in bee products decompose rapidly, their quantity in honey is low and they do not have an adverse effect on the health of consumers (21). Although in small amounts, essential oils and organic acids are normally contained in various types of honey. According to some authors their use as alternative means for prevention and control of bee diseases guarantees ecologically clean bee products (22).

This study showed antileishmanial effects of *Kelussia odoratissima* Mozaff essential oil on promastigot form of *Leishmania major.* The current treatment regimens for leishmaniasis, which are based on chemotherapy, are limited and are not ideal because they are often associated with severe side effects (23). In a case report from France, successful treatment of a 10-year-old boy with cutaneous leishmaniasis (*L. major*) was reported with oral azithromycin (24).

Pentavalent antimonials remain the drug of choice for the treatment of cutaneous and mucocutaneous leishmaniasis. Despite its availability in health facilities, its high toxicity and its parenteral use are limiting factors for the proper treatment of cases of CL. It should be noted that most of these cases occur in areas of difficult access, in rural areas, which complicates the parenteral application of the drug and monitoring of its side effects. Treatment of CL with the drugs currently available represents an obstacle to proper clinical handling of the cases of leishmaniasis, and efforts should be made in order to add the promising drugs to clinical trials and investigate the use of new alternative drugs (25)

Traditional alternatives to antimonials used in unresponsive cases are amphotericin B, which cause serious, toxic side-effects (26,27), and the emergence of drug-resistant parasites is a major problem (17). These limitations and factors emphasize the urgent need for new, inexpensive, safe and easy-to-administer substances for the treatment of this infectious disease, possibly through the form of traditional medicines which represent the accumulation of practices based on theories, beliefs and experiences of different cultures over a wide period of time (28).

Amphotericin B is the second drug of choice when antimonials fail or cannot be used. However, they are toxic and expensive drugs, which often require hospitalization for their administration (29). An alternative to the treatment with conventional amphotericin B is the use of liposomal amphotericin B, which has higher peak plasma levels and lower toxicity (30).

Traditional medicines are used for the maintenance of health and in the prevention, diagnosis, improvement and treatment of illnesses (31). Based on traditional medicine, new drugs of herbal origins discovered through ethnopharmacological studies have shown promising results.

Conclusion

By considering an increase in drug resistance against leishmania, it is possible to use the essential oil of *Kelussia odoratissima* instead of chemical drugs. The use of any concentration of essential oil of *Kelussia odoratissima* controlled *L. major* more effectively by increasing in essential oil concentration. Future research would assess the effect of this essential oil on the amastigote form of *L. major*.

Acknowledgments

Work in the laboratory was supported by University of Shahrekord. I would like to thank all of persons who help us to do this research.

Authors' contributions
All the authors wrote the manuscript equally.

Conflict of interests
The authors declared no competing interests.

Ethical considerations
Ethical issues (including plagiarism, misconduct, data fabrication, falsification, double publication or submission, redundancy) have been completely observed by the authors.

Funding/Support
This research was financially supported by Shahrekord University, Shahrekord, Iran.

References

1. Kelmanson JE, Jager AK, Van Staden J. Zulu medicinal plants with antibacterial activity. J Ethnopharmacol 2000; 69: 2416.
2. Srinivasan D, Sangeetha N, Suresh T, Perumalsamy PL. Antimicrobial activity of certain Indian medicinal plants used in folkloric medicine. J Ethnopharmacol 2001; 74: 217-20.
3. Fazeli MR, Amin GH, Ahmadian AM, Ashtiani H, Jamalifar H, Samadi N. Antimicrobial activities of Iranian sumac and avishan-e-shirazi (Zataria multiflora) against some food-borne bacteria. Food Control 2007; 18: 646-9.
4. Ahmadi F, Kadivar M, Shahedi M. Antioxidant activity of Kelussia odoratissima Mozaff. in model and food systems. Food Chem 2007; 105: 57-64.
5. Tehrani Z. Phytochemical chemical study on Kelussia odoratissima Mozaffarian: Pharmacy thesis. School of Pharmacy, Isfahan University of Medical Sciences. 1999; 42-48.
6. Gandomkar M. Phytochemistry of the essential oil of wild celery plant: Pharmacy thesis. School of Pharmacy, Isfahan University of Medical Sciences. 1999; 37-41.
7. Asgari S, Naderi GA, Garipour M, Dashti G, Sadjadian RA. Effect of Amirkabiria odoratissima on the development and progression of atherosclerosis in hypercholesterolemic rabbits. Iranian Journal of Diabetes and Lipid Disorders 2003; 3(1): 88-3.
8. Hashemi V, Ghannadi A, Soltani RL. Analgesic and anti-inflammatory effects of Amirkabiria odoratissima. Journal of Research in Medical Sciences 2003; 7(4): 121-5.
9. Asgari S, Naderi GA, Jafariyan A, Askari N, Behagh AR. Fibrinolytic activity of Amirkabiria odoratissima Mozaffarian. Journal of Medicinal Plants 2005; 4(13): 19-25.
10. Roghani M, Baluchnejadmojarad T, Ramazani M. The effect of chronic oral feeding of Apium graveolens on learning and memory in diabetic rats. Journal of Medicinal Plants 2008; 7(27): 98-105.
11. Cao YX, Zhang W, He JY, He LC, Xu CB. Ligustilide induces vasodilatation via inhibiting voltage dependent calcium channel and receptor- mediated Ca2+ influx and release. Vascul Pharmacol 2006; 45: 171-6.
12. Craker LE. Herbs species and medicinal plants. Encanto. Oxyx Press 1984; 2: 15-6.
13. Beck J. Investigation of the bioactive constituents of several herbal medicines [Doctoral dissertation]. Colorado State University; 1996.
14. WHO. Leishmaniasis. The global trend. [Accessed 30 January 2009]. http:// www.who.into /neglected_ disease/ integrated-media_ Leishmaniasis/ en/ index. html
15. Desjeux P. Leishmaniasis: Current situation and new perspectives. Comp. Immunol Microbiol Infect Dis 2004; 27: 305-18.
16. Noazin S, Khamesipour A, Moulton LH, Tanner M, Nasseri K, Modabber F. Efficacy of killed whole-parasite vaccines in the prevention of leishmaniasis-A meta-analysis. Vaccine 2009; 27: 474-5.
17. Croft SL, Sundar S, Fairlamb AH. Drug resistance in leishmaniasis. Clin Microbiol Rev 2006; 19: 111-26.
18. Hadighi R, Boucher P, Khamesipour A, Meamar AR, Roy G, Ouellette M, *et al.* Glucantime- resistant Leishmania tropica isolated from Iranian patients with cutaneous leishmaniasis are sensitive to alternative antileishmania drugs. Parasitol Res 2007; 101: 1319-22.
19. Sandhu DS, Heinrich M. The use of health foods, spices and other botanicals in the Sikh community in London. Phytother Res 2005; 19: 633-42.
20. Adams RP. Identification of Essential Oil Components by Gas Chromatography/Quadruple Mass Spectroscopy. 3rd ed. Carol Stream, IL: Allured Publishing Corporation; 2001. p. 456,.
21. Nozal MJ, Bernal JL, Jiménez JJ, González MJ, Higes M. Extraction of thymol, eucalyptol, menthol, and camphor residues from honey and beeswax. Determination by gas chromatography with flame ionization detection. Journal of Chromatography A 2002; 19: 207-15.
22. Zhelyazkova I, Gurgulova K, Malinova K, Ali AS. Investigation on the sti-mulating effect of plant preparations "Green TM" and "Ecophyl-P" upon bee families development. In: Proceedings of the International Scientific Conference. 2009; Union of Scientists Stara Zagora.
23. Tasdemir D, Kaiser M, Brun R, Yardley V, Schmidt TJ, Tosun F, Rüedi P. Antitrypanosomal and antileishmanial activities of flavonoids and their analogues: in vitro, in vivo, structure-activity relationship, and quantitative structure-activity relationship studies. Antimicrob. Agents Chemother 2006; 50(4): 1352-64.

24. Minodier P, Zambelli L, Mary C, Faraut F, Garnier JM, Berbis P. Cutaneous leishmaniasis treated with azithromycin in a child. Pediatr Infect Dis J 2008; 27 (1): 80-1.
25. Basano AS, Camargo LM. [American cutaneous leishmaniasis: history, epidemiology and prospects for control]. Rev Bras Epidemiol 2004; 7: 328-37.
26. Sereno D, Holzmuller P, Lemesre JL. Efficacy of second line drugs on antimonyl-resistant amastigotes of Leishmania infantum. Acta Trop 2000; 74: 25-31.
27. Croft SL, Seifert K, Yardley V. Current scenario of drug development for leishmaniasis. Ind J Med Res 2006; 123: 399-410.
28. Fennel CW, Makunga NP, Van Staden J. Medicinal plants and biotechnology: An integrated approach to healthcare. In: Teixeira da Silva JA, (Ed.). Floriculture, Ornamental and Plant Biotechnology: Advances and Topical Issues. 1st ed. Isleworth, UK: Global Science Books, Ltd.; 2006. p. 41-53.
29. Machado-Pinto J, Pinto J, da Costa CA, Genaro O, Marques MJ, Mobabber F. Immunochemotherapy for cutaneous leishmaniasis: a controlled trial using killed Leishmania (Leishmania) amazonensis vaccine plus antimonial. Int J Dermatol 2002; 41: 73-8.
30. Berman JD. Human leishmaniasis: clinical, diagnostic, and chemotherapeutic developments in the last 10 years. Clin Infect Dis 1997; 24: 684-703.
31. Firenzuoli F, Gori L. Herbal Medicine Today. Clinical and Research 2007; 4(S1): 37-40.

13

Salicylic acid and methyl jasmonate enhance drought tolerance in chamomile plants

Hossein Nazarli[1*], Ali Ahmadi[1], Javad Hadian[2]

[1]Department of Agronomy and Plant Breeding, University College of Agriculture and Natural Resources, University of Tehran, Karaj, Iran
[2]Medicinal Plants and Drugs Research Institute, University College of Agriculture, University of Shahid Beheshti, Tehran, Iran

ARTICLE INFO

Keywords:
Chamomile
Drought stress
Salicylic acid
Methyl jasmonate

ABSTRACT

Introduction: The dried flowers of chamomile contain many terpenoids and flavonoids contributing to its medicinal properties. Salicylic acid (SA) and methyl jasmonate (MeJA) have antioxidant properties and function as direct radical scavengers. Two *Matricaria chamomilla* cultivars (Bodgold and Hungary breed seeds) were used in this study to investigate the effects of exogenous application of SA and MeJA on protection against drought stress as well as on changes of malone dialdehyde (MDA) and electrolyte leakage index (ELI), and the fluctuation of proline and soluble sugars content in the leaves under drought stress.
Methods: The experiment was conducted in a factorial design based on randomized complete blocks with three replicates. Chamomile plants were treated by two levels of drought stress as well as two different levels of MeJA (i.e., 0.0 and 100 μM) and SA (i.e., 0.0 and 0.5 mM) solutions.
Results: There was a dramatic drought induced increase in the MDA content (128%) and ELI (49%) in the leaves. Deleterious effect of drought stress was more severe in untreated plants than in treated ones. Treatments with SA and MeJA significantly improved drought tolerance in chamomile plants. These treatments effectively maintained membrane integrity, thereby retarding electrolyte leakage and membrane lipid peroxidation (MDA). Treatments with SA and MeJA were also effective in enhancing the antioxidant concentrations of proline and soluble sugars.
Conclusion: The production of these antioxidants could have been part of a defence system against drought damage, reducing MDA and ELI and maintaining membrane stability.

Implication for health policy/practice/research/medical education:
The results indicate that SA and MeJA were found to individually enhance compatible solutes production in leaves but when administered in combination there was no further enhancement in compatible solutes production.

Introduction

Chamomile (*Matricaria chamomilla* L.) is one of the important medicinal plant species from the Asteraceae family and represented by two common varieties viz. German Chamomile (*Chamomilla recutita*) and Roman Chamomile (*Chamaemelum nobile*). The flowers of chamomile contain terpenes, flavonoids, coline, coumarin, malic acid, proteins, sugars, lipids and mineral elements. About 120 chemical compounds have been identified in the oil, including 28 terpenes (the more important being α-bisabolol, chamazulene, bisabolol oxide, etc.), 36 flavonoids (apigenin, etc.) and other 52 substances that are organic acids, coumarins, coline, etc. (1).

Drought stress is often related to the production of oxygen radicals that play an important role in cell signaling, but at the same time is cytotoxic and need to be detoxified (2). Reactive oxygen species (ROS) acts as signaling molecules that triggers the cascade of protective reactions in plants (3), including activation of antioxidant enzymes and production of compatible solutes. Plant cells contain a repertoire of ROS scavenging enzymes and lipid-related substances like carotenoids (4), the putative compatible

***Corresponding author**: Hossein Nazarli, University College of Agriculture and Natural Resources, University of Tehran. Karaj, Iran.
Email: H_Nazarli@ut.ac.ir

osmolytes including sorbitol, mannitol, myo-inositol and proline (5). A stress response is initiated when plants recognize stress at the cellular level. Plants produce jasmonic acid (and its volatile methyl ester methyl jasmonate (MeJA) and salicylic acid (SA) in response to many biotic and abiotic stresses.

In plants, SA plays an important role in signaling both local and systemic defense responses. SA is an endogenous growth regulator of phenolic nature, which participates in the regulation of different physiological processes in plants. SA has been recognized as a regulatory signal mediating plant response to abiotic stresses such as drought (6) and osmotic stress (7). Also, SA action is tightly related to the generation of various ROS (8).

The role of jasmonic acid (JA) and its volatile MeJA as signalling molecules in biotic and abiotic stresses (9) is well known, having either inhibitory or promoting effects, in the different form of morphological, physiological changes or in defence metabolism (10). In summary, it is clear that JA signaling exert its functions via interaction with multiple plant hormones; however the crossroads of these interactions still remain to be explored. We need the information for understanding the mechanisms of the anti-stress effects of SA and MeJA in medicinal plants under drought stress which are prerequisite to justify the use of these natural growth regulators for increasing *Matricaria Chamomilla* resistance to drought.

It was hypothesized that treatments with MeJA and SA may enhance drought tolerance in chamomile plants by enhancing the synthesis of biochemical compounds such as proline, ascorbic acid and soluble sugars. These biochemical compounds are thought to be involved in the response of chamomile plants to drought conditions and the signaling cascade are mediated with MeJA and SA.

This study is aimed to answer whether MeJA and SA can function as stress molecules and how MeJA and SA mediate a stress response to diverse physiological and physical stresses.

Materials and Methods

Current investigation was conducted under greenhouse condition at the University of Tehran, Iran, from April to August 2013, to investigate the effects of MeJA, SA and different irrigation regimes on the synthesis of biochemical compounds (proline and soluble sugars content), cell membrane stability, determination of lipid peroxidation i.e., malone dialdehyde (MDA) in the leaves of two chamomile cultivars (Bodgold and Hungary breed seed). The seeds of two chamomile cultivars were kindly provided by Pakanbazr Institute, Isfahan, Iran. Subsequent to initial germination of the seeds in the pots supplemented with loamy soil and sand (3:1), the 30-day old seedlings were transferred into the new plastic pots (with the ratio of 3 loamy soil and 1 perlite) containing six ones. In the following, two out of which were thinned in providing suitable feeding conditions.

For the two months, pots were weighed every other day, and all plants were watered to field capacity (FC), supplying an amount of water equal to transpiration losses; to ensure the establishment of seedlings and to allow adaptation to surround conditions before water stress was imposed. By the end of this period, watering was discontinued.

Plants were watered to field capacity for about two months until roots were established and shoot system was in a reasonable size.

Experimental treatments applied as a combination of visual symptom appearance in plant (normal to severe wilting) and soil moisture. So, treatments irrigated in 20.1 and 10.4% of soil moisture content (w/w) that are created in greenhouse situation with irrigation of 4 and 10 days interval, respectively. Also chamomile plants were treated with the two different levels of MeJA (i.e., 0.0 and 100 μM) and SA (i.e., 0.0 and 0.5 mM) solutions. The first MeJA and SA treatments were applied after two months from transplanting and the process was repeated every other 10 days.

For proline determination, the last fully expanded leaves were detached from the plants after the drought treatment. Leaf samples (0.5 g) were homogenized in 5 mL of sulfosalicylic acid (3%) using mortar and pestle. The mixture was centrifuged at 9000 g for 10 min at 4 °C and the supernatant was recovered. About 2 mL of extract was taken in test tube and 2 mL of glacial acetic acid and 2 mL of ninhydrin reagent were added to it. The reaction mixture was boiled in water bath at 100 °C for 60 min. The reaction was stopped by placing the test tubes in cold water. After cooling the reaction mixture, 6 mL of toluene was added and then transferred to a separating funnel. After thorough mixing, the chromophore containing toluene was separated and absorbance read at 520 nm in spectrophotometer against toluene blank. Concentration of proline was estimated by referring to a standard curve of proline (11).

To measure the content of soluble sugars, 0.5 g of dry leaves was homogenized with 5 ml of 95% ethanol. One-tenth ml of alcoholic extract preserved in refrigerator mixed with 3 ml anthrone (150 mg anthrone, 100 ml of 72% sulphuric acid, W/W). The samples placed in boiling water bath for 10 min. The light absorption of the samples was estimated at 625 nm using a PD-303 model spectrophotometer. Contents of soluble sugar were determined using glucose standard and expressed as mg g^{-1} DW of leaves.

Oxidative damage to leaf lipids, resulting from drought stress, was measured in terms of MDA content using thiobarbituric acid (TBA)-reactive substances (12). Leaf samples of 0.5 g were homogenized in 10 mL of 0.1% trichloroacetic acid (TCA). The homogenate was centrifuged at 15,000 g for 5 min. Four milliliter of 0.5% TBA in 20% TCA was added to 2 mL of aliquot of the supernatant. The mixture was heated at 100 °C for 30 min and then quickly cooled in an ice bath. After centrifugation at 10,000 g for 10 min, the absorbance of supernatant was recorded at 532 nm. The value for non-specific absorption at 600 nm was subtracted. The following formula was applied to calculate malondialdehyde content using its absorption coefficient (ε) and expressed as nmol malondialdehyde g^{-1} fresh mass following the formula: MDA (nmol g^{-1} FM) = [(A532-A600) ×V×1000/ε] ×W where ε is the specific extinction coefficient (=155 mM cm^{-1}), V is the volume of crushing medium, W is the fresh weight of leaf, A600 is the absorbance at 600 nm wavelength and A532 is the absorbance at 532 nm wavelength.

In the middle of flowering stage cell membrane stability was analyzed. Leaf tissue (three plants/ replicate) was cut in segments of 1 cm^2 with cork-borer. Samples collected were washed three times in deionized water to remove electrolytes adhered on the surface (13). The samples were then kept in a capped vial (20 ml) containing 10 ml of deionized water and incubated in the dark for 24 h at 10±1 °C. The conductance was measured with a conductivity meter. After the first measurement the vials were autoclaved for 15 min to kill the leaf tissue and release the electrolytes. After cooling, the second conductivity reading was taken. These two measurements were carried out individually for all the samples from both the control and stress treatments. ELI was calculated as the reciprocal of cell membrane stability (CMS) (13): ELI% =1-[1-(T2-T1))/ (1-(C2-C1))]′100, where T and C refer to the stress and control samples, respectively; the subscripts 1 and 2 refer to the initial and final conductance readings, respectively.

The experiment was conducted in a factorial design based on randomized complete blocks with three replicates. Graphs were drawn using Microsoft Office Excel 2013 software.

Results

Data analysis showed that the factors including irrigation regimes, SA and MeJA (except MDA and soluble sugars) appear to influence the activity of proline, soluble sugar content, MDA and ELI. Also, interaction effect among three factors is significant at 1% level (Table 1). As in Table 1 is shown, interaction effect between SA and MeJA exhibited significant effects on all the aforementioned measured variables ($P<0.01$). In addition, a significant association was observed among irrigation regimes, SA and MeJA in terms of proline content ($P<0.01$), and ELI ($P<0.05$).

The free proline and soluble sugar contents were significantly enhanced in the stressed plants over control plants in both cultivars (Bodgold and Hungary breed seed). There was a considerable increase in free proline accumulation (19.72%) and soluble sugars (17.69%) with increasing drought stress. The results showed that the highest level of proline (24.05 n mol g^{-1} FW) and sugar (34 mg. g^{-1} DW) contents were achieved by applying SA under the condition of restrictive irrigation regime (I2) in Hungary breed seed, whereas the lowest amounts were related to the treatment of normal irrigation (I1) without using SA and MeJA (Table 2).

Table 1. Variance analysis for proline, soluble sugars content, MDA and ELI as effected by different irrigation regimes, SA and MeJA

S. O. V.	df	MS			
		Pro	MDA	ELI	Soluble sugar
Rep	2	2.1^{ns}	267.53**	2.39^{ns}	85.93**
Irrigation regimes (I)	1	71.72**	302.65**	1002.37**	95.34**
MeJA	1	7.55**	8.34^{ns}	9.45**	0.14^{ns}
SA	1	105.44**	19.21*	58.83**	270.55**
Cultivar	1	3.65*	29.5^{ns}	161.5**	0.69^{ns}
I * MeJA	1	24.97**	4.47^{ns}	12.42**	66.67**
I * SA	1	10.64**	5. 5^{ns}	7.53*	36.29*
I * C	1	0.67^{ns}	0.03^{ns}	0.03^{ns}	1.93^{ns}
MeJA * SA	1	30.38**	62.76**	74.17**	22.4*
MeJA * C	1	4.84*	5.98^{ns}	9.43**	1.66^{ns}
SA * C	1	25.95**	0.13^{ns}	0.54^{ns}	64.04**
I * MeJA * SA	1	45.75**	53.9**	43.27**	113.98**
I * MeJA * C	1	1.45^{ns}	2.95^{ns}	2.81^{ns}	1^{ns}
I * SA * C	1	8.64**	1.75^{ns}	6.06*	0.22^{ns}
MeJA * SA * C	1	4.56*	5.16^{ns}	0.05^{ns}	6.81^{ns}
I * MeJA * SA * C	1	0.83^{ns}	4.45^{ns}	0.16^{ns}	2.55^{ns}
Error	30	0.89	7.55	1.22	4.95
CV%		15	8	15	14

Pro: Proline content, MDA: Malone dialdehyde, ELI: Electrolyte leakage index, SA: salicylic acid, MeJA: methyl jasmonate, C: cultivar, df: degree of freedom; MS: mean of square; *,** significant at 0.05 and 0.01 probability levels, respectively. ns; non-significant.

Table 2. Mean proline content (µmol/g^{-1} F. W), soluble sugars (mg/g D.W), malondialdehyde (nmol g^{-1} F.W) and electrolyte leakage index (%) in chamomile under different irrigation regimes with or without SA and MeJA applications.

Irrigation regimes	Methyl jasmonate	Salicylic acid	Cultivar	Pro	Soluble sugars	MDA	% ELI
Normal	Control	Control	Bodgold	15.1 ± 0.93	23.06 ± 1.2	5.53 ± 1.52	23.71± 0.25
			Hungary breed seed	14.1 ± 0.12	20.40 ± 1.2	7.68 ± 2.8	28.71 ± .031
		0.5 mM	Bodgold	17.15 ± 0.35	25.1 ± 1.2	5.1 ± 1.42	22.68 ± 0.31
			Hungary breed seed	19.15 ± 0.35	27.91 ± 1.2	6.61 ± 2.55	25.73 ± 0.24
	100 µM	Control	Bodgold	15.81 ± 0.35	23.22 ± 1.2	5.4 ± 1.45	23.71 ± 0.31
			Hungary breed seed	17.15 ± 0.35	21.31 ± 3.6	7.04 ± 2.6	27.80 ± 0.29
		0.5 mM	Bodgold	20.34 ± 1.0	29.27 ± 2.23	5.2 ± 1.51	23.75 ± 0.25
			Hungary breed seed	21.15 ± 0.35	31.67 ± 3.03	6.39 ± 2.51	26.09 ± 0.24
Severe wilting	Control	Control	Bodgold	19.15 ± 0.35	27.91 ± 1.23	13.29 ± 4.74	36.85 ± 0.17
			Hungary breed seed	15.81 ± 0.35	23.22 ± 1.23	16.78 ± 6	41.26 ± 0.28
		0.5 mM	Bodgold	22.04 ± 0.35	31.98 ± 1.74	7.72 ± 2.58	28.78 ± 0.28
			Hungary breed seed	24.05 ± 0.35	34.07 ± 0.76	9.66 ± 2.95	34.55 ± 0.32
	100 µM	Control	Bodgold	20.71± 0.35	28.02 ± 2.23	9.911 ± 3.16	31.75 ± 0.28
			Hungary breed seed	20.04 ± 0.35	27.08 ± 2.23	8.46 ± 2.13	33.78 ± 0.25
		0.5 mM	Bodgold	17.22 ± 0.35	25.62 ± 0.74	10.63 ± 1.34	32.82 ± 0.57
			Hungary breed seed	20.49 ± 0.35	26.6 ± 2.03	12.68 ± 1.08	35.48 ± 0.45

Pro: Proline content, MDA: Malone dialdehyde, ELI: Electrolyte leakage index, Means followed by different lower-case letters are significantly different at ($P < 0.05$) by the Duncan's Multiple Range Test.

The treatment of seedlings with SA caused a significant increase in the concentrations of proline and soluble sugars in seedlings, which induced 24.3% and 34% growth in terms of proline content and 22% and 29.26% in terms of sugars under normal (I1) and severe drought stress (I2), respectively, compared with the control (Table 2).

Our results showed that lipid peroxidation (MDA) and electrolyte leakage index (ELI) were influenced by drought stress in leaves of chamomile. There was a dramatic drought induced increase in the MDA content (128%) and ELI (49%) in the leaves. The highest MDA content (16.78 n mol g^{-1} FW) and ELI (41.26%) were observed under the condition of restrictive irrigation regime (I2) in Hungary breed seed (without SA and MeJA treatments) (Table 2). The treatment of chamomile plants with SA caused a significant reduction in the content of MDA and ELI in seedlings, which induced 12.45% and 72.95% decrease in terms of MDA content and 8.3% and 23.34% in terms of ELI under normal (I1) and severe drought stress (I2), respectively, compared with the control. Pretreatment with MeJA brought about a 6.11% decrease in the ELI under water stress condition (Table 2).

Discussion

Plants have to cope with various environmental stresses and thus protect themselves using different strategies such as chemical defences. In general, concentrations of proline and soluble sugars of leaves increased with the decline in irrigation water, suggesting that the production of these solutes is probably a common response of chamomile under drought conditions. Non-enzymatic antioxidant system (low molecular metabolites) plays an important role in the process of neutralization of the after effects of oxidative stress.

The role of proline in adaptation and survival of plants under drought stress have been reported by many researchers (14,15). The accumulation of sugars in response to drought is also quite well documented (15,16). Proline accumulation may contribute to osmotic adjustment at the cellular level in many plants, suggesting it as one of the possible means for overcoming osmotic stress caused by the loss of water (17).

An imbalance between ROS production and antioxidant concentration (which resulted from stress condition) in a cell may cause damage to membranes leading to the increase in membrane permeability. However, ROS are not only produced as a toxic by-product but also play a role in plant response to stress. These responses to stress include hormone signalling, gene activation and stomatal regulation (18). Enhanced ROS production can act positively to signal or induce protective mechanisms, such as accumulation of proline, soluble sugars, tocopherols and phenolic compounds. Induction of defences is mediated by phytohormones like JA and SA.

Because of low cost and good effects on secondary metabolites accumulation, MeJA and SA are considered as effective chemicals for large-scale cultures. Our study showed that SA and MeJA treatments increased proline and sugars concentrations whether plants were under stress or not. However, the most effects of mentioned hormones on compatible metabolites were more pronounced in stressed than that in non-stressed plants. Increasing the amount of proline and sugars in the plants would lead to the resistance against loosing water, protect turgor, reduce the membrane damage and accelerate the growth of plants in stress conditions (19).

Clearly, SA induced an increase in Abscisic acid (ABA) content that might be contributed to preadaptation of plants to different stressful influences of abiotic nature (20).

Exogenous application of methyl jasmonate is transported through phloem and xylem pathways (21). Through cell membranes MeJA is probably transported by the same or a similar carrier as sucrose, due to enhancement of the energy of the plasma membrane (21). Exogenously applied JA induced anthocyanin accumulation in different plants (22,23). Adding jasmonic acid to culture medium of sour cherry stimulated cyanidin 3-glucoside synthesis (24).

Our data show that SA and MeJA are involved in the regulation of proline and sugars production, these solutes may function as typical osmoprotectants, stabilizing cellular membranes and maintaining turgor pressure. Therefore, it is safe to suggest that these osmoprotectants contribute to the preadaptation effect of SA and MeJA on chamomile plants.

Plants drought tolerance was assessed by MDA content and ELI in tissues damaged by drought treatments. Estimation of MDA amount, which is a secondary end product of polyunsaturated fatty acid oxidation, is widely used to measure the extent of lipid peroxidation as indicator of oxidative stress (25). The lower membrane stability index reflects the extent of lipid peroxidation, which in turn is a consequence of higher oxidative stress due to water stress conditions.

Drought stress is well-known to cause a shift in the balance of plant cells. This shift is due to an increase in the rate of generation of ROS, which induce lipid peroxidation (LPO) in the membrane structures of the cells (26).

The treatment with SA and MeJA dramatically decreased MDA content and ELI in the leaves. This could be the consequence of the preadaptation effect of SA and MeJA on chamomile plants, in which hormone-induced events leading to activation of the low molecular metabolites were initiated before the exposure of the seedlings to severe drought stress. This may facilitate the strengthening of cell walls and effectively neutralize excessive (damaging) increase in the level of ROS during further exposure to the stress-factor, thereby preventing the damage of cellular membrane structures and changes in their permeability under stress conditions (27).

Finally, SA and MeJA were found to individually enhance compatible solutes production in leaves (especially SA), but when administered in combination there was no further enhancement in compatible solutes production. The combination treatment was also found to result in high MDA and ELI. The highest levels of compatible solutes were produced in the treatment with SA applied alone. The JA signal acts co-operatively with other plant hormones. The cross-talk between JA and SA can be synergistically or antagonistically, depending on particular stress (28).

Conclusion

Drought stress caused dramatic increase in MDA content and ELI in both cultivars. Deleterious effects of drought stress were more severe in untreated plants than in treated plants. Treatments with 100 μM MeJA and 0.5 mM SA enhanced seedling total antioxidant capacity. The enhancement of antioxidant capacity in chamomile plants could have contributed to the drought tolerance. This treatment effectively maintained membrane integrity, thereby retarding electrolyte leakage and membrane lipid peroxidation (MDA).

Authors' contributions

All the authors wrote the manuscript equally.

Conflict of interests

The authors declared no competing interests.

Ethical considerations

Ethical issues (including plagiarism, misconduct, data fabrication, falsification, double publication or submission, redundancy) have been completely observed by the authors.

Funding/Support

This work was financially supported by University of Tehran, Iran.

References

1. Lawrence MB, Tobacco RJ. Progress in essential oil. Perfum Flavor 1996; 21(3): 55-68.
2. Mittler R. Oxidative stress, antioxidants and stress tolerance. Trends Plant Sci 2002; 7(9): 405–10.
3. Tarchevskii LA. Signal'nye sistemy kletok rastenii (Signal Systems of Plant Cells). Moscow: Nauka;2002.

4. Liebler DC, McClure TD. Antioxidant reactions of beta-carotene: identification of carotenoid-radical adducts. Chem Res Toxicol 1996; 9(1):8-11.
5. Smirnoff N, Cumbes Q. Hydroxyl radical scavenging activity of compatible solutes. Phytochem 1989;28: 1057-60.
6. Munné-Bosch S, Peñuelas J. Photo and antioxidative protection, and a role for salicylic acid during drought and recovery in field grown Phillyrea angustifolia plants. Planta 2003; 217(5):758-66.
7. Borsani O, Valpuesta V, Botella A. Evidence for a role of salicylic acid in the oxidative damage generated by NaCl and osmotic stress in Arabidopsis seedlings. Plant Physiol 2001; 126(3):1024-30.
8. Kawano T, Muto S. Mechanism of peroxidase actions for salicylic acid-induced generation of active oxygen species and an increase in cytosolic calcium in tobacco cell suspension culture. J Exp Bot 2000; 51 (345):685-93.
9. Creelman RA, Mullet JE. Jasmonic acid distribution and action in plants: Regulation during development and response to biotic and abiotic stress. Proc Natl Acad Sci USA 1995; 92: 4114–9.
10. Gundlach H, Muller MJ, Kutchan TM, Zenk MH. Jasmonic acid is a signal transducer in elicitor-induced plant cell cultures. Proc Natl Acad Sci USA 1992; 89(6): 2389–93.
11. Bates LS, Waldran RP, Teare ID. Raipid determination of free proline for water studies. Plant Soil 1973; 39: 205-8.
12. Sairam RK, Desmukh PS, Saxena DC. Role of antioxidant systems in wheat genotypes tolerant to water stress. Biol Plant 1998; 41:387–94.
13. Blum A, Ebercon A. Cell membrane stability as a measure of drought and heat tolerance in wheat. Crop Sci 1981; 21:43–7.
14. Saruhan N, Terzi R, Kadioglu A. The effects of exogenous polyamines on some biochemical changes during drought stress in Ctenanthe setosa. Acta Biol Hung 2006; 57:221-9.
15. Watanabe S, Kojima K, Ide Y, Satohiko S. Effects of saline and osmotic stress on proline and sugar accumulation in Populus euphratica in vitro. Plant Cell Tiss Org 2000; 63(3):199-206.
16. Izanloo A, Condon AG, Langridge P, Tester M, Schnurbusch T. Different mechanisms of adaptation to cyclic water stress in two South Australian bread wheat cultivars. J Exp Bot 2008; 59(12):3327-46.
17. Caballero JI, Verduzco CV, Galan J, Jimenz ES. Proline accumulation as a symptom of drought stress in maize: A tissue differentiation requirement. J Exp Bot 2005; 39(7):889-97.
18. Sharma P, Jha AB, Dubey RS, Pessarakli M. Reactive oxygen species, oxidative damage, and antioxidative defense mechanism in plants under stressful conditions. J Bot 2012; 2012: 217037.
19. Amin B, Mahleghah G, Mahmood HMR, Hossein M. Evaluation of interaction effect of drought stress with ascorbate and salicylic acid on some of physiological and biochemical parameters in okra (Hibiscus esculentus L.). Res J Biol Sci 2009; 4(4):380-7.
20. Rock CD. Pathways to abscisic acid-regulated gene expression. New Phytol 2000;148:357-96.
21. Thorpe MR, Ferrieri AP, Herth MM, Ferrieri RA. C-imaging: methyl jasmonate moves in both phloem and xylem, promotes transport of jasmonate, and photo assimilate even after proton transport is decoupled. Planta 2007; 226:541-51.
22. Saniewski M, Horbowicz M, Puchalski J, Ueda J. Methyl jasmonate stimulates the formation and the accumulation of anthocyanins in Kalanchoe blossfeldiana. Acta Physiol Plant 2003;25:143-9.
23. Saniewski M, Horbowicz M, Puchalski J. Induction of anthocyanins accumulation by methyl jasmonate in shoots of Crassula multicava Lam. Acta Agrobot 2006; 59:43–50.
24. Blando F, Scardino AP, Debellis L, Nicoletti I, Giovinazoo G. Characterization of in vitro anthocyanin-producing sour cherry (Prunus cerasus L.) callus cultures. Food Res Int 2005; 38(9): 937–42.
25. Lin CC, Kao CH. Effect of NaCl stress on H2O2 metabolism in rice leaves. Plant Growth Regul 2000; 30(2):151-5.
26. Zenkov NK, Lankin VE, Menshchikova EV. Okislitel'nyi stress (Oxidative Stress). Moscow: Nauka;2001. p. 280.
27. Hayat S, Ahmad A. Salicylic Acid: A Plant Hormone. Springer;2007. p. 69–89.
28. Beckers GJ, Spoel SH. Fine-tuning plant defence signalling: salicylate versus jasmonate. Plant Biol 2006;8:1-10.

The effect of aqueous Elaeagnus angustifolia extract on acute non-inflammatory diarrhea in 1-5 year old children

Abofazl Khoshdel[1*], Fatemeh Famuri[2], Elham keivani[3], Masoud Lotfizadeh[2], Karam-Ali Kasiri[2], Mortaza Rafieian[4]

[1]Clinical Biochemistry Research Center, Shahrekord University of Medical Sciences, Shahrekord, Iran
[2]Medical Plants Research Center, Shahrekord University of Medical Sciences, Shahrekord, Iran
[3]Student Research Committee, Shahrekord University of Medical Sciences, Shahrekord, Iran
[4]Isfahan Governor Office, Isfahan, Iran

ARTICLE INFO

Keywords:
Aqueous extract
Diarrhea
Non-inflammatory diarrhea
Children
Elaeagnus angustifolia
Medical plants

ABSTRACT

Introduction: Acute diarrhea is one of the most important causes of global childhood mortality and morbidity. The most common complication of acute diarrhea is dehydration. The aim of this study was to evaluate the use of aqueous Elaeagnus angustifolia extract in controlling non-inflammatory diarrhea in a hospital setting.
Methods: In this case–controlled randomized double blind clinical trial 80 children in age range of 1-5 years were admitted in pediatric ward with diagnosis of non-inflammatory diarrhea. The patients were randomly divided into two equal groups of 40 cases. The subject in the first group received aqueous Elaeagnus angustifolia extract, 1.2 ml/Kg single dose for 4 days duration and the second group (control group) 1.2 cm/Kg distilled water single dose for 4 days duration. Data analysis were performed by Chi-square and t-tests, using SPSS software.
Results: The groups were similar regarding gender, mean age, and frequency, and consistency of defecation ($p > 0.05$). Although the children seemed better in regard to frequency and consistency of defecation, however the results showed that aqueous extract of Elaeagnus angustifolia was not significantly effective in the treatment of non-inflammatory diarrhea.
Conclusion: The results of this study demonstrated that the use of aqueous extract of Elaeagnus angustifolia was not effective in the treatment of non-inflammatory diarrhea in children.

Implication for health policy/practice/research/medical education:
The results of this study demonstrated that the use of aqueous extract of Elaeagnus angustifolia might not be significantly beneficial in the treatment of non-inflammatory diarrhea.

Introduction

Acute gastroenteritis is a major cause of mortality and morbidity in the world so that more than 2.5 million deaths are reported annually in children younger than five years (1). It is often caused by an infection. Rotavirus causes 75 to 90% of diarrhea infections in children. Bacterial pathogens cause another 10 to 20% and parasites cause less than 5% of infections (2). Acute gastroenteritis in children is presented with or without abdominal pain, fever, nausea or vomiting (3). It is the major cause of hospitalization in children under age of five (1).

Diarrhea is usually defined as increase in vomiting or fluidity of stool, change in consistency, and increased frequency of defecation. World health organization (WHO) defines diarrhea as the passage of loose or watery stools at least three times in 24 hours period but this definition emphasizes the important of change in stool consistency rather than frequency (4).

Diarrhea disorder can be divided into inflammatory and non-inflammatory ones (5). Inflammatory diarrhea causes bloody stools that are usually full of white blood cells. It involves the large intestine, and may be accompanied by fever, vomiting and colicky abdominal pain or tenderness. But, non inflammatory diarrhea is watery without blood and mucus and usually without fever (6). It often involves small bowel and does not cause destruction of mucosa (7).

*Corresponding author: Abofazl Khoshdel,
Email: Nikakhosh@gmail.com

Management of non-inflammatory diarrhea is supportive until the mucosa heals. This support includes fluid therapy and preventing nutritional damage (8).

Medical plants have been used for the management of various conditions for thousands of years (9). Elaeagnus angustifolia (Russian olive, Oleander) is one of the traditional medicines used in the management of diarrhea (9). In herbal medicine oleaster fruit or flower extract are used for management of nausea, vomiting, asthma and flatulence (10).

Extract of Elaeagnus (E) angustifolia is used as anti-inflammatory agent, muscular relaxant, antiulcerogenic agent and antipyretic in traditional medicine (11-14). In Iranian traditional medicine, fruit of E. angustifolia have been used to relief pain in patients with rheumatoid arthritis (14). Also, it has been reported that the use of the fruit of E. angustifolia is beneficial in the treatment of dysentery and diarrhea (15).

In this research we evaluated the effect of aqueous E, angustifolia extract on non-inflammatory diarrhea in 1-5 age group children.

Materials and Methods

In this experimental double blind randomized clinical trial 80 children with non-inflammatory diarrhea were divided into two equal groups. The study was conducted in Pediatric ward of Hajar hospital in Shahrekord, Iran, during the period from September 2013 to May 2014.

The study protocol was approved by the Ethical Committee of Shahrekord University of Medical Sciences, Iran. Written informed consents were obtained from all parents of children. The children with severe diarrhea, chronic diarrhea and/or intractable vomiting were excluded from the study. For preparation of the aqueous extract of E. angustifolia 150 grams of E. angustifolia with cores were grinded and added 1200 ml of distilled water. The resulting solution was boiled for 20 minutes. When the volume of the solution reached to one liter, the solution was filtered after cooling. The extract was frozen in –20 °C.

Placebo was made of distill water in syringes, the same as the extract. After preparation, one code was given for placebo and other code was given to drug by a third person. For diagnosis of non-inflammatory diarrhea, stool exam was done for all the patients. This study was double blind in which the code of the drug or placebo was undefined for the patients or their parents, as well as for the doctor. In case group aqueous extract of E. angustifolia with dose of 1.2 ml/Kg, one time per day, was used for 4 days. In control group, the same volume of distilled water was used as placebo. Demographic data, frequency, volume and consistency of stool of both groups were recorded in first and fifth days of admission. The data were analyze using SPSS software, by Chi square and t-tests.

Results

In this study 80 children were enrolled and entered the trial. Seventeen children (8 subjects from the control group and 9 subjects from the case group) were excluded from the study because of non-compliance. The mean age in the study population was 18.65±9.13 years. The mean age in case group was 19.43±10.6 and in control group was 17.83±7.3 years. The mean weight in the study population was 10.76±2.01 Kg (10.93±2.07 Kg, in case group and 10.59 ±1.9 Kg, in control group) ($p>0.05$; Table 1).

The mean frequency of defecation in case group before E. angustifolia usage was 8.5 ± 4 times and after usage, it was 3.5±1.84 times and in control group it was 7.6±3.5 times and 3.4±2, respectively. Statistical analysis showed no significant difference in decrease of frequency of defecation between the two groups ($p>0.05$; Table 2). Also, there was no difference in decrease of volume and consistency of stool in two groups ($p>0.05$; Table 3).

Table 1. Demographic information of study population

	Weight (Kg)			Age (month)			Gender
	Total	Case	Control	Total	Case	Control	
Mean	10.76	10.93	10.59	18.65	19.43	17.83	-
Std. Deviation	2.01	2.07	1.9	9.13	1.06	7.3	-
Minimum	7	7	8	12	12	12	-
Maximum	16	15	16	60	60	50	-
P-value (Case & Control)		0.63			0.49		0.06

Table 2. Frequency of defecation

Group	Stool (first visit)					Stool (second visit)				
	Mean	Std. Deviation	Minimum	Maximum	P-value	Mean	Std. Deviation	Minimum	Maximum	P-value
	8.5	4	4	20	0.37	3.5	1.84	4	16	0.72
	7.6	3.5	4	16		3.4	2	1	9	

Table 3. Percent of recovery following drug or placebo consumption

	Complete recovery	Relative recovery	Without recovery (no change)	p-value
Extract group	62.5%	34.4%	3.1%	0.31
Control group	51.6%	41.9%	6.5%	

Discussion

Despite widespread use of oral rehydration therapy (ORT) and an increased understanding of the pathogenesis of diarrhea, the illness has still high mortality, especially in developing countries (16).

In folk medicine E. angustifolia has been used for diarrhea. The results of this study indicated that aqueous extract of E. angustifolia had no effect in improvement of consistency of stool and decreased volume, as well as the frequency of defecation in children with non-inflammatory diarrhea.

The findings of current study are in consistent with those of a previous study which reported that this drug had no effect in decrease of consistency of mice stool (17).

In one study, Galves *et al.* (18) showed that tannins of the E. angustifolia decreased motility of gastrointestinal tract of mice and decreased volume of defecation in mice with diarrhea. The discrepancy of this study with our results may be due to the usage of one of the ingredients of E. angustifolia but in our study all of components in aqueous extract were used. Also, in another study lactoferrin of E. angustifolia had good effect in the treatment of diarrhea (19). But in this study all of the patients had diarrhea with iron deficiency anemia and this improvement probably was due to improvement of anemia.

In Rozhon study on mice infected with vibrio cholera showed that procyanidin, one of the ingredients of E. angustifolia was effective in diarrhea (20), but in our study we did not examine specific pathogen and a wide range of viral and bacterial infections that cause non-inflammatory diarrhea were included.

In a study in patients with allergic rhinitis, intradermal injection of extract of E. angustifolia caused positive skin test (21). Therefore, children with non-inflammatory diarrhea and simultaneously food allergy might get no beneficial effects and even worsen their conditions.

Authors' contributions

All the authors wrote the manuscript equally.

Conflict of interests

The authors declared no competing interests.

Ethical considerations

Ethical issues (including plagiarism, misconduct, data fabrication, falsification, double publication or submission, redundancy) have been completely observed by the authors.

Funding/Support

None.

References

1. Walker WA. Pediatric gastrointestinal disease. 3rd edition. Hamilton, Ontario: BC Decker;2000.
2. Acute Gastroenteritis Guideline Team, Cincinnati Childrens Hospital Medical Center. Evidence-based care guideline for prevention and management of acute gastroenteritis in children age 2 months to 18 years. [updated December 21, 2011; Accessed January 20, 2012]. Available from: http://www.Cincinnatichildrence.org/service/j/Anderson-center/evidence-based-care/gastroenteritis/
3. Children Mercy Hospitals and Clinics, Kansas City. Acute gastroenteritis (AGE) clinical practice guideline. Accessed July 11, 2010. Available from: http://www.childrensmercy.org/content/view.aspx?id=8990
4. World Health Organization. The treatment of diarrhea: A manual for physicians and other senior health workers, WHO/CDR/95.3. Geneva: WHO; 1995.
5. World Health Organization. The management of bloody diarrhea in young children: WHO/CDD/94.49. Geneva: WHO; 1994.
6. World Health Organization. Persistent diarrhea in children: CCD/DDM/85.1. Diarrheal disease control. Geneva: WHO; 1985.
7. Udayakumar N, Ralph AG. Mechanisms of infectious diarrhea. Nat Rev Gastroenterol Hepatol 2008; 5: 637-647.
8. Centers for Disease Control and Prevention. Managing acute gastroenteritis among children: Oral rehydration, maintenance, and nutritional therapy. MMWR Morb Mortal Weekly Rep 2003; 52: 1-13.
9. Ramezani M, Hosseinzadeh H, Daneshmand N. Antinociceptive effect of Elaeagnus angustifolia fruit seeds in mice. Fitoterapia 2001; 72(3): 255-62.
10. Mirheydar H. Encyclopedia of plants: Indications of plants in the prevention and treatment of diseases, Vol. 2. Tehran: Islamic Farhang Press; 1998. p.163-4 .
11. Ahmadiani A, Hosseiny J, Semnanian S, Javan M, Saeedi F, Kamalinejad M, *et al.* Antinociceptive and anti-inflammatory effects of Elaeagnus angustifolia fruit extract. J Ethnopharmacol 2000; 72(1- 2): 287- 92.
12. Hosseinzadeh H, Ramezani M, Namjo N. Muscle relaxant activity of Elaeagnus angustifolia L. Fruit seeds in mice. J Ethnopharmacol 2003; 84 (2-3): 275–8.

13. Gurbuz I, Ustum O, Yesilada E, Sezik E, Kutsal O. Antiulcerogenic activity of some plants used as folk remedy in Turkey. J Ethnopharmacol 2003;88(1): 93–7.
14. Farahbakhsh S, Arbabian S, Emami F, Rastegar-Moghadam B, Ghoshooni H. Inhibition of cyclooxygenase type 1 and 2 enzyme by aqueous extract of Elaeagnus angustifolia in mice. Basic Clin Neurosci 2011;2(2):31-7.
15. Lev E, Amar Z. Ethnopharmacological survey of traditional drugs sold in the Kingdom of Jordan. J Ethnopharmacol 2002;82:131-145.
16. Nikhil T, Lan RS. Diarrhoea in children: an interface between developing and developed countries. Lancet 2004;21:(363):641-652 .
17. Ganan ZH, Zhihua H, Yaxian W. An inquiry in to preparing diarrhea model of mice and application of diarrhea index. Chinese Trad Herb Drugs 1994;4.
18. Galvez J, Zarzulo A, Cresp ME. Anti diarrhoeic activity of sclerocarya birrea bark extract and its active tannin constituent in rats. Pharmacol Pharmacent Med 1991; 5 (6): 276-278.
19. Delia R, Huang B, Huang J. Recombinant human laectoferin treatment for global health issue: Iron deficient and acute diarrhea. Biometals 2004; 17: 337-342.
20. Rozhan EJ, Khandwala AS, Sabouni A. Method of threating secretory diarrhea with enteric formulations of pro-anthocyanidin polymer. Google Patents, 2008.
21. Kernerman SM, Mccullough J, Green J. Evidence of cross- reactivity between olive, ash, privet, and Russian olive tree pollen allergens. Ann Allergy 1992;69(6): 493-496.

Development of a validated HPLC method for the determination of sennoside A and B, two major constituents of Cassia obovata Coll

Nasrollah Ghassemi-Dehkordi[1], Mustafa Ghanadian[1*], Sajjad Arabha[2]

[1]Department of Pharmacognosy, School of Pharmacy, Isfahan University of Medical Sciences, Isfahan, Iran
[2]Isfahan Pharmaceutical Sciences Research center, Isfahan University of Medical Sciences, Isfahan, Iran

ARTICLE INFO

Keywords:
Cassia obovata
Sennoside A
Sennoside B
High Pressure Liquid Chromatography

ABSTRACT

Introduction: *Cassia obovata* Coll is the only *Senna* species which grows wild in Iran. In the present study, an optimised reverse High Performance Liquid Chromatography (HPLC) validated method was established for quantification of sennosides A and B, the major constituents of *C. obovata* with a simple and accurate method.
Methods: HPLC analysis was done using Waters 515 pump on a Nova-Pak C18 (3.9 × 150 mm). Millennium software was used for the determination of the sennoside A and B in *Cassia* species and processing the information. The method was validated according to USP 32 requirements.
Results: The solvent impact on the selectivity factor and partition coefficient parameters evaluated. Using a conventional RP-18 L1 column, 3.9 × 150 mm, the mobile phase was selected after several trials with different mixtures of water and acetonitrile. Sennosides A and B were determined using the external standard calibration method. Using USP 35-NF 30, the LOD and LOQ were calculated. The reliability of the HPLC-method for analysis of sennoside A + B was validated through its linearity, reproducibility, repeatability, and recovery. Finally ethanol:water (1:1) extracts of *Cassia obovata* and *Cassia angustifolia* were standardized by assay of sennoside A and B through above HPLC validated method.
Conclusion: Through the above method, determination of sennosides in *Cassia* species are completely possible. Moreover, through comparing the results, even though sennosides are rich in *Cassia angustifolia* but, the results shows that *C. obovata* could be considered as an alternative source for sennosides A and B.

Implication for health policy/practice/research/medical education:

In the present study, and for the first time, we developed a validated High Performance Liquid Chromatography (HPLC) method for the determination of sennoside A and B, two major constituents of *Cassia obovata* Colladon. Through the above HPLC method, assay of sennosides in different *Cassia* species and *Cassia* adultrations as well as single or combined formulations containing *Cassia* extracts are completely possible.

Introduction

Medicinal herbs are normally supplied in the shops without standardization. Herbalists sometimes unintentionally, supply closed morphological medicinal herbs instead of each other. So, control of herbal bulk drugs is necessary to avoid adulterations or unwanted mistakes. *Cassia angustifolia* known as senna and *Cassia acutifolia* known as senna Mackie are widely applied in the Iranian traditional medicine to treat intestinal complications (1). One of the frequently reported adultrations of the *C. angustifolia* or

***Corresponding author**: Mustafa Ghanadian, Department of Pharmacognosy, School of Pharmacy, Isfahan University of Medical Sciences, Isfahan, Iran.
E-mail: ghannadian@gmail.com

C. acutifolia are with *C. obovata* due to their similarities. Dog senna or kaspind in Persian in the Iranian herbal Pharmacopeae is ascribed to the dried leaflets of *Cassia obovata* Coll., or its synonym name, *Cassia italica* (Mill.) Lam., containing at least 1.0-1.15% of anthraquinone derivatives (2,3). This plant is the only *Senna* species grows wild in the Hormozgan and Sistan Baluchestan provinces in the south east of Iran. It is also endemic to tropical Africa, the Middle East countries, and Pakistan (3). *C. obovata* is also cultivated in Italy from the sixteenth century (3). *Cassia Italica* is commercially available as a laxative drug in Mali and African countries (3). It is one of the plants of the Sudan used to treat intestinal complications, circulatory problems, urinary stones and sexually transmitted diseases (4). Previous phytochemical studies of *C. italica* have resulted in the isolation of β-sitosterol, stigmasterol, α-amyrin and 1,5-dihydroxy-3-methyl anthraquinone, physcion, chrysophanol and 10,10′-chrysophanol bianthrone (5-7) which could occur also as their 1,1′-diglucosides. Bianthrones are compounds with two identical or different anthrone molecules like sennidin A and B which are present in the *Cassia* species. They also could form by artifact from the converting of the monoanthrones enzymatically by drying between 20 and 50 °C (3). They have two chiral centres at C-10 and C-I0′, and for a compound having two identical anthrone moieties like sennidin A, two forms (the 10S,1 0′S and l0R, 10′R) are possible together with the meso form sennidin B (Figure 1). Anthraquinone compounds suggested being responsible for the purgative effects of the plant. So, their contents should be quantified and used as an index for the valuation or even its detection in the bulk powder form. According to pharmacopeias guideline, before marketing the plant drugs, if the active constituents are known and quantifiable, the amount in which they are present in the herbal drug should be detected. In the case of lack of knowledge of active constituent(s), other tests like spectroscopic and/or chromatographic fingerprints and process validation especially for the drug substance are required for authentication and control (8).

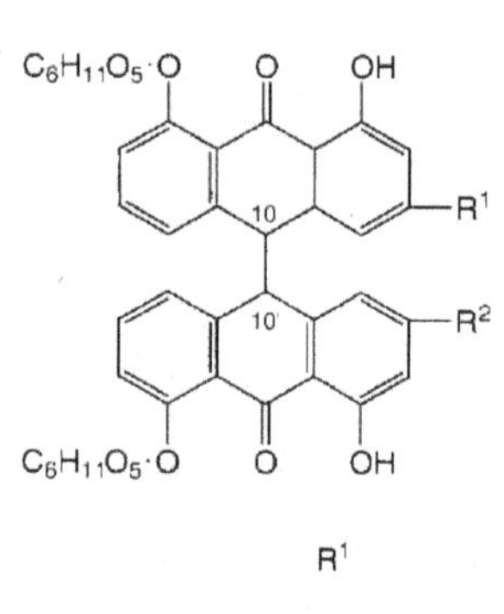

	R^1	R^2
Sennoside A	COOH	COOH
Sennoside B	COOH	COOH
Sennoside C	CH_2OH	COOH
Sennoside D	CH_2OH	COOH

Figure 1. Chemical structures of sennosides A-D in the *Cassia obovata* Coll

To the best of our knowledge, there is no report on the HPLC method development and determination of dianthrones like sennosides for the *Cassia obovata*. Thus, the purpose of this work was to develop a High Performance Liquid Chromatography (HPLC) validated method for determination of sennosides A and B of Cassia obovata with a simple, rapid and precise method.

Materials and Methods

Plant Material

The aerial parts of *Cassia obovata* Colladon (Caesalpiniaceae) were supplied from the Bandar Abbas, Iran and was identified by Dr. L. Ghaem-maghami, Department of biology, Faculty of Science, University of Isfahan. A herbarium specimen (No 1541) was deposited in the herbarium of the Faculty of Pharmacy, Isfahan University of Medical Sciences (Iran).

Instrumentation

HPLC analysis was done on the 515 HPLC pump, waters 2487 dual wavelength absorbance detector (Waters, Milford, MA, USA). The column was a Nova-Pak C18, 3.9 × 150 mm (Waters, Milford, MA, USA) and Millennium software was used for the determination of compounds and processing the data.

Chemicals

Methanol and acetonitrile HPLC-grade solvents were purchased from Caledon Company (Canada). Sennoside A and B, as analytical standards, were purchased from Sigma-Aldrich Corporation, USA.

Determination of Sennosides

Using high pressure liquid chromatography, sennosides were determined through external standard calibration method.

Solvent Effect

For evaluating the solvent impact on the selectivity factor and partition coefficient parameters which affecting on the extraction of sennosides from plant matrix, hot water and ethanol: water (50%) with different strength and selectivity's were selected.

Sample Preparation

In a volumetric flask, 1 g of the leaflets powder was weighed and 10 mL of the solvent were added to the sample powder. It was extracted, filtered, and washed three times with 10 milliliter of the solvent. Using the rotary evaporator under vacuum and at a 40 °C temperature, the filtrates were combined and evaporated till dryness. The rotary evaporated extract was washed 3 times with 2 ml HPLC-grade acetonitrile: water (1:1).

Preparation of the Standard Solutions

800 μg analytical standards were diluted in 1 ml of HPLC-grade acetonitrile: water (1:1) to prepare the stock solution

of 800 μg/ml. Different standard solutions were made by serially diluting the stock solution to concentrations of 400, 200, 100, and 50 μg/ml.

Limit of Detection and Limit of Quantification

Limit of detection (LOD) and Limit of Quantification (LOQ) were counted on using equations, LOD = 3 × S/N and LOQ = 10 × S/N. USP 35-NF 30 defines S/N = 2h/hn, where h is the height of the peak corresponding to the interest component from the peak apex to the midpoint of the noise, and hn is the difference between the largest and smallest background noise value observed over a distance equal to five times the width at the half-height of the peak of interest. The USP definition from S/N is useful in the gradient systems, in which a drift in the baseline is present. Differently, in the event of using signal to noise ratio, noise will be overestimated when drift is present (9).

Validation

The reliability of the HPLC-method for analysis of sennoside A + B was validated through its linearity, reproducibility, repeatability, and recovery (10).
The linearity means how well a calibration plot of response versus concentration approximates a straight line. It was performed by linear squares regression. Correlation coefficient (r^2) in addition to plot slope and intercept provided desired information on linearity. A linearity correlation coefficient greater than 0.999 for p-value<0.1 or greater than 0.99 for p-value<0.05 is thought to be acceptable (10).
Precision is the level of agreement among individual test results, when a series of determinations for the same analyte are done repeatedly. Repeatability and reproducibility could be measured as the parts of precision through intra-day, and inter-day assays followed by determination of coefficient of variance. CV is calculated utilizing the equation CV, %= (Stdev/X) × 100, where Stdev is the standard deviation, and X is the mean of HPLC responses. In the in-vitro systems, with easy isolation, CV less than 3% is needed (10).

Intra-day Precision

Instrumental precision is evaluated through several times injection of the same sample within the selected range. Intra–day precision was found out by injecting two replications of different concentrations (800, 400, 200, 100, and 50 μg/ml), three times in the same day (n= 6). Peak area was measured and CV % was calculated (10).

Inter-day Precision

Inter-day precision was found by injecting of two replicates of different concentrations (800, 400, 200, 100, and 50 μg/ml) on three sequential days in a week (n= 6). Peak area was measured and % CV was calculated (10).

Recovery

Recovery assures you that the real quantity of substances in the real sample has been evaluated. One method of determining the recovery is adding a certain amount of analytical standards to a blank matrix lacking standard. The samples are extracted as mentioned in the sample preparation method, and volumized to 6 ml. The added standard is determined through a validated HPLC method by three times and the recovery percentage is calculated in every case (10,11).

Statistical Analysis

Data analysis were performed using Waters Millennium Chromatography Software (Build 1154, Waters Corporation, Milford, USA). Data were reported as Mean ± SD and the results were analyzed statistically by Excel 2007 software.

Results

The HPLC method carried out in this study was aimed to optimize the resolution, reduce runtime and the limit of quantification of sennosides in the crude plant material.

Optimizing the extraction method

Two extraction methods consisted of ultrasonic radiation (60 min), and maceration overnight was compared to check the effect of the procedure on the extraction (Table 1).

Method development

Using a conventional RP-18 column, 3.9×150 mm (Waters, Milford, MA, USA), the mobile phase was selected after several trials with different mixtures of water and acetonitrile. At the first using gradient method from 10% to 100% acetonitrile in water, the solvent composition which the sennosides are eluted was detected. Then shorter gradient times from 0% to 50% were selected to reduce run times and improve peaks. The water is nonabsorbing and 0-50 % ACN-water was a solvent mix with low UV absorbance and low background noise (<0.0005 at 280 nm). Finally, a gradient system of water with 0.1% phosphoric acid (A), and ACN:H2O (50:50) with 0.1% phosphoric acid (B) was selected. It was started with A: B (100:0) for 2 min, then 0–30% B in 12 min, A: B (70:30) for 10 min, then 30→50% B in 20 min, and A: B (50:50) for 5 min following with equilibrating with A: B (100:0) for 10 min. The flow rate was 1 ml/min and

Table 1. The effect of solvents and extraction procedures for determination of sennosides in *Cassia obovata*

Sample	Extraction method		Solvent	
	Maceration overnight	Ultrasonication (60 min)	Ethanol: Water (1:1)	Hot Water (60 °C)
Sennoside A	0.28 ± 0.011	0.19 ± 0.008	0.28 ± 0.011	0.064 ± 0.0021
Sennoside B	0.26 ± 0.010	0.18 ± 0.007	0.26 ± 0.010	0.069 ± 0.0018

temperature was kept constant at 30 °C to eliminate the temperature variations. UV detector time constant was set to 0.1 and the detector sample rate to 10 pts/Sec in the single wavelength mode at 280 nm to increase the signal to noise ratio. Smaller volume of the sample was injected by reducing the loop to 5 μL to have sharp peaks with good resolution.

Determination of sennosides

Using high pressure liquid chromatography, sennosides A and B was determined using the external standard calibration method. The retention time for sennoside B and A was observed to be 19.07, and 28.35 min (Figures 2 and 3).

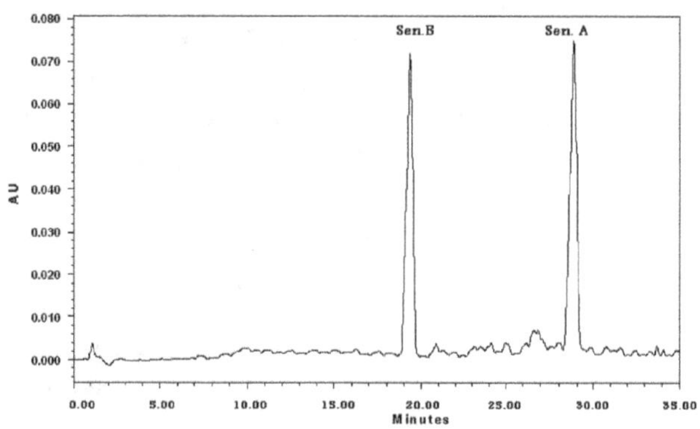

Figure 2. HPLC chromatogram of sennoside B and A (50 μg/mL) at 280 nm. The retention time for sennoside B and A was observed to be 19.07, and 28.35 min.

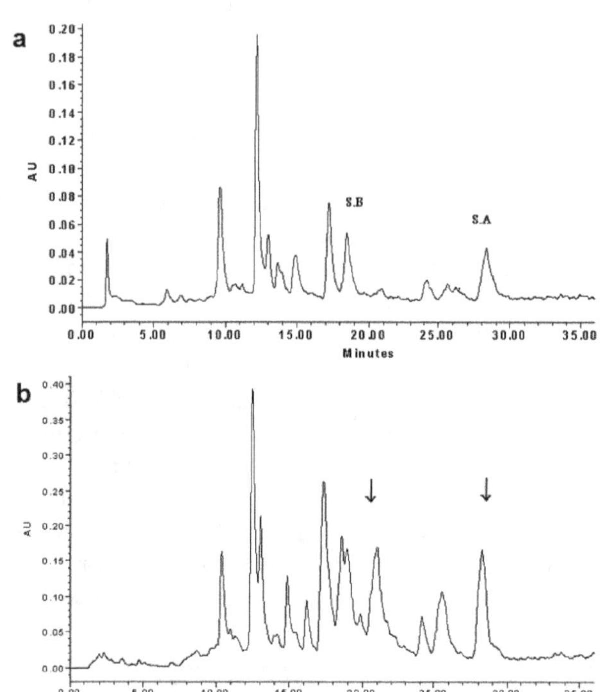

Figure 3. High performance liquid chromatography chromatograms of a) *Cassia obovata* and b) *Cassia angustifolia*. Chromatograms were carried out at 280 nm on a reversed-phase HPLC column (RP-18, 150 mm × 3.9 mm, 5 μm particle size, waters, US) using water with H_3PO_4 (0.2%) as solvent A and acetonitrile : water (50:50) as solvent B with gradient elution at 30 °C and flow rate of 1 ml.min^{-1}.

Signal, Noise, and Assay precision

Using USP 35-NF 30 definition of signal to noise ratio: S/N=2h/hn, the LOD and LOQ were calculated as 2.2 μg/mL and 7.5 μg/mL for sennoside B, and 3.75 μg/mL and 12.5 μg/mL for sennoside A, respectively (9,12). The LOD and LOQ values could be reduced more in the case of using isocratic mobile phase system, but the current gradient mobile phase system possessed better selectivity (Table 2). The instrumental precision by intra-day results and intermediate precision through inter-day results of repetitive standards quantitation in the different concentrations in the selected linear range, 50 to 800 μg/mL, as is presented in Table 3.

Recovery

The accuracy of the validated method describes the extent to which test results quantified by the method and the real amount. In this method, accuracy was evaluated as recovery test after spiking of 800 μg of sennoside B standard to 2 g of the *Myrtus communis* L. powder plant as blank sample matrix. After extraction as is mentioned in the sample preparation method it was volumized to 2 mL in each additional level. Three determinations were carried out and the recovery percentage was calculated in every case was found to be 83.69 ± 3.28%.

Discussion

HPLC validated method was established for quantification of sennosides A and B, the major constituents of *C. obovata* with a simple and accurate method. The retention time for sennoside B and A was observed to be 19.07, and 28.35 min. By the aid of the Millennium software, the calibration curve was determined by linear regression in the range of 50 to 800 μg/mL. The regression equation was y= 4351.x – 28210 with the correlation co-factor (R2) of 0.999 for sennoside A and y= 3572.x + 10685 with R^2=0.998 for sennoside B, where x is the concentration of standard in μg/mL (Figure 4).

Ethanol:water (1:1) extract obtained from 1 gram *Cassia obovata* dried powder diluted to 4 mL was standardized to contain 722.05 ± 24.30, and 790.70 ± 29.35 μg/mL sennoside A and B. It is equivalent to % 0.29 of sennoside A and 0.32% of sennoside B in the dried plant. The extract obtained from *Cassia angustifolia* dried powder was standardized also to yield % 0.83 of sennoside A and 1.49% of sennoside B. Comparing the results shows that the amounts of both sennosides in *Cassia angustifolia* are more than *C. obovata*, even though *C. obovata* is also considered as an alternative source for sennosides A and B.

Cassia species are freely administrated without controlling the main constituents. Sennosides A and B are the main active constituents of senna or its related formulations. The validated HPLC method described in this article allowed the assay of sennosides in *cassia* extracts or pharmaceutical formulations containing these

Table 2. Linearity, LOD, and LOQ parameters of Sennoside A, and B standards

Compound	LOD µg/mL	LOQ µg/mL	R^2 square	Equation	Linear range (µg/mL)
Sennoside A	3.75	12.5	0.999	y = 4351.x – 28210	50-800
Sennoside B	2.2	7.5	0.998	y= 3572.x + 10685	50-800

Table 3. Repeatability and intermediate precision assays of standards and real sample

Analytes	Concentrations (µg/mL)	inter-day n=6	RSD% (inter-day)	RSD% (intra-day)
Sennoside A	50	208215±8051	3.87	3.80
	100	425023±12201	2.87	2.71
	200	829363±20145	2.43	2.21
	400	1664790±45012	2.70	2.01
	800	3476863±125014	3.60	3.12
Sennoside B	50	263262±11820	4.00	2.80
	100	475446.5±20940	3.98	2.67
	200	843383±35343	3.76	2.06
	400	1524978±54948	3.44	1.41
	800	3111968±110862	3.20	2.34

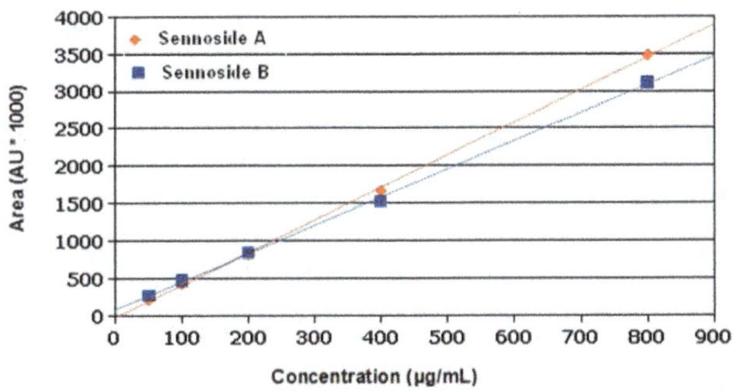

Figure 4. Calibration curve of sennoside A and B using HPLC method and acetonitrile:water as mobile phase with pH adjusted to 2.3 at 280 nm. Using the millennium processing software, the calibration curve was determined by linear regression in the range of 50-800 µg/mL. The regression equation was y= 4351.x – 28210 with the correlation co-factor (R2) of 0.999 for sennoside A and y= 3572.x + 10685 with R^2=0.998 for sennoside B, where x is the concentration of standard (µg/mL).

two compounds in accordance with USP requirements. In comparison with previous validated HPLC methods on sennosides, the LOD and LOQ in this method were decreased to lower amounts and the linear range was optimized to a larger range from 50 to 800 µg/mL (13,14). Previous reports on determination of sennosides by the HPLC method was done on *Cassia angustifolia* while this method was optimized on both *C. angustifolia* and *C. obovata*.

Authors' contributions

NGD co-ordinated the study and participated in most of the experiments. MG carried out the design and contributed in data analysis and writing and finalizing the manuscript. SA participated in most of the experiments and in manuscript preparation.

Conflict of interests

The authors declared no competing interests.

Ethical considerations

Ethical issues (including plagiarism, misconduct, data fabrication, falsification, double publication or submission, redundancy) have been completely observed by the authors.

Funding/Support

It has been supported by Isfahan Pharmaceutical Sciences Research Center, Isfahan University of Medical Sciences.

References

1. Aghili-Alavi MH. Gharabadin Kabir. 10th ed. Tehran: Marvi; 1996.
2. Ghasemi-Dehkordi N. Herbal Pharmacopeia of Iran. Tehran: Research Vice Chancellor of Ministry of Health of Iran, Drug and Food Vice Chancellor; 1992.
3. Trease GE, Evans WC. Pharmacognosy. 12th ed. London: Bailliere Tindall; 1983. 385-94.
4. Yagi S, El-Tigani S, Ali M, Elkhidir I, Mohammed AM. Chemical constituents and insecticidal activity of Senna italica mill. from the sudan. International letters of chemistry, Physics and Astronomy 2013; 9: 146-51.
5. Kazmi MH, Malik A, Hameed S, Akhtar N, Noor-Ali S. An anthraquinone derivative from Cassia italica. Phytochemistry 1994; 36: 761-3.
6. Wu YB, Zheng CJ, Qin LP, Sun LN, Han T, Jiao L, *et al.* Antiosteoporotic activity of anthraquinones from Morinda officinalis on osteoblasts and osteoclasts. Molecules 2009; 14: 573-83.
7. Alemayehu G, Abegaz B, Snatzke G, Duddeck

H. Bianthrones from Senna longiracemosa. Phytochemistry 1993; 32: 1273-7.
8. US Food and Drug Administration. FDA Guidance for Industry: Botanical drug products. U.S. Food and Drug Administration, Center for Drug Evaluation and Research, Rochville, 2004. p. 5-20.
9. Snyder RA, Tarpley MJ, Tarpley JL, Davidson M, Brophy C, Dattilo JB. Teaching in the operating room: results of a national survey. J Surg Educ 2012; 69: 643-9.
10. Hajimehdipoor H, Kondori BM, Amin GR, Adib N, Rastegar H, Shekarchi M. Development of a validated HPLC method for the simultaneous determination of flavonoids in Cuscuta chinensis Lam. by ultra-violet detection. Daru 2012; 20: 57-62.
11. Häkkinen S, Auriola S. High-performance liquid chromatography with electrospray ionization mass spectrometry and diode array ultraviolet detection in the identification of flavonol aglycones and glycosides in berries. J Chromatogr A 1998; 829: 91-100.
12. Ghassemi N, Ghanadian M, Ghaemmaghami L, Kiani H. Development of a Validated HPLC/Photodiode Array Method for the Determination of Isomenthone in the Aerial Parts of Ziziphora tenuior L. Jundishapur J Nat Pharm Prod 2013; 8: 180-6.
13. Sun SW, Su HT. Validated HPLC method for determination of sennosides A and B in senna tablets. J Pharm Biomed Anal 2002; 29: 881-94.
14. Verma RK, Uniyal GC, Singh SP, Sharma JR, Gupta MM. Reverse-phase high performance liquid chromatography of sennosides in Cassia angustifolia. Phytochem Anal 1996; 7: 73-5.

16

Antiepileptic activity of hydroalcoholic extract of basil in mice

Mehrdad Modaresi[1*], Arezoo Pouriyanzadeh[2], Majid Asadi-Samani[3]

[1]Biology Faculty, Khorasgan (Isfahan) Branch, Islamic Azad University, Isfahan, Iran
[2]Payam-e-Noor University, Isfahan Center, Isfahan, Iran
[3]Medical Plants Research Center, Shahrekord University of Medical Sciences, Shahrekord, Iran

ARTICLE INFO

Keywords:
Epilepsy
Seizure
Ocimum basilicum
Hydro alcoholic extract
Pentylenetetrazole

ABSTRACT

Introduction: Epilepsy has been always considered as one of the most prevalent disorders of nervous system and despite various drugs available, there are still some patients who have drug resistance. In traditional medicine, basil (*Ocimum basilicum*) has been used in treating epilepsy. To achieve an effective antiepileptic drug with few side effects, the antiepileptic effect of *O. basilicum* was investigated in pentylenetetrazole (PTZ)-induced epilepsy model.
Methods: In this experimental research, 48 laboratory female mice (for removing gender factor) were designated in 6 equal groups. The experimental groups comprised control, sham, and four treatment groups receiving the extract at 100, 250, 300, and 350 mg/kg doses (intraperitoneally; ip), 65 minutes before PTZ injection and the factors of epilepsy symptoms and the symptoms frequency were studied.
Results: The obtained results of using different doses (100, 250, 300, 350 mg/kg) of the extract indicated that the mice in 100 mg/kg dose group exhibited the highest frequency of epileptic attacks. The samples receiving the extract at 100 and 250 mg/kg doses exhibited the highest and lowest frequency of myoclonic twitches, respectively. In the group treated with 250 mg/kg dose, the symptoms of epilepsy, frequency of epilepsy, and mortality rate respectively increased, decreased, and decreased ($p<0.05$).
Conclusion: By the obtained results, the hydroalcoholic extract of *O. basilicum* at 250 mg/kg dose could be recommended as an effective drug for preventing epilepsy in the animal model.

Implication for health policy/practice/research/medical education:
The hydroalcoholic extract of *Ocimum basilicum* is able to prevent the attacks in the animal epilepsy model and might be beneficial in epileptic patients.

Introduction

In traditional medicine, there is an attempt to introduce suitable alternatives to synthetic drugs by means of the chemical compounds existing in plants or through combining different parts of a number of plants. In other words, the purpose in traditional medicine is to improve the function of a system in relation to other systems and hence herbal medicines enjoy a more extensive range of effects than existing synthetic ones in pharmacotherapy (1). Use of antiepileptic drugs can lead to numerous complications including decreased white blood cells and hepatic toxicity. Also, taking these drugs in pregnancy can have teratogenic effects and cause fetal anomalies. Therefore, herbal medicines with fewer complications could be a very appropriate alternative for treating this disease (2).

Ocimum basilicum has long been used as sedative, analgesic, and anticonvulsant (3). *O. basilicum* is a herbaceous, annual, and aromatic plant, reaching a height of 60 cm (4). In a study by Li et al, 1-8 cineole, linalool, and geraniol together comprising 93% of the essential oils were introduced as the main components of *O. basilicum* (3,5). In India, *O. basilicum* leaves are used as smoothing and their sap as febrifuge and drug bust in bronchitis. The powder of its dried leaves is blown into the nose for atrophic rhinitis which is manifested by excessive dryness of the nose, ample and smelly scabs, and broad nasal cavity

***Corresponding author**: Mehrdad Modaresi,
Email: mehrdad_modaresi@hotmail.com

(3). The boiled root of the plant is taken as diaphoretic in malaria fever cases. The leaves and stems of this plant are crushed and put on the mosquito bite. Its essence is applied as disinfectant, insecticide, and insect repellent especially at the onset of typhus. This plant is also anti *Bacillus typhosus* (3). Epilepsy is one of prevalent disease (6) as more than 50 million people are suffering from it worldwide (7).
Epilepsy is a chronic and mainly progressive disorder and is manifested as an unpredictable and periodical attack, developed by abnormal discharge of brain neurons (8). Regarding that no study has been yet conducted on antiepileptic effect of *O. basilicum* in pentylenetetrazole (PTZ) model, the present study was designed and conducted to study the antiepileptic effect of *O. basilicum* in an animal model to take a small step in treatment of epilepsy, and relief of pain, suffering, and concerns of human.

Materials and Methods

This experimental research was conducted in 2010-2011 in Payam-e-Noor University of Isfahan, Iran. In this research, we used small female Balb/C mice weighing 30±5 gr. The adult female mice under study were kept in laboratory conditions for one week to get adapted to the environment. The animals were kept in a room with normal light conditions and 24-26 °C temperature and water and food were freely placed at their disposal. The laboratory mice under this study comprised 48 mice randomly assigned into six groups of eight each and each group was kept in a separate cage.
To prepare the hydroalcoholic extract of O. basilicum, we divided the supplied leaves into small pieces and pulverized them using mill. 30 gr of this powder was poured into a sterile erlen and 40 ml ethyl alcohol was introduced. The mixture was kept in a cool environment for 24 hours and then the contents of the erlen were completely mixed using a shaker for five minutes. After the sample was filtrated using Whatman paper and the remaining extract in the solution (2.34 gr) was calculated, *O. basilicum* concentration was determined in the mother solution and the required doses were prepared through diluting by injectable normal saline. The hydroalcoholic extract was intraperitoneally injected to the experimental groups as follows:
A) Control group received injectable normal saline intraperitoneally at 0.5 ml.
B) Sham group: For comparison between the extract's effect and diazepam, this group received injectable diazepam at 2 mg/kg dose.
C) The group receiving injection at 100 mg/kg
D) The group receiving injection at 250 mg/kg
E) The group receiving injection at 300 mg/kg
F) The group receiving injection at 350 mg/kg
All samples were injected with the epilepsy-causing PTZ at 130mg/kg dose, 65 minutes after receiving the extract at determined doses (9-11). Then, the factors of epilepsy symptoms and symptoms frequency were investigated. In this research, the mice were checked for one hour after the extract and PTZ injection and all manifested movements were recorded by a camera, so that the type of movements could be closely interpreted and measured. Epileptic responses were classified as follows:
Stage zero: no response, stage one: immobility, stage two: body stretching, stage three: myoclonic twitches, and stage four: general tonic-clonic seizures. The obtained data were analyzed by SPSS 11.5 using Tukey's test, Duncan's test, and ANOVA.

Results

The control and C groups developed body stretching most frequently. The sham and D groups developed fewest attacks of body stretching ($p<0.05$). The control and C groups developed myoclonic twitches most frequently. Also, the D group developed the fewest myoclonic twitches ($p<0.05$; Table 1).
The effect of 250 mg/kg dose on absence of various attacks was greater than that of other doses. In addition, none of the used doses had a significant effect on absence of immobility ($p>0.05$). The 250 mg/kg dose could be introduced as the best dose with a function similar to that observed in the B group. The highest reduction in mean frequency of myoclonic twitches was noted in the F group. The 300 mg/kg dose had the greatest effect, after diazepam, on decreasing mean frequency of general tonic-clonic seizures. Also, the 350 mg/kg dose had the highest effect on decreasing mean frequency of myoclonic twitches compared to the other doses ($p<0.05$). There was no significant difference in mean frequency of general tonic-clonic seizures between the A group and other groups ($p>0.05$; Table 1).

Discussion

The analysis of the data obtained in this study indicated that intraperitoneal injection of *O. basilicum* hydroalcoholic extract was effective on the epileptic behaviours parameters in the mice and confirmed the antiepileptic property of this plant leaves. The obtained data indicated that the effect of *O. basilicum* extract is dose-dependent and different concentrations could exert inhibitory effect on or delay a different series of epileptic behaviors.
Herbal medicines have long been addressed as therapeutic compounds with fewer complications and used as very appropriate alternatives for treating diseases (2). *O. basilicum* has been much used as a very suitable sedative, analgesic, and anticonvulsant herbal medicine (3). The important issue in using herbal medicines is determination of the appropriate dose with the fewest complications; therefore we studied the effect of 100, 250, 300, and 350 mg/kg dose of *O. basilicum* hydroalcoholic extract on treating the epilepsy induced by PTZ injection in this research project. It has been well confirmed that PTZ has adverse effects on neuronal membrane. PTZ affects potassium and calcium channels and discharges the intracellular repertoires of calcium ions. In addition, PTZ decreases the neurotransmitter-induced chloride conductance (9).

Table 1. Comparison of effect of basil hydro-alcoholic extract against pentylenetetrazole-induced seizure in mice

Parameters	Groups					
	A	B	C	D	E	F
The number of attacks (stretching)	6.80±0.20	6.65±0.33	6.80±0.30*	3.80±0.20*	3.70±0.30	4.75±0.30
The number of myoclonic contractions	6.90±0.50	3.90±0.54	6.60±0.33*	3.70±0.23*	4.80±0.60	4.85±0.20
The absence of attacks	6.80±0.60	6.90±0.50	6.80±0.30	3.60±0.40*	6.80±0.40	6.90±0.70
Frequency of myoclonic contractions	3.60±0.20	2.50±0.20	2.60±0.70	2.50±0.20	2.60±0.30	1.50±0.20*
Frequency of generalized tonic-clonic seizures	6.40±0.70*	3.10±0.50	6.40±0.80*	6.60±0.20*	3.81±0.30	6.50±0.20*

A: Control, B: Sham, C, D, E, and F: The groups receiving the extract at doses of respectively 100, 250, 300, and 350 mg/kg; The data are shown as Mean±SD; * significant at $p<0.05$.

As the drugs effective on PTZ-induced epilepsies are clinically very useful in treating small epilepsy or absence (10,11). Therefore, the extract of *O. basilicum* leaves has also exhibited good effects on inhibiting the PTZ-induced epilepsies and could be effective on absence seizure treatment (12).

Since seizure mechanism is thought to be associated with decreased cerebral GABA levels, Castor *et al.* studied the effect of benzene ethyl acetate fraction of *Sesbania grandiflora* on the cerebral GABA contents in the mice after demonstrating antiepileptic property of this fraction in the PTZ-induced seizure animal model. The results indicated an increase in cerebral GABA content (13). Analysis of *O. basilicum* essential oil indicated that terpenes were the main existent compounds in this extract, with linalool, (44.18%), cineole (13.65%), eugenol (8.59%), isocaryophyllene (3.10%), and methyl cinnamate (4.26%) as the main terpenes (14). As linalool is one of the main components of *O. basilicum*, the mechanism of linalool effect has been mentioned on modulation of GABAergic system (15). Therefore, the antiepileptic effect of *O. basilicum* extract is likely to be exerted also in the PTZ-induced seizure model thanks to increased cerebral GABA content.

Linalool is a monoterpene which is present in many aromatic oil essences as a main component and could be a candidate for antiepileptic effect of *O. basilicum*. Many of the plants containing linalool are used as antiepileptic agents in traditional medicine, of which juniper, scientifically named *Aeollanthus* from family Labiatae, could be mentioned. Also, oil essence of *Laurus nobilis* leaves containing linalool was demonstrated to be effective on PTZ-induced seizure. Linalool exerts its antiepileptic effect through inhibiting glutamate binding in rats' cortex and impacting GABAergic and glutamatergic connections (16). Linalool is one of the main components of the extract and has dose-dependent effects. This component has been used for dyspepsia and epilepsy, which its effects were attributed to its local anesthetic activity (2, 17). The local anesthesia developed by linalool is attributed to its inhibitory effect on discharging acetylcholine and the duration within which the channel remains open in muscular neural functions. One of the causes of this dose's toxicity is increased linalool which disrupts vital functions of the cells because of excessive inhibition of acetylcholine transmission and leads to the animal death (18).

Conclusion

In view of the obtained results, the effect *O. basilicum* hydroalcoholic extract at 250 mg/kg dose on developing myoclonic twitches is more pronounced than that of this extract at other doses and this dose is recommended as the best one, with a function similar to that observed in the sham group. Therefore, the notable point, in view of the effect's dose-dependency, in using this herbal medicine is to select the exact dosage based on the need. This should be further investigated in complementary works.

Acknowledgments

Appreciate and thanks to all persons in biology department of Payam-Noor University of Isfahan who helped us in implementing this project.

Authors' contributions

All the authors wrote the manuscript equally.

Conflict of interests

The authors declared no competing interests.

Ethical considerations

Ethical issues (including plagiarism, misconduct, data fabrication, falsification, double publication or submission, redundancy) have been completely observed by the authors.

Funding/Support

None.

References

1. Van V. The most important medicinal plants of the world. Mashhad: Green Farm Training Complex; 2009. p. 234
2. Rabani M, Jafarian A, Hasanzadeh F, Hashemi S, Haghirabadi A, Sabet S. Evaluation of anti-epileptic effect of conjugated form of valproic acid and phenytoin in mice. J Shahrekord Univ Med Sci 2004; 6(2): 22-30.
3. Kasture VS, Deshmukh VK, Chopde CT. Anxiolytic

and anticonvulsive activity of Sesbania grandiflora leaves in experimental animals. Phytother Res 2002; 16(5):455-60.
4. Hirtz D, Thurman DJ, Gwinn-Hardy K, Mohamed M, Chaudhuri AR, Zalutsky R. How common are the 'common' neurologic disorders? Neurology 2007; 68(5):326-37.
5. Lee SJ, Umano K, Shibamoto T, Lee KG. Identification of volatile components in basil (Ocimum basilicum L.) and thyme leaves (Thymus vulgaris L.) and their antioxidant properties. Food Chem 2005;91:131-7.
6. Rogawski MA. KCNQ2/KCNQ3 K+ channels and the molecular phathogenesis of epilepsy: imlications for therapy. TINS 2000;23:393-8.
7. White HS. Comparative anticonvulsant and mechanistic profile of the established and newer antiepileptic drugs. Epilepsia 1999;40(5):S2-10.
8. Loscher W. New visions in the pharmacology of anticonvulsion. Eur J Pharmacol 1998;342:1-13.
9. Atapour N, Kalantaripour TP, Nourpanah M, Niazi M. Chemical kindling and seizure susceptibility in morphine dependent rats. Eur Neuropsy Chopharmacol 2000;10:483-7.
10. Steven LP. Glycine potentiation of anticonvulsant drugs in pentylenetetrazol seizures in rats. Brain 1991; 26: 43-7.
11. Namvaran-Abbasabad A, Tavakkoli-Ghazani F. The effect of Salvia officinalis hydroalcoholic extract on PTZ-induced seizure threshold in Vincristine injected mice. J Shahrekord Univ Med Sci 2012; 13(6): 47-55.
12. Malawska B. Application of pharmacophore models for the design and synthesis of new anticonvulsant drugs. Mini Rev Med Chem 2003;3:341-8.
13. Kasture VS, Deshmukh VK, Chopde CT. Anxiolytic and anticonvulsive activity of Sesbania grandiflora leaves in experimental animals. Phytother Res 2002; 16 (5):455-60.
14. Smail M. Central properties and chemical composition of Ocimum basilicum essential oil. Pharma Biol 2006; 44(8): 619-26.
15. Brum LF, Elisabetsky E, Souza D. Effects of linalool on [(3)H] MK801 and [(3)H] muscimol binding in mouse cortical membranes. Phytother Res 2001;15(5): 422-5.
16. Elisabetsky E, Marschner J, Souza DO. Effects of linalool on glutamatergic system in the rat cerebral cortex. Neurochem Ress 1995;20(4):461-5
17. Rafieian-Kopaei, M, Hosseini-asl K. Effects of Ocimum basilicum on functional dyspepsia. IJMS 2005;30(3): 134-7.
18. Re L, Barocci S, Sonnino S, Mencarelli A, Vivani C, Paolucci G, *et al.* Linalool modifies the nicotinic receptor – ion channel Kineties at the mouse neuromuscular. Junction Pharmacol Res 2000; 42(2): 177-82.

17

Histomorphometric study on the effects of *Artemisia sieberi* extract in mice skin

Jahangir Kaboutari[1*], Mohammad Saeed Haydarnejad[2], Rahmat allah Fatahian Dehkordi[1], Sedigheh Raeisi Vanani[2]

[1]Department of Basic Sciences, Faculty of Veterinary Medicine, Shahrekord University, Shahrekord, Iran
[2]Department of Biology, Faculty of Basic Sciences, Shahrekord University, Shahrekord, Iran

ARTICLE INFO

Keywords:
Artemisia sieberi
Histomorphometry
Skin

ABSTRACT

Introduction: Skin as the biggest single body organ is always exposing to various injuries, therefore health and healing of its injuries is vital. *Artemisia sieberi* is a valuable medicinal plant with a long history of indication in folk and modern medicine. Due to different chemical components and antioxidant, anti-inflammatory, antimicrobial and cytoprotective properties of *Artemisia*, this study was conducted to study the histomorphometric effects of *Artemisia sieberi* (*A. sieberi*) extract on mice skin.
Methods: Ninety adult mice were randomly divided in 3 groups. In the treatment group *A. sieberi* extract dissolved in ethanol & distilled water, in the positive control ethanol & distilled water, and in negative control only distilled water were applied on the shaved dorsum twice daily for 21 days. Mean thickness of epidermis, hypodermis & dermis layers, percentage of collagen fibers and histological evaluation of skin layers were studied in 1, 3, 5, 14 and 21days post treatment. Data were presented as mean± SD and analyzed using one way ANOVA and LSD post hoc tests. The $P<0.05$ was considered as statistically significant.
Results: *A. sieberi* extract significantly increased epidermis thickness in day 1, hypodermis, dermis and percentage of collagen fibers in day 3 in comparison to positive and negative control groups. Histology study revealed normal structure of skin and no abnormality was seen.
Conclusion: *A. sieberi* extract can be effective for health and healing of skin injuries by increasing thickness of the skin layers and amount of collagen fibers.

Implication for health policy/practice/research/medical education:
It seems that *A. siebri* extract via antimicrobial, anti-inflammatory and anti-oxidant properties and increasing fibroblast activity increases thickness of skin layers and improves integrity and healing of its injuries. Therefore, it might be beneficial for skin health.

Introduction

Skin involves about 16% of body weight and is the first physical defense barrier between internal and external body environment against microbial, physical and chemical infectious agents and also via its lymphatic system participates in the primary immune reactions (1). Skin has basic role in the homeostasis and thermoregulation and as a sensory organ it has numerous nerve terminals and sensory receptors. Skin especially facial skin is very important in beauty and social-emotional communications and due to the extensive area and different functions, it is always exposing to various injuries, therefore skin health and integrity is vital (1). So from ancient times human had great attention toward remedies and medications for beauty and repairing skin injuries e.g. dressings made of milk of mothers of baby boys, honey, tea leaves, wine and myrrh, pig fat and vinegar, aloe vera, red Ginseng root, and henna (2).

Medicinal plants existed long before human life and although it is not known that when does human discover their therapeutic property, but in all civilizations trace of their indication has been seen. Since medicinal plants

*Corresponding author: Dr. Jahangir Kaboutari, Discipline of Pharmacology, Department of Basic Sciences, School of Veterinary Medicine, University of Shahrekord, POB 115, Postcode 88186/34141, Shahrekord, Iran.
E-mail: Kaboutari-j@vet.sku.ac.ir

possess suitable therapeutic efficacy and lesser side effects than chemical drugs, there is increasing tendency toward them so that nowadays they are valuable source of natural health keeping products and about 80% of people in developed countries use remedies derived from medicinal plants (3). *Artemisia* is one of these valuable medicinal plants with long history of indication in the traditional medicine especially in China as tonic, appetizer, disinfectant, analgesics, antipyretic, anti-rheumatoid and anti-helminthes (4-7). Chemical analyses have shown presence of active compounds e.g. flavonoids, coumarins, caffeoylquinic acids, sterols, satonins, sesquiterpene lactones (artemisinin & dehydroleucodine) in different species of *Artemisia*, thus, antimicrobial, antifungal, antiviral, anti-diabetic, analgesic, anti-inflammatory, anti-parasitic, anti-oxidant, antipyretic, antispasmodic, anti-tumor, anti-complementary and anti-ulcerogenic properties have been attributed to *Artemisia* plant in the modern medicine (3,8-18). In the 1990 decade anti-ulcerogenic activity of *A.annua* in peptic ulcers was shown for the first time (19). Anti-ulcerogenic effects of ethanolic extract and some component of aerial part of *Artemisia* has also been shown (20). Biochemical and histopathological study of *A. sieberi* extract has shown its suitable effects on wound healing in experimental dermal injuries (21). Hydro alcoholic extract of *A. aucheri* can accelerate wound healing and decrease healing time in experimental dermal injuries (22). Also suitable therapeutic effects of *A. sieberi* extract on healing of second degree burn injuries have been shown (23). So, due to antioxidant, anti-inflammatory, antimicrobial and cytoprotective efficacies of *Artemisia* and its therapeutic effects on healing of dermal injuries, this study was conducted to evaluate the effects of *A. sieberi* extract on histomorphometric parameters of skin in mice.

Material and Methods

Animals

Ninety adult healthy mice (20-30 g BW) were prepared and housed under standard laboratory conditions in accordance with the European community guidelines for laboratory animals (12 h. light/dark cycle, ambient temperature of 22±1°C, 60% humidity) and under supervision of the Ethical Committee of the Shahrekord University. During experiments chow pellet and water were freely available.

Plant extraction

Aerial parts of *A. Sieberi* were collected from Yazd province of Iran, in the late summer and beginning of autumn, dried at room temperature, grounded and sieved. Artemisinin extraction was done by using petroleum ether based on the previously published method (21-25).

Animal experiment

After one week for acclimatization, animals were randomly divided into three groups. In the negative control group only distilled water and in the positive control group distilled water plus ethanol were administered. In the treatment group, *A. sieberi* extract dissolved in distilled water and ethanol was administered. Before any experiment, animals dorsum were shaved and depicted carefully and local medication was done twice daily with sterile swab. In the days 1, 3,5,14 and 21 post treatments, 5 animals of each group were randomly selected and after euthanasia, a full thickness skin flap of the experimental area was taken and fixed in the 10% buffer formalin. Tissue processing was done by Autotechnicon tissue processor (Citadel 1000, Thermoshanon, UK), 20 slides were prepared from each paraffin block and Hematoxylin - Eosin (H&E) staining was done. By using an ocular micrometer lens, tackiness of epidermis, dermis and hypodermis layers were measured and registered. Percentage of collagen fibers was determined by using a gridding graticule as a percentage of tissue matrixes. Histological changes of skin were studied on different sampling days by using light microscope.

Statistical analysis

Data were demonstrated as mean± SD. One-way analysis of variance (ANOVA) followed by LSD post hoc test were used for analysis of data ($p<0.05$).

Results

Epidermis layer

As the Table 1 shows, while there was no significant difference in the average thickness of epidermis layer between positive and negative control groups ($p>0.05$), in the treatment group, it was significantly higher than control groups at day 1 post treatment ($p<0.05$), meanwhile this difference in the rest of days was not significant ($p>0.05$).

Dermis and hypodermis layers

Despite that there was no significant difference in the average thickness of dermis & hypodermis layers between positive and negative groups ($p>0.05$), but in the treatment group it was significantly higher than control groups at day 3 post treatment ($p<0.05$), although in other days this difference was not significant ($p>0.05$; Table 1).

Percentage of collagen fibers

Comparison between negative and positive control and treatment groups revealed that only in the day 3 post treatment, percentage of collagen fiber in the treatment groups was significantly higher than that of control groups ($p>0.05$), but in the other days such a significant difference was not seen ($p>0.05$; Table 1).

Histological survey

Histological survey showed that in the control and treatment groups, skin tissue had natural structure and no injury or abnormality was seen. Epidermis was composed of stratified squamous cells with acidophil cytoplasm and basophil nucleus (Figure 1A & D). In the dermis, a loss

Table 1. Mean± standard deviation of thickness of skin layers (Micrometer) and percentage of collagen fibers in the control and treatment groups during different days.

	Sampling day	Group		
		Negative control	Positive control	Treatment
Mean thickness of epidermis	1	2.49±0.41	2.48±0.24	3.46±0.14[a]
	3	2.71±0.32	2.68±0.31	2.81±0.36
	5	2.84±0.18	2.63±0.28	2.21±0.23
	14	2.12±0.24	2.21±0.32	2.72±0.48
	21	2.36±0.72	2.30±0.36	2.29±0.64
Mean thickness of dermis	1	25.24±2.23	28.74±1.24	29.56±5.4
	3	24.16±4.1	25.19±3.04	65.24±8.13[a]
	5	28.36±3.4	26.47±3.81	32.18±2.5
	14	31.18±1.4	30.24±2.73	38.11±4.2
	21	35.47±5.2	31.21±4.29	40.02±2.61
Mean thickness of Hypodermis	1	24.74±6.4	22.36±6.4	21.02±4.3
	3	31.42±7.1	28.13±7.1	46.65±8.6[a]
	5	24.68±5.1	23.76±5.1	24.58±7.2
	14	27.45±2.7	25.27±2.7	22.50±3.5
	21	21.58±4.9	21.17±4.9	23.75±6.7
Percentage of collagen fibers	1	86.35±7.2	89.41±7.2	91.69±4.3
	3	90.43±6.5	88.59±6.5	108.42±4.2[a]
	5	96.4±3.9	93.62±3.9	89.76±6.1
	14	87.28±6.8	89.48±6.8	93.21±5.3
	21	92.73±5.4	90.15±5.4	92.57±4.5

[a]Significantly different at ($P<0.05$) in comparison to control groups (LSD test).

connective tissue was seen that support the epidermis and connected to the underlying tissue (Figure 1B and C). Papillary layer invaginated between dermis papilla and fibroblasts and other cells could be seen. In the connective tissue blood vessels and hair follicles were seen clearly (Figure 1A). Hypodermis with its loss connective tissue and adipocytes was directly connected with underlying muscular structure, and it had properties of connective tissue (Figure 1A).

Discussion

Different *Artemisia* species are widely distributed in Iran which among them *A. sieberi* is the most valuable (7). Various indications of *Artemisia* have been reported in the folk and modern medicine, so that nowadays, Artemisinin isolated form *Artemisia* is the best medication for malaria especially cerebral and drug resistant with excellent efficacy, high therapeutic index and rapid action (6,26,27). Additionally, some researches indicated suitable effects of *Artemisia* extract on the healing of dermal injuries and burns (19-23). Results of this research showed that *A. sieberi* extract increases thickness of the epidermis, dermis and hypodermis layers and also percentage of collagen fibers.

Oil essence of *Artemisia is* composed of a mixture of terpenes (7). Chemical analysis of *Artemisia* extract revealed presence of compounds such as verbenol, camphor, α & β thujone, cineole, linaleole, borneol, cymene, sabinene and 1, 8-Cineole, thus it has anti-bacterial activity against bacteria such as: *Staphylococcus aurous, streptococcus, E. coli, Bacillus subtilis, Pseudomonas aeruginosa* and *dermatophyte* fungi (3,10,11,14,16,17,28). Wound infection is one the major reasons of delaying wound healing, so it seems that *Artemisia* can prevent growth of bacteria and fungi on the skin, hinder, and control infection following skin injuries, boosts skin defense against microorganisms' invasion and colonization, therefore accelerates wound healing. In addition anti-oxidant and anti-inflammatory properties of many *Artemisia* species have been shown (15,18). It is reported that sesquiterpene lactone compound dehydroleucodine interacts with production of nuclear factor κB(NF-κB) and inhibits release of inflammatory mediators and thus possess anti-inflammatory activity (9,15). Additionally, scoparone of the plant extract inhibits nitric oxide synthase and cyclooxygenase II and thus inhibits production of inflammatory mediators in macrophages (18,21). *Artemisia* extract hinders proliferation and activation of T lymphocytes and exerts immunosuppressive activity, so it can be effective in the inflammatory conditions such as contact hyper sensitivity (18,21). *Artemisia* extract contains some compounds e.g. flavonoids, coumarins, tannin, xanthines, copper, zinc and manganese with high anti-oxidant and frees radical scavenger potential which prevent lipids peroxidation (21). Beside this, it is reported that aqueous extract of *Artemisia* increases superoxide dismutase, catalase and glutathione S-transferase activity which are among the most important anti-oxidant mechanisms of the body (18,21). Therefore, it seems that anti-oxidant and anti-inflammatory activity of *Artemisia* decrease the impact of free radicals and inflammatory reactions and associated diseases on the skin and also during skin injuries predispose healing process. In this study similar to previous studies significant increase in

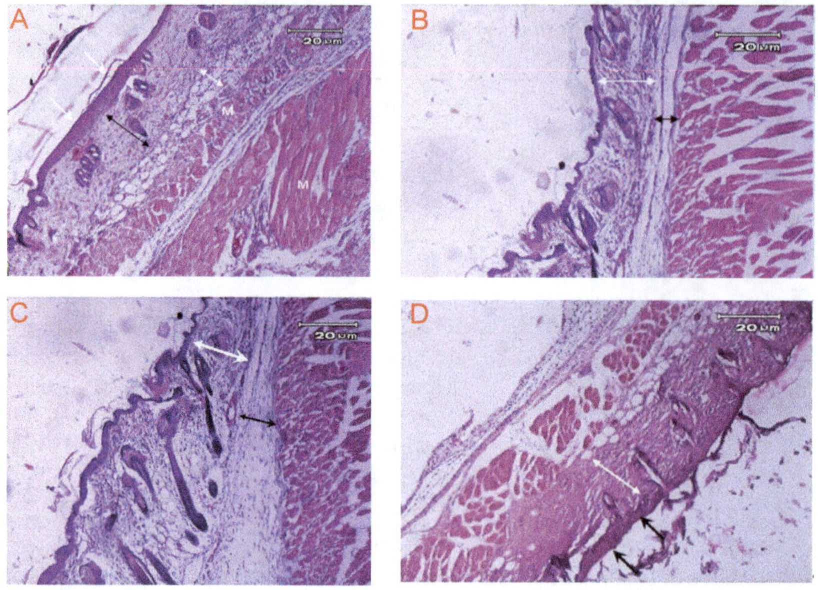

Figure 1. A) Light microscope structure of the skin in the control group. Epidermis (white arrow) Dermis (black double head arrow), hypodermis (white double head arrow), Muscle layers (M). H&E staining, magnification ×20. B) Light microscope structure of the skin day 1 after treatment. Dermis structure is completely seen. (White double head arrow), muscle layer (M). H&E staining, magnification ×20. C) Light microscope structure of the skin days 3 after treatment. Attention to the different thickness of dermis (white double head arrow) which is located on the hypodermis (black double head arrow). Muscle layer (M). H&E staining, magnification ×20. D) Light microscope structure of the skin days 14 after treatment. Attention to the hypodermis (white double head arrow) and dermis (black arrows); H&E staining, magnification ×20.

the percentage of collagen fibers were seen. Significant increase of collagen fibers and capillary buds following treatment with *A. sieberi* extract has previously been reported (21). In another study significant improvement in healing of second degree burn healing and increase of hydroxyproline as an indicator for collagen production has been reported (23). Collagen has a basic role in the remodeling stage of healing process and increases tensile of skin tissue and its resistance against pressure and tension (1). Increased number of fibroblast may be due to mitogenic activity of the *Artemisia* plant leading to increase synthesis of collagen and further durability of healing tissue. Also increasing capillary buds can accelerate granulation tissue formation and thus decrease healing time (21).

Conclusion

It seems that *Artemisia* by utilizing different mechanisms such as antimicrobial, anti-inflammatory and anti-oxidant properties, decreasing inflammation, increasing defense against free radicals, free radical scavenging, preventing bacteria and fungi colonization and infection, increasing fibroblast activity and collagen synthesis boosts skin health and improve its healing following injuries.

Authors' contributions

JK and MSH: designing study; RF: histological examination and statistical analysis; SR: performing animal experiment and histological examination; JK: manuscript preparation.

Conflict of interests

All authors declare that they have no conflict of interests.

Ethical considerations

Authors have been entirely regarded ethical issues such as: plagiarisms, data assembly, fraud, double publication or submission. Also all animal experiments had been approved by the institutional ethical committee and carried out according to the International Guide for the Care and Use of Laboratory Animals.

Funding

This study was financially supported by Research Council of Shahrekord University, Shahrekord, Iran.

References

1. Mescher AL. Junqueira's Basic Histology: Text and Atlas. New York: McGraw-Hill; 2010.
2. Herndon D. Total burn care: A brief history of acute burn care management. 4th ed. Edinburgh Scotland: Saunders. 2012. p. 1-30.
3. Ihsan-ul-Haq A, Ahmed I, Hussain I, Jamil M, Mirza B. Antibacterial activity and brine shrimp toxicity of *Artemisia dubia* extract. Pak J Bot 2012; 44(4): 1487-90.
4. Kaboutari J, Arab HA, Ebrahimi K, Rahbari S. Prophylactic and therapeutic effects of a novel granulated formulation of *Artemisia* extract on broiler coccidiosis. Trop Anim Health Prod 2013; 46(1): 43-48.
5. Mino J, Moscatelli V, Hnatyszyn O, Gorzalczany S, Acevedo C, Ferraro G. Anti-nociceptive and anti-inflammatory activities of *Artemisia copa* extracts. Pharmacol Res 2004; 50(1): 59-63.
6. Woodrow CJ, Haynes RK, Krishna S. Artemisinins.

Postgrad Med J 2005; 81: 71.
7. Zargari A. Medical plants. Tehran; Tehran University Publication; 2011.
8. Al-Soqeer A. Antioxidant activity and biological evaluation of hot-water extract of *Artemisia monosperma* and *Capparisspinosa* against lead contamination. Res J Bot 2011; 6: 11-20.
9. Guardia T, Juarez A, Guerreiro E, Guzman J, Pelzer L. Anti-inflammatory activity and effect on gastric acid secretion of dehydroleucodine isolated from *Artemisia douglasiana*. J Ethnopharmacol 2003; 88(2): 195-8.
10. Hakimi M, Afkhami M, Jalili B. Biologic activity of *Artemisia sieberi* extract in Iran. Pajohesh and Sazandegi 2002; 16: 2-5.
11. Jan G, Khan MA, Jan F. Medicinal Value of the Asteraceae of DirKohistan Valley, NWFP, Pakistan. Ethno leaflets 2009; 2009(13): 1205-15.
12. Keiser J, Shu-Hua X, Jian X, Zhen-San C, Odermatt P, Tesana S, *et al.* Effect of artesunate and artemether against Clonorchissinensis and *Opisthorchis viverrini* in rodent model. Int J Antimicrob Agents 2006; 28(4): 370-3.
13. Nofal SM, Mahmoud SS, Ramadan A, Soliman G, Fawzy R. Anti-Diabetic effect of *Artemisia judaica* extracts. Res J Med Sci 2009; 4(1): 42-8.
14. Nofal SM, Mahmoud SS, Ramadan A, Soliman G, Fawzy R. Anti-Diabetic effect of *Artemisia judaica* extracts. Res J Med Sci 2009; 4(1): 42-8.
15. Reddy AM, Lee JY, Seo JH, Kim BH, Chung EY, Ryu SY, *et al.* Artemisolide from *Artemisia asiatica*: Nuclear Factor-κB (NF-κB) inhibitor suppressing prostaglandin E2 and nitric oxide production in macrophages. Arch Pharm Res 2006; 29(7): 591-7.
16. Setzer WN, Vogler B, Schmidt JM, Leahy JG, Rives R. Antimicrobial activity of *Artemisia douglasiana* leaf essential oil. Fitoterapia 2004; 75(2): 192-200.
17. Vahdani M, Faridi P, Zarshenas MM, Javadpour S, Abolhassanzadeh Z, *et al.* Major compounds and antimicrobial activity of essential oils from five Iranian endemic medicinal plants. Pharmacognosy J 2011; 3(22): 48-53.
18. Yin Y, Gong FY, Wu XX, Sun Y, Li YH, Chen T, *et al.* Anti-inflammatory and immunosuppressive effect of flavones isolated from *Artemisia vestita*. J Ethnopharmacol 2008; 120(1): 1-6.
19. Foglio MA, Cirrea Dias P, Antonio MA, POssenti A, Rodrigues RA, *et al.* Anti-ulcerogenicactivity of some sesquiterpene lactones isolated from *Artemisia annua*. Planta Med 2002; 68: 515-8.
20. Dias PC, Foglio MA, Possenti A, Christian Fachim Nogueira D, Ernesto de Carvalho J. Anti-ulcerogenic activity of crude ethanol extract and some fractions obtained from aerial parts of *Artemisia annua* L. Phytother Res 2001; 15(8): 670-5.
21. Derakhshanfar A, Oloumi MM, Kabootari J, Arab H. Histopathological and biomechanical study on the effect of *Artemisia sieberi* extract on experimental skin wound healing in rat. Iran J Vet Surg 2006; 1(1): 36-42.
22. Âllahtavakoli M, Ârab Banissad F, Mahmoudi M, Jafari Naveh HR, Tavakolian V, *et al.* Effect of Hydro-Alcoholic Extract of *Artemisia Aucheri* on Healing of Skin Wound in Rat. J Mazandaran Uni Med Sci 2010; 20: 70-6.
23. Karimi baba Ahmadi B. Effects of *Artemisia sieberi* extract on the second degree burn healing [Thesis]. Shahrekord: Faculty of Veterinary Medicine, Shahrekord University; 2012.
24. Arab HA, Rahbari S, Rassouli A, Moslemi MH, Khosravirad F. Determination of artemisinin in *Artemisia sieberi* and anticoccidial effects of the plant extract in broiler chickens. Trop Anim Health Prod 2006; 38(6): 497-503.
25. Liersch R, Soicke H, Stehr C, Tullner HU. Formulation of artemisinin in *Artemisia annua* during one vegetation period. Planta Med 1986; 52: 387-90.
26. Meshnick SR, Tsang TW, Lin FB, Pan HZ, Chang. Activated oxygen mediates the oxygen mediates the antimalarial activity of qinghaosu. Prog Clin Biol Res 1989; 313: 95-104.
27. Weinberg ED, Moon J. Malaria and iron: history and review. Drug Metab Rev 2009; 41: 644-62.
28. Farzaneh M, Ghorbani-Ghouzhdi H, Ghorbani M, Hadian J. Composition and antifungal activity of essential oil of *Artemisia sieberi Bess*. On soil-borne phytopathogens. Pak J Biol Sci 2006; 9(10): 1979-82.

18

Antibacterial effects of *Arctium lappa* and *Artemesia absinthium* extracts in laboratory conditions

Reza Habibipour[1], **Mohsen Rajabi**[2*]

[1]Department of Microbiology, Faculty of Basic Sciences, Hamedan Branch, Islamic Azad University, Hamedan, Iran
[2]Young Researchers and Elite Club, Hamadan Branch, Islamic Azad University, Hamadan, Iran

ARTICLE INFO

Keywords:
Arctium lappa
Artemesia absinthium
Haemophylus influenza
Antibacteria drugs

ABSTRACT

Introduction: *Arctium lappa* (Great burduck) and *Artemesia absinthium* are medicinal plants that some of their antibacterial and antivirus properties have been suggested in nutritional industries. The objective of this research was to study the effects of *A. lappa* and *A. absinthium* on some microorganisms including *Pseudomonads aeraginosa, Haemophilus influenza, Bacillus subtilis, Bacillus cereus, Klebsiella pneumonia* and *Staphylococcus aureus.*
Methods: Extracts were prepared by maceration method and tested on Mueller Hinton agar medium based on disc diffusion method. The minimum inhibitory concentration (MIC) and minimum bactericidal concentration (MBC) were determined by micro-dilution method. Antibiotic disks used for controlling and standardizing the examination.
Results: The extracts of *A. lappa* and *A. absinthium* had significant effect on *S. aureus*. The MIC and MBC concentrations of the extract of *A. lappa* on *B. subtilis* were respectively 600 and 750 mg/ml. Also, these values were 230 and 540 mg/ml for *H. influenza.* Extract of *A. absinthium* showed more inhibitory effect on *B. subtilis.* All extracts showed inhibitory effect on *B. cereus*. The extracts of *A. lappa* and *A. absinthium* had inhibitory effects on *H. influenza and P. aeraginosa.* Among antibiotics, only *Ofloxacin* and *Ciprofloxacin* had effects on *H. influenza.* Extract of *A. lappa* showed flimsy effect on *K. pneumonia,* while extract of *A. absinthium* had no effect on this bacterium.
Conclusion: Due to the effects of *A. lappa* and *A. absinthium* on some bacteria, they might be good substitutes for synthetic substances.

Implication for health policy/practice/research/medical education:
Extracts of *Arctium lappa* and *Artemesia absinthium* have good antibacterial properties against some gram positive and negative bacteria. Nevertheless, more investigations need for identification of the active chemical compositions of these extracts responsible for their antibacterial properties as well as their certain mechanisms of accomplishment.

Introduction

Herbal remedies utilization in order to treat diseases goes back to thousands of years in Iran and there are several scientific documents in this era (1). Medicinal plants have considerable antimicrobial activities that can be used for preventing or inhibiting growth of infectious microorganisms and degeneration factors. High interest in replacing chemical materials with natural ones caused performing thousands of studies on natural resources researches on different plants extracts resulted in discovery of suitable natural substances of treatment of various diseases (2). The therapeutic properties of extracts and essential oils against microbial and non-microbial diseases have been known from many years ago and many positive effects have been reported from different plant species against microorganisms (3,4). In recent decades, antimicrobial properties of herbal products have attracted many researchers because of a rapid increase in antibiotic resistance to microorganisms (5). Many members of the genus *Artemisia* are important medicinal plants. Previously, the

***Corresponding author:** Mohsen Rajabi, Madani Town, Moosivand Professor Boulevard, Islamic Azad University, Young Researchers and Elite Club, Hamedan, Iran.
Email: m.rajabi@iauh.ac.ir

antibacterial effects of some *Artemisia* species have been reported (6,7). *Artemisia* is one of the various genera of Asteraceae family with many important medicinal properties (8). Essential oils of *Artemisia* spp. have been widely used for different medicinal purposes for several years (9,10). *Artemisia* species have been used in folk medicine as antipyretic, antiseptic, anthelmintic, tonic and diuretic remedy (11). *A. lappa* was brought from Japan and acclimated in Brazil. It is widely used in popular medicine all over the world for its well-known therapeutic applications. It has anti-bacterial, antifungal (12), diuretic (13), anti-oxidant (14) anxiolytic (15), anti-platelet aggregating (16) and HIV-inhibitory properties (17). Bacterial resistant to antibiotics is increasing, requiring introduction of new and safe antibacterial substances. The present investigation was undertaken to evaluate the antibacterial activity of hydro-alcoholic extracts of *A. lappa* and *Artemesia absinthium* on *P. aeruginosa, H. influenza, B. subtilis, B. cereus, Klebsiella pneumonia* and *Staphylococcus aureus* in laboratory conditions.

Materials and Methods

In this research, *A. lappa* and *A. absinthium* were collected from Dare-Moradbeig region and Buali-Sina garden of Agriculture and Natural Research Center of Hamedan in June 2012, respectively. Herbarium samples were prepared and authenticated by Dr. Kalvandi (Botanist of Agriculture and Natural Research Center). Aerial parts of *A. absinthium* (including flower, leaf and stem) and *A. lappa* (including leaf and stem) were dried in shade and powdered (18). Hydro-alcoholic (70%) extracts were prepared by Maceration method. Microorganisms (including *P. aeruginosa* PTCC1599, *H. influenza* PTCC1623, *B. subtilis* PTCC1156, *B. cereus* PTCC1247, *Klebsiella pneumonia* PTCC1290 and *Staphylococcus aureus* PTCC1337) were obtained from Fungi and Industrial Bacterial Collection of Iran (Scientific Industrial Researches Center of Iran). Standard medium was used for microorganism culture. Antibiotics (such as *Penicillin, Gentamicin, Ciprofloxacin, Ofloxacin* and *Erythromycin*) were obtained from Padtan Teb Company of Tehran. The microorganisms were transferred to tubes containing sterile distilled water and their turbidities were analyzed with McFarland Turbidity Standards through optic method. Then, they were inoculated in optimum mediums (19,20). Antibacterial activity was assessed by diffusion disk method. Extracts were used in different concentrations (0, 45, 90, 166, 230, 285, 333, 500, 600, 666, 714 and 750 mg/ml). Blank disks were soaked into the extract solutions and incubated in 37°C at incubator for 30 minutes. Then, the disks containing extracts were placed on culture medium in equal distances and were incubated in 37°C at incubator for 24 hours. Mean of inhibitory halos diameter of bacterial growth was measured and recorded by Murray et al (21). Minimum Inhibitory Concentration (MIC) and Minimum Bactericidal Concentration (MBC) were determined by micro dilution method (22). In order to compare the means of inhibitory halos diameter of bacterial growth, values were compared with the antibiotics ones and each test was carried out with 4 replications (21). Statistical analysis was performed using analysis of variance by SPSS version 18.0 software. Data considered significant when $P \leq 0.05$.

Results

Results showed that extract of *A. lappa* had inhibitory effect on *H. influenza* and *P. aeruginosa* (16.4 mm and 11.4 mm, respectively) (Figure 1A). Also, extract of *A. absinthium* showed inhibitory effect on *H. influenza* and *P. aeruginosa* (18.4 mm and 11.9 mm, respectively) (Table 2; Figure 2A). The MIC and MBC of *A. lappa* on *H. influenza* were obtained 230 mg/ml and 540 mg/ml, respectively. These values for extract of *A. absinthium* were 45 mg/ml and 90 mg/ml, respectively. Among antibiotics just *Ofloxacin* had effect on *H. influenza* (16.4 mm). MIC and MBC of *A. absinthium* against *P. aeruginosa* were 285 and 430 mg/ml, respectively. These values for *A. lappa* were 500 and 750 mg/ml, respectively. Ofloxacin and Gentamicin showed higher inhibitory halos diameter of bacterial growth on *P. aeruginosa*. Extract of both medicinal plants showed inhibitory effects against *B. cereus* in low concentration (166 mg/ml) and increased inhibitory effect with increasing the concentration. All antibiotics were effective on *B. cereus*, so that the highest effect was related to gentamicin (32.4 mm) and the lowest effect was related to *Penicillin* (10.4 mm). The MIC of *A. lappa* against *B. cereus* was obtained in 166 mg/ml and inhibitory effect increased with higher concentrations. Extract of *A. lappa* did not show MBC in studied concentrations. The MIC and MBC of *A. absinthium* were obtained to be 166 and 440 mg/ml, respectively. *A. lappa* showed inhibitory effect on *B. subtilis* less

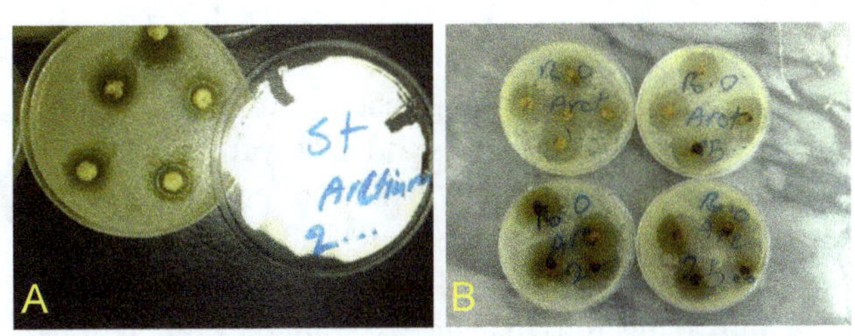

Figure 1. Effect of *Arctium lappa* on (A) *Haemophilus influenza* and (B) *Staphylococcus aureus.*

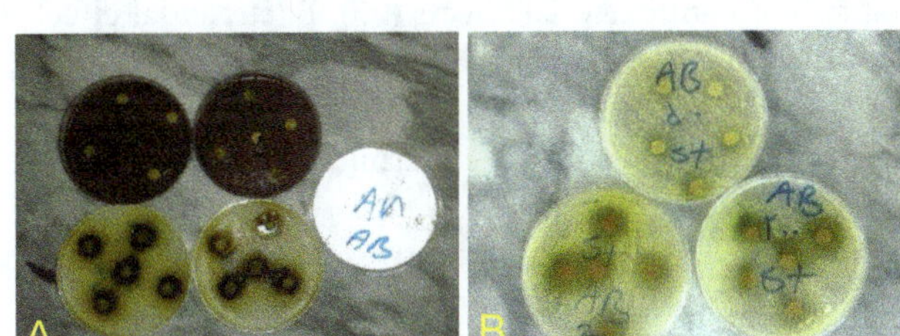

Figure 2. Effect of *Artemisia absinthium* on (A) *Haemophilus influenza* and (B) *Staphylococcus aureus.*

Table 1. Mean of inhibitory halos diameter of Bacteria growth based on used antibiotic in this study

Bacteria	Antibiotic				
	P	GM	CP	OF	ER
Haemophilus influenzae	-	-	26.4	16.4	-
Pseudomonads aeraginosa	-	26.4	36.4	20.4	-
Staphylococcus aureus	-	-	22.4	14.4	-
Klebsiella pneumoniae	-	-	16.4	18.4	-
Bacillus subtilis	-	20.4	32.4	18.4	-
Bacillus cereus	10.4	32.4	30.4	28.4	30.4

P: Penicillin (10 μg), GM: Gentamicin (10 μg), CP: Ciprofloxacin (5 μg), OF: Ofloxacin (5 μg), ER: Erythromycin (5 μg).

than *A. absinthium* (based on inhibitory halos diameter of bacteria growth). The MIC and MBC of *A. absinthium* on *B. subtilis* were 600 and 750 mg/ml, respectively, obtained by micro dilution method. These values for *A. absinthium* were 166 and 430 mg/ml, respectively. *Gentamicin* (20.4 mm), *Ofloxacin* (18.4 mm) and *Ciprofloxacin* (32.4 mm) had effect on *B. subtilis*, but *Penicillin* and *Erythromycin* had no effect. *A. lappa* and *A. absinthium* showed significant effect on *Staphylococcus aureus* ($P<0.01$) (Figures 1 and 2B). MIC of *A. absinthium* on *Staphylococcus aureus* was 230 mg/ml. *Ofloxacin* developed 14.4 mm inhibitory halos diameter of bacterial growth, while extract of *A. absinthium* in concentration of 666 mg/ml (14.9 ± 1.91) and 750 mg/ml (17.4 ± 1.15) showed higher inhibitory halos diameter (Tables 1 and 2). Different concentrations of *A. absinthium* extract had no effect on *Klebsiella pneumonia*, while MIC and MBC of *A. lappa* against *Klebsiella pneumonia* were obtained 666 and 750 mg/ml, respectively. *Ofloxacin* and *Ciprofloxacin* were able to inhibit this *bacterium* (18.4 mm and 16.4 mm, respectively) (Table 2).

Discussion

From past decades, anything that was used as drug, obtained from natural resources and mainly from plants. Using of chemical drugs developed acute problems such as auto safety due to continues taking and without caring of certain taking drug and beside effects that some of them were more dangerous than diseases. On the other hand, in recent years, microorganism resistance to chemical drugs and undesirable beside effects resulted to has been attended using of extracts and essential oils of medicinal plant that showed antibacterial effects (23). Bactericidal effects of studied plants extracts against *H. influenzae* were equal to *Ofloxacin*.

Based on the results, it was determined that sensitivities of gram positive bacteria like *Staphylococcus aureus* and *B. cereus* compared with gram negative bacteria such as *P. aeruginosa* and *Klebsiella pneumonia* to plants extracts were higher (Table 1). It has been demonstrated that *A. lappa* has antimicrobial activity against oral microorganisms. Three forms of the extract of this plant (20% tincture, extract concentrated by rotary-evaporation and lyophilized extract) were examined and reported that the lyophilized extract was the most effective against *B. subtilis* and *C. albicans* (24). In another research study it was shown that essential oil of *S. amanica* affected on all positive gram bacteria except *Staphylococcus epidermidis*. Also, these components just inhibited 2 negative gram bacteria like *Chryseomonas luteola* MU 65 and *Stenotrophomonas maltophilia* MU 64 (25). Similar results were obtained in this research from *A. absinthium* against this bacterium (Table 1).

Higher resistance in gram negative bacteria can be attributed to external phospholipid membrane that is infiltrated to lipophilic components. Lack of this membrane in gram positive bacteria causes easier entrance of the essential oil and extract components to bacterium. This process may cause increase in ionic permeability and permeation of vital inner cellular components which finally result in damage to enzyme system of bacterium. Other researchers have proved inhibition of growth of *Staphylococcus aureus, B. cereus, Klebsiella pneumonia sub sp. Pneumonia, Pseudomonas aeruginosa* and *B. subtilis* by medicinal plants (26,27). The higher effect on *H. influenza* was obtained by extract of *A. absinthium*. Extract of *A. lappa* had effect on this bacterium similar to *Ofloxacin*, while *A. absinthium* was better than *Ofloxacin*. Similar results about *A. lappa* have been obtained showing inhibitory effect on *P. aeruginosa, B. cereus* and *B. subtilis* (28). In comparison with studied medicinal plants, the effects of essential oil of different medicinal plants have been evaluated which showed positive effects on different microorganisms (29). Therefore, these plants might be suitable to be used instead of synthetic drugs. However, more studies are needed to establish the effective and safe use of these plant extracts.

Acknowledgements

The authors would like to thank Ms. Sara Vesaghati Ezatpoor, Ms. Safura Vesaghati Ezatpoor, Ms. Marjan Pirmohammadain and Ms. Leila Moradi Haghgoo for their professional assistance during this research project.

Authors' contributions

MR contributed to the conception of the work, conducting the study, revising the draft, approval of the final version of the manuscript, and agreed for some aspects of the work. RH contributed to the conception of the work, approval of the final version of the manuscript, and agreed for some aspects of the work.

Conflict of interests

Authors declare no conflict of interests.

Ethical considerations

Ethical issues (including plagiarism, misconduct, data fabrication, falsification, double publication or submis-

Table 2. Average diameter (mm) of inhibition halos produced by *Arctium lappa and Artemesia absinthium* Extracts on the target microorganisms

Medicinal plant (Extract)	Bacterium	Concentration (mg/ml)											
		0	45	90	166	230	285	333	500	600	666	714	750
Arctium lappa	*Haemophilus influenzae*	0±0	0±0	0±0	0±0	4.7±1.63	9.9±1.91	10.4±1.63	11.9±1.00	13.4±2.00	14.4±0.00	14.4±0.00	16.4±0.00
	Pseudomonads aeraginosa	0±0	0±0	0±0	0±0	0±0	0±0	0±0	2.1±1.00	8.4±0.00	9.4±1.15	10.9±1.00	11.4±1.15
	Staphylococcus aureus	0±0	0±0	0±0	0±0	0±0	0±0	6.3±1.00	9.9±1.00	11.4±1.15	14.9±1.91	16.9±1.00	17.4±1.15
	Klebsiella pneumoniae	0±0	0±0	0±0	0±0	0±0	0±0	0±0	0±0	0±0	4.2±0.50	8.4±0.00	9.9±1.00
	Bacillus subtilis	0±0	0±0	0±0	0±0	0±0	0±0	0±0	0±0	4.2±0.50	6.3±1.00	8.4±0.00	9.4±1.15
	Bacillus cereus	0±0	0±0	0±0	4.2±1.00	5.2±1.00	9.4±1.15	11.4±1.15	13.9±1.00	17.4±1.15	18.9±1.00	19.4±1.15	21.4±1.15
Artemesia absinthium	*Haemophilus influenzae*	0±0	2.1±0.00	2.1±0.00	6.3±0.60	9.4±1.15	9.4±1.15	9.4±1.15	10.9±1.00	16.4±0.00	16.9±1.00	17.4±1.15	18.4±1.63
	Pseudomonads aeraginosa	0±0	0±0	0±0	0±0	0±0	4.2±0.50	6.8±1.00	10.4±1.15	11.9±1.00	11.9±1.00	11.9±1.00	11.9±1.00
	Staphylococcus aureus	0±0	0±0	0±0	0±0	2.1±0.50	9.4±1.15	10.4±0.00	11.9±1.00	13.4±1.15	13.9±1.91	15.4±2.00	15.9±1.00
	Klebsiella pneumoniae	0±0	0±0	0±0	0±0	0±0	0±0	0±0	0±0	0±0	0±0	0±0	0±0
	Bacillus subtilis	0±0	0±0	0±0	0±0	2.1±0.50	2.1±0.50	8.4±0.00	9.4±1.15	10.4±0.00	11.4±1.15	13.4±1.15	14.4±0.00
	Bacillus cereus	0±0	0±0	0±0	4.2±0.50	8.9±1.00	9.4±1.15	10.9±1.00	15.4±1.15	16.4±1.63	16.4±1.63	20.4±1.63	20.4±1.00

sion, redundancy) have been completely observed by the authors. This work has been performed in culture medium; so ethical committee approval was not needed.

Funding/Support

Personal funding.

References

1. Saad B, Azaizeh H, Said O. Tradition and perspectives of Arab herbal medicine: a review. Evid Based Complement Alternat Med. 2005;2:475-9.
2. Weinstine RA. Controlling antimicrobial resistance in hospitals: Infection control and use of antibiotics. Emerg Infect Dis. 2001;7(2):188-192.
3. Arrieta J, Reyes B, Calzada F, Cedillo-Rivera R, Navarrete A. Amoebicidal and giardicidal compounds from the leaves of Zanthoxylum liebmannianum. Fitoterapia. 2001;72(3):295-297.
4. Ciani M, Menghini L, Mariani F, Pagiotti R, Menghini A, Fatichenti F. Antimicrobial properties of essential oil of Satureja montana L. on pathogenic and spoilage yeasts. Biotechnol Lett. 2000;22(12):1007-1010.
5. Guangrong H, Jiaxin J, Dehui D. Antioxidative and antibacterial activity of the methanol extract of Artemisia anomala S. Moore. Afr J Biotechnol. 2008;7:1335-1338.
6. Hedi M, Hajlaoui H, Akrout A, Najjaa H, Neffati M. Antimicrobial and antioxidant activities of Artemisia herba-alba essential oil cultivated in Tunisian arid zone. CR Chim. 2010;13:380-386.
7. Karabegovic I, Nikolova M, Velickovic D, Stojicevic S, Veljkovic V, Lazic M. Comparison of antioxidant and antimicrobial activities of methanolic extracts of the Artemisia sp. recovered by different extraction techniques. Chin J Chem Eng. 2011;19:504-519.
8. Zia M, Mannan A, Chaudhary MF. Effect of growth regulators and amino acids on Artemisinin production in the callus of Artemisia absinthium. Pak J Bot. 2007;39(2):799-805.
9. Ahameethunisa AR, Hopper W. Antibacterial activity of Artemisia nilagirica leaf extracts against clinical and phytopathogenic bacteria. BMC Complement Altern Med. 2010;10:6.
10. Yano Y, Satomi M, Oikawa H. Antimicrobial effect of spices and herbs on Vibrio parahaemolyticus. Int J Food Microbiol. 2006;111:6-11.
11. Ramezani M, Fazli-Bazzaz BS, Saghafi-Khadem F, Dabaghian A. Antimicrobial activity of four Artemisia species of Iran. Fitoterapia. 2004;75 (2):201-203.
12. Silva RC. Plants as Medicinals na Saúde Bucal. Vitória: Artgraf; 2001.
13. Holetz FB, Pessini GL, Sanches NR, Cortez DA, Nakamura CV, Dias-Filho BP. Screening of some plants used in the Brazilian folk medicine for the treatment of infectious diseases. Mem Inst Oswaldo Cruz. 2002;97:1027-1031.
14. Maruta Y, Kawabata J, Niki R. Antioxidative caffeoylquinic acid derivatives in the roots of burdock. J Agric Food Chem. 1995;43:2592-2595.
15. Sbolli KC, Rieck L, Oliveira BH. Estudo Farmacológico da atividade depressora do sistema nervosa central (SBC) do extrato bruto da A. lappa. In: XIV Simpósio de Plantas Medicinais do Brasil. Livro de Resumos: Florianópolis, SC; 1996.
16. Iwakami S, WU J, Ebizuka Y. Platelet activating factor antagonists contained in medical plants ligants and sesquiterpenes. Chem Pharm Bul Tokyo. 1992;40:196-197.
17. Ito M, Nakashima H, Baba M, et al. Inhibitory effect of glycyrrhizin on the in vitro infectivity and cytopathic activity of human immunodeficiency virus. Antiviral Res. 1987;7:127-137.
18. Arunkumar S, Muthuselvam M. Analysis of phytochemical constituents and antimicrobial activities of Aloe vera L. against clinical pathogens. World J Agr Sci. 2009;5(5):572-576.
19. Nejatzadeh-Barandozi F. Antibacterial activities and antioxidant capacity of Aloe vera. Org Med Chem Lett. 2013; 3(5): 1-8.
20. Thiruppathi S, Ramasubramanian V, Sivakumar T, Thirumalai Arasu V. Antimicrobial activity of Aloe vera L. Burm Against Pathogenic Microorganisms. J Bio Sci Res. 2010;1(4):251-258.
21. Murray PR, Rosenthal KS, Pfaller MA. Medical Microbiology. Elsevier Health Sciences press; 2009:947.
22. Rasooli I, Mirmostafa SA. Bacterial susceptibility and chemical composition of essential oils from Thtmus Kotschyanus and Thymus persicus. J Agr Food Chem. 2003;51(8):2200-2205.
23. Chitsaz M, Barton M, Bazargan M, Kamali Nejad M. Essential oil components and antibacterial effect of Ziziphora clinopodioides. Int J Antimicrob Agents. 2007; 29(suppl 2):S512-S513.
24. Perin FM, França SC, Saquy PC, Sousa-Neto MD. In vitro antimicrobial of aqueous herbal extracts for Endodontics. J Dental Res. 2002;81:157.
25. Ugur A, Sarac N, Varol O. Antimicrobial activities of the essential oils of endemic Stachys rupestris and Stachys amanica against multi-resistant bacteria. Indian J Pharmacol. 2013;45:201-202.
26. Heidari Sureshjani M, Tabatabaei Yazdi F, Mortazavi SA, Alizadeh Behbahani B, Shahidi F. Antimicrobial effects of Kelussia odoratissima extracts against food borne and food spoilage bacteria "in vitro". Journal of Paramedical Sciences. 2014;5(2):115-120.
27. Sengula M, Ercislib S, Yildizb H, Gungorc N, Kavaza A, Çetina B. Antioxidant, Antimicrobial Activity and Total Phenolic Content within the Aerial Parts of Artemisia absinthum, Artemisia santonicum and Saponaria officinalis. Iran J Pharm Res. 2011;10(1):49-56.
28. Pereira JV, Bergamo DC, Pereira JO, França Sde C, Pietro RC, Silva-Sousa YT. Antimicrobial activity of A. lappa constituents against microorganisms commonly found in endodontic infections. Braz Dent J. 2005;16(3):192-196.
29. Roussis V, Chinou I, Perdetzog L, Loukis A. Identification and bacteriostatic activity of the essential oil of Lamium graganicuml, Spp, Laevigatum Arcangeli. J Essential Oil Research. 1996;8:291-293.

19

Protective effect of date palm pollen (*Phoenix dactylifera*) on sperm parameters and sexual hormones in male NMRI mice exposed to low frequency electromagnetic field (50 Hz)

Javad Baharara[1*], Elaheh Amini[2], Farzaneh Salek-Abdollahi[3], Najme Nikdel[3], Majid Asadi-Samani[4]

[1]Research Center for Animal Development Applied Biology & Department of Biology, Mashhad Branch, Islamic Azad University, Mashhad, Iran
[2]Department of Animal Biology, Faculty of Biological Sciences, Kharazmi University, Tehran, Iran
[3]Faculty of Biological Science, Mashhad Branch, Islamic Azad University, Mashhad, Iran
[4]Medical Plants Research Center, Shahrekord University of Medical Sciences, Shahrekord, Iran

ARTICLE INFO

Keywords:
Electromagnetic field
Testes
Sperm parameters
Sexual hormones
Infertility
Date palm pollen

ABSTRACT

Introduction: Exposure to electromagnetic fields (EMFs) induces harmful effects on testis and reproductive activities. In traditional medicine, date palm pollen (DPP) which has remarkable nutritional values is used for curing male infertility and impotency. The aim of this study was to investigate the protective effect of DPP in preventing the detrimental effects of low frequency electromagnetic field (50 Hz) on sperm parameters and sexual hormones.
Methods: Adult male mice were randomly divided into 7 groups of 8 and exposed to EMF 4 h/day for 10 days. In this study experimental groups received DPP with doses of 25, 50, 100 and 200 mg/kg, respectively before exposure. At the end of the experiment each group were tested for sperm parameters including: motility, count, morphology, viability and the level of luteinizing hormone (LH) and testosterone.
Results: Our results revealed that exposure to EMF induced significant reduction ($P<.001$) in sperm count, viability and progressive motility in comparison with control group. EMF caused abnormalities in sperm and significant decrease in testosterone level while there was no significant difference in level. Administration of DPP before exposure improved the sperm count, viability, motility and testosterone level in experimental groups. In addition, pretreatment with DPP prevented the sperm abnormality induced by EMF.
Conclusion: The results indicate the protective effect of DPP against EMF adverse effects on sperm parameters and sexual hormones in male mice.

Implication for health policy/practice/research/medical education:
Date palm pollen (DPP) has protective effects against EMF adverse effects on sperm parameters and sexual hormones in male mice and might be beneficial in human sexual dysfunction.

Introduction

Nowadays, the widespread use of various electrical and telecommunication appliances that produce electromagnetic fields is increasing rapidly and results in daily exposure of humans to electromagnetic fields (EMFs), more than past few decades (1). Modern societies are pervaded by Non-ionizing 50-60 Hz low frequency electromagnetic field exposure. The probable health effects of different electromagnetic spectrum produced by electrical instruments have resulted in performance of researchers in this field (2).

Testes have 2 critical functions: spermatogenesis and male sex hormone production. However, the Leydig cells secrete testosterone which regulates the spermatogenesis also the pituitary gland secretes luteinizing hormone (LH) and follicle stimulating hormone (FSH) that regulate male reproduction. So LH stimulates Leydig cells to produce testosterone and maintains their functions (3). Male fer-

***Corresponding author**: Javad Baharara, Professor, Dept. of Biology & Research Center for Animal Development Applied Biology, Mashhad Branch, Islamic Azad University, Mashhad, Iran,
Email: baharara@yahoo.com

tility depends on the semen quality that contains normal spermatozoa (quality) in the adequate number (quantity). Nevertheless different risk factors may be associated with male fertility problems such as genetic disorders, genital duct obstruction, varicocele, decreased sperm production, decreased semen quality parameters, erectile dysfunction and male impotence (4). It has been also proved that EMF has adverse effects on gonads, liver and brain. Moreover, many studies have shown that testis are very sensitive to electromagnetic fields and can be damaged by extremely low frequency irradiation exposure in which decreased number of sperms and reproductive activities may result in infertility (5). Electromagnetic fields can intensify the generation of oxidative stress and cause an imbalance between the production of reactive oxygen species (ROS) and their antioxidant defense system, inducing cellular damage (6). In testis the rates of metabolism and cell replication is high and oxidative stress can be harmful in seminiferous tubules because electromagnetic exposure and heat can affect the blood-testis barrier and cause spermatogonial degeneration. On the other hand, several studies have shown that antioxidants provide protective barrier by breaking the oxidative chain reaction in the sperm cellular content (7,8).

Herbal medicines have been popular for prevention and treatment of diseases from ancient times and in recent years herbal remedies are used as primary health care with minimum side effects around the world (9). The use of natural antioxidants from plant is increasing day by day. In addition, numerous natural antioxidants such as, vitamins C, E and their derivatives, Vitamin A, β-carotene, curcumin, *Allium cepa*, quercetin, caffeine, chlorogenic acid, ellagic acid, bixin, flavonoids, epigallocatechin and other polyphenols consumption before or after radiation exposure can protect cells against radiation induced damage (10,11). *Phoenix dactylifera* commonly known as the date palm belongs to Arecaceae or palm family. Its various parts such as leaves, barks, pits, fruits and pollens have anticancer, antioxidant, hepatoprotective, antidiabetic, antihypertensive, antiulcerative, anti-inflammatory, antiproliferative, antimutagenic, antidiarrheal, antibacterial, antifungal and antiviral potential (12,13). Date palm pollen (DPP) has been used for curing male and female infertility and impotency for thousands of years as a traditional herbal medicine. DPP contains various types of phytochemicals such as estrone, α-amirin, triterpenoidal saponins, flavonoids estrone, estradiol and estriol and a crude gonadotrophic substance (14). DPP is a good source of natural antioxidants and has remarkable health benefits and nutritional values. Many studies have shown that DPP can enhance spermatogenesis, increase sperm count and concentration of testosterone, FSH and LH (15).

Therefore, the aim of this study was to evaluate the possible protective effect of DPP in preventing the harmful effects of 50 Hz low frequency electromagnetic field on sperm parameters such as sperm count, viability, motility, morphology and sexual hormones in male NMRI mice.

Materials and Methods

Collection and administration of date palm pollen

DPP grains samples were collected from the botanical garden in Bushehr city (South of Iran). Pollen grains were washed with distilled water and then dried. The extract was prepared by mixing palm pollen grain powder with normal saline as solvent by shaking and vortexin. It was administered to mice via oral gavage before each exposure to EMF.

Animals

Adult male NMRI mice, 6-8 weeks old and weighing 25±2 g obtained from Razi Vaccine and Serum Research Institute, Mashhad, Iran. These animals were housed in the animal house under standard conditions of temperature (25°C) and 12 hours light: 12 hours dark, as well as fed pellets and water ad libitum.

Experimental design

Mice were randomly divided into 7 groups, each group consisting of 8 animals as follows: Control group (kept in normal conditions in animal house), sham exposed group (exposed to a power off EMF), EMF group (exposed to 50 Hz electromagnetic field 4 h/day for 10 days without any treatment), experimental groups (1 to 4) (received DPP with doses of 25, 50, 100 and 200 mg/kg respectively before exposure to EMF).

At the end of the experiment, animals were weighed and anesthetized with ether. Blood samples were collected from the heart. The serum was obtained by centrifugation at 3000 rpm for 10 minutes. The sera were separated and preserved in -20°C until analysis.

Then, the epididymis was carefully separated and fragmented in Dulbecco's modified Eagle's medium (DMEM) containing 5% FBS. The sperm suspension was used for the analysis of sperm parameters including motility, count, morphology, and viability. To count the sperms, after putting the sperm suspension on Neubauer's chamber, the sperms on the 4 corners of the central square were counted by light microscope (16). The sperm morphology was examined using the Papanicolaou staining method and sperm viability was evaluated by application of eosin staining (17). Sperm motility was evaluated microscopically and categories as progressive motility (rapid and slow), nonprogressive motility and immotility (18).

Statistical analysis

Data were analyzed by one-way analysis of variance (ANOVA), using the statistical package of SPSS version 16. In all tests $P<.05$ was considered as statistically significant.

Results

Our experimental results revealed that exposure of mice

to electromagnetic field significantly decreased ($P<.001$) the sperm count and administration of DPP before exposure increased sperm count against deleterious effects of EMF (Figure 1).

The eosin staining evaluates the viability of spermatozoa which is based on the ability of the cell membrane to exclude dyes. In this method, dye enters a nonvital (dead) cell due to the damaged plasma membrane. Our results indicated that the percentage of stained cells increased under exposure to 50 Hz electromagnetic field while pretreatment with DPP elevated the percentage of unstained spermatozoa live cells (Figure 2). Therefore the viability of sperms with intact membrane was significantly decreased ($P<.001$) in EMF group while the rates of viability enhanced in all experimental groups, although only in experimental group 4 the percentages of viability returned to the normal control value.

Figure 3 shows that sperm progressive motility had a significant reduction ($P<.001$) in EMF and increasing the concentration of DPP improved sperm progressive motility. Furthermore, electromagnetic field significantly increased ($P<.001$) immobility and nonprogressive motility in mice. However, in experimental group 4 the percentages of progressive motile sperm as well as nonprogressive and immotile spermatozoa were enhanced similar to control group. Meanwhile, there were no significant differences in the percentage of motile sperm between the sham and control groups.

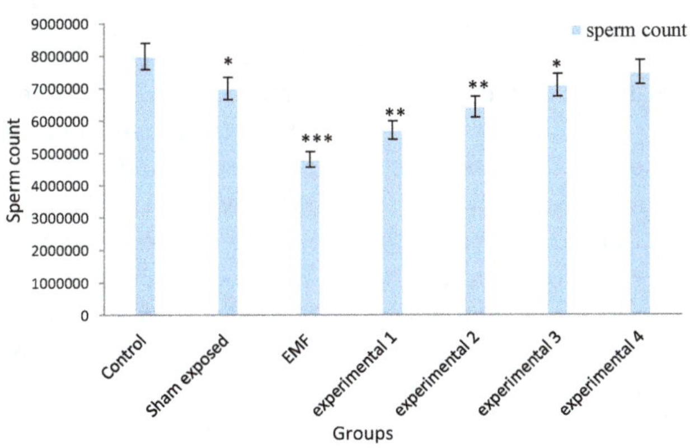

Figure 1. Effect of electromagnetic field (50 Hz) and date palm pollen treatment on total sperm count in mice. * $P<.05$, ** $P<.01$, *** $P<.001$.

In current study we used Papanicolau staining method to examine the morphology of spermatozoa. As shown in Figure 4 our results demonstrated a significant increase in the percentage of sperm with abnormal morphology in EMF and sham groups as compared to control. In addition the rates of normal sperm morphology were improved in treated groups while the best improvement for sperm morphology was observed in experimental group 4.

The experimental data show that exposure to EMF induced significant reduction of testosterone level in EMF group (0.47±0.92 nmol/L) ($P<.05$) while there was no significant difference in sham exposed group (1.21±1.09 nmol/L) compared to control (1.5±0.46 nmol/L). In addition the amounts of testosterone hormone in experimental groups (1-4) were 0.69±1.41, 0.98±1.33, 1.07±1.24, and 1.39±0.18 nmol/L, respectively. However, the levels of this hormone in experimental groups 3 and 4 increased nearly similar to the value of control group. The amounts of LH in sham exposed and EMF groups were 1.24±1.47 and 1.1±0.74 IU/L. In addition, in experimental groups (1-4) the levels of LH were 1.35±1.23, 1.21±2.5, 1.33±1.47, and 1.27±0.39 IU/L, respectively. Therefore there were no significant changes of LH level ($P>.05$) in all groups compared to control group (1.3±1.22 IU/L).

Discussion

Our study showed that low frequency electromagnetic field has negative effects on sperm parameter such as viability, morphology and motility characteristics. Exposure to EMF leads to significant decrease in LH and testosterone levels which can change the hormonal balance of sex hormones and affects the reproductive activity. Daily exposure of humans to electromagnetic fields has grown concerns over the public health. Low frequency EMFs induced tissue damage and had adverse effects in organs

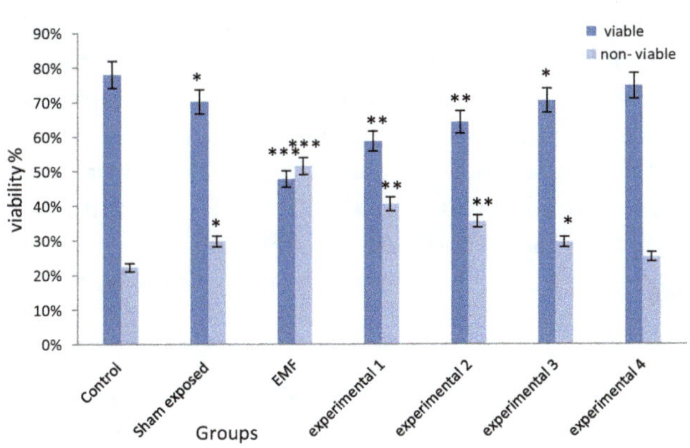

Figure 2. Effect of electromagnetic field (50 Hz) and date palm pollen treatment on sperm viability in mice. * $P<.05$, ** $P<.01$, *** $P<.001$.

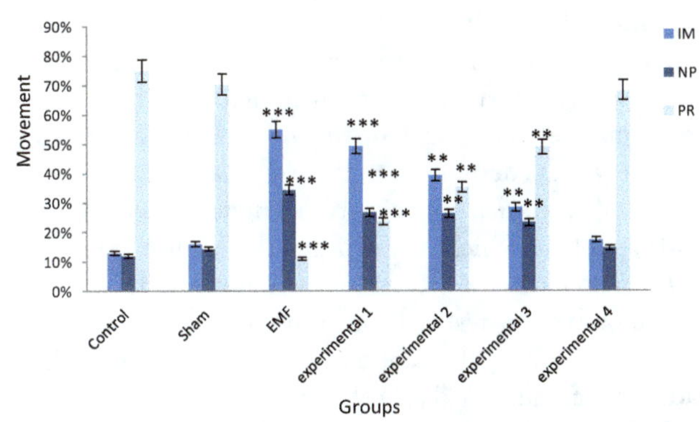

Figure 3. Effect of electromagnetic field and date palm pollen treatment on sperm motility in mice. Abbreviations: PR, Progressive motility; NP, nonprogressive motility; IM, immotility. * $P<.05$, ** $P<.01$, *** $P<.001$.

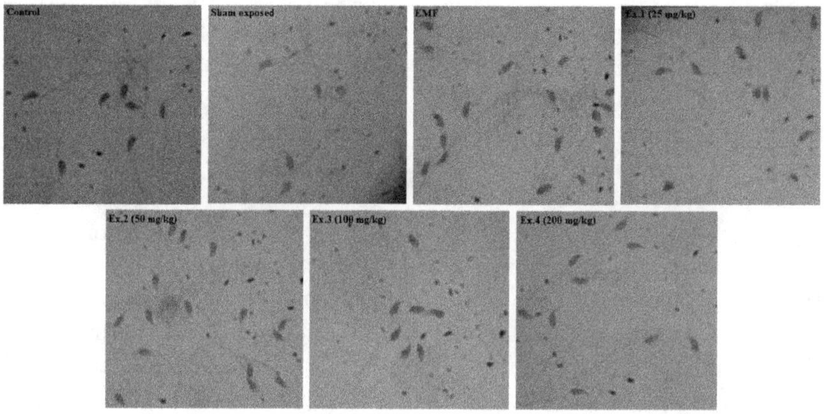

Figure 4. The protective effect of date palm pollen pretreatment in reducing sperm abnormality induced by electromagnetic field (40X) (Papanicolau staining).

particularly on testis and spermatogenesis (11). The results achieved in this study revealed that administration of DPP before exposure could prevent the detrimental effects of EMF on reproductive parameters and sex hormones in mice. The protective role of DPP may be attributed to its antioxidant contents and free radical scavenging activities. In recent years natural medicines particularly herbal medicines are extensively used to improve health conditions due to their minimum side effects, being readily accessible and inexpensive price. Herbs are an important source of phytochemicals, too (19).

There are several reports related to the protective effect of natural based substances in prevention and treatment of deleterious effects induced by electromagnetic radiation which are similar to our results. *Alstonia scholaris* is a tree belonging to family Apocyanaceae. Gupta et al (20) investigated the radioprotective potential of the *Alstonia scholaris* extract and noted that this extract could be efficient against radiation-induced biochemical alterations. So the protective effect of this extract might prove the beneficial use of plants as radio-protector. Green tea (*Camellia sinensis*) has various benefits in human health in prevention and treatment of different diseases like cancer. Accordingly in 2015 a study about the inhibitory effects of green tea on electromagnetic waves damages showed that the antioxidant property of green tea might decrease the genotoxic effects of electromagnetic radiation (21). *Ocimum basilicum* (Basil) belongs to Lamiaceae family which has been used since ancient times as an herbal remedy. Khaki et al (11) designed a study to evaluate the protective effects of *O. basilicum* on electromagnetic fields effects on testis apoptosis which revealed that the administration of *O. basilicum* may reduce the reproductive toxicity of EMF and apoptosis in testis. L-carnitine and coenzyme Q10 (CoQ10) are 2 effective antioxidants which scavenge free radicals. Ramadan et al (22) reported the protective effects of these compounds on testicular toxicity in mice induced by exposure to magnetic field.

In 2014 Arfat et al (23) revealed that DPP could enhance the reproductive activity and the levels of serum testosterone, FSH and LH in rats which might be due to the presence of gonadotropin like substances in the DPP. Cadmium is an extremely toxic heavy metal which has adverse health effects in various organs particularly testes. Prolonged exposure to cadmium caused reproductive disorder including histological alterations, reduced sperm count and motility, increased rates of sperm abnormalities, high generation of ROS and decreased serum testosterone level. El-Neweshy et al (24) reported that administration of DPP efficiently improved the spermatogenesis and sperm characteristics. Another study in 2012 examined the protective effect of DPP against testicular damages caused by cadmium toxicity in male rats and indicated the significant protective effect of DPP against testicular dysfunction through enhancing estradiol level, normalization of testosterone level and sperm function parameters (25). *P. dactylifera* pollen has various types of phytochemicals and nutrients such as carotenoids, flavonoids and phytosterols. A study revealed the preventive role of DPP against adverse side effects of chemotherapy induced infertility in male subjects. So DPP treatment decreased sperm abnormalities and improved the sperm parameters (26). DPP contains a wide range of bioactive compounds and may be efficient in prevention and treatment of oral microsites caused by radiation and chemotherapy. So, DPP may have the potential protective effect to block oxidative free radicals, prevent DNA damage, and neutralize inflammatory reactions (27). Cisplatin is a potent chemotherapy drug which induces testicular dysfunction. The impact of cisplatin on reproductive parameters of male rats was ameliorated by administration of DPP and *P. ginseng* through increasing the level of serum testosterone, sperm count, motility and viability as well as genital organs weight (28).

Conclusion

The results of the present study showed that exposure to low frequency electromagnetic field (50 Hz) can induce deleterious effects on reproductive parameters such as sperm count, viability, motility, morphology, and testosterone level which lead to decreased male fertility. In addition, pretreatment with DPP improved these parameters to normal control value. Accordingly, it is concluded that medicinal plants such as DPP can be used as efficient electromagnetic protective agent to reduce the adverse effects of EMFs on sperm parameters and sexual hormones in male mice.

Acknowledgments
The authors would like to thank Research Center for Animal Development Applied Bilogy, Islamic Azad University, Mashhad, Iran.

Authors' contributions
All authors had role in design, work, statistical analysis and manuscript writing.

Conflict of interests
The authors declared no competing interests.

Ethical considerations
Ethical issues (including plagiarism, misconduct, data fabrication, falsification, double publication or submission, redundancy) have been completely observed by the authors.

Funding/Support
This work was financially supported by the Research Center for Animal Development Applied Biology, Mashhad Branch, Islamic Azad University, Mashhad, Iran.

References

1. Hamidian Jahromi M, Kargar Jahromi H, et al. Investigating 500 micro-tesla electromagnetic field effects on testicular tissue changes and hormones lh and testosterone in syrian mice race balb/c. Int J Biol Phar Allied Sci. 2014;3(3):296-303.
2. Bayat P, Darabi M, Ghanbari A. Effects of prenatal exposure to extremely low electro-magnetic field on in vivo derived blastocysts of mice. Iran J Reprod Med. 2012;10(6):555-560.
3. Agarwal A, Singh A, Hamada A, Kesari K. Cell phones and male infertility: a review of recent innovations in technology and consequences. Int Braz J Urol. 2011;37(4):432-454.
4. Mohammadi F, Nikzad H, Taherian A, Mahabadi JA, Saleh M. Effects of herbal medicine on male infertility. Anat Sci. 2013;10(4):3-16.
5. Luo Q, Li J, Cui X, Yan J, Zhao Q, Xiang C. The effect of Lycium barbarum polysaccharides on the male rats' reproductive system and spermatogenic cell apoptosis exposed to low-dose ionizing irradiation. J Ethnopharmacol. 2014;154(1):249-258.
6. Baharara J, Zafar-Balanejad S, Kamareh E, Asadi-Samani M. The effects of green tea extract on teratogenicity induced by low frequency electromagnetic field on bone marrow Balb/C mice embryo. J Herbmed Pharmacol. 2014;3(1):47-51.
7. Vaez A, Mardani M, Razavi S. Impact of saffron on rat sperm membrane integrity and spermatogenesis status. Adv Biomed Res. 2014;3:146.
8. Sowa P, Sieron-Stoltny K, Cieslar G, Sieron A. Impact of electromagnetic field generated by mobile phone on prooxidant-antioxidant balance in selected internal organs of rats. PIERS Proc. 2013;1903-1937.
9. Pan S, Litscher G, Gao S, et al. Historical perspective of traditional indigenous medical practices: the current renaissance and conservation of herbal resources. Evidence-Based Complement Altern Med. 2014;2014:20.
10. Rifat F, Sharma A, Srivastava P, Patni S, Sisodia R. Protective effects of Prunus avium extract on 10 GHz induced damages in the spleen of swiss albino mice. Indian J Appl Res. 2013;3(8):680-684.
11. Khaki A, Fathiazad F, Nouri M, Khaki A. Effect of Ocimum basilicum on apoptosis in testis of rats after exposure to electromagnetic field. Afr J Pharm Pharmacol. 2011;5(12):1534-1537.
12. Mallhi TH, Qadir MI, Ali M, Ahmad B, Khan YH, Rehman A. Ajwa Date (Phoenix dactylifera): An emerging plant in pharmacological research. Pak J Pharm Sci. 2014;27(3):607-616.
13. Abedi A, Parviz M, Karimian SM, Sadeghipour Rodsari HR. The effect of aqueous extract of Phoenix dactylifera pollen grain on sexual behavior of male rats. J Physiol Pharmacol Adv. 2012;2(6):235-342.
14. Abedi A, Karimian SM, Parviz M, Mohammadi P, Reza H, Roudsari S. Effect of aqueous extract of Phoenix dactylifera pollen on dopamine system of nucleus accumbens in male rats. Neurosci Med. 2014;5(1):49-59.
15. Salman I, Munazza A, Hina MA, Tahir S, Yasir A, Gul EN. Evaluation of spermatogenesis in prepubertal albino rats with date palm pollen supplement. Afr J Pharm Pharmacol. 2014;8(2):59-65.
16. Lotfi N, Khazaei M, Shariatzadeh SM, Mehranjani MS, Ghanbari A. The effect of cannabis sativa hydroalcoholic extract on sperm parameters and testis histology in rats. Int J Morphol. 2013;31(1):82-86.
17. Avendaño C, Mata A, Sanchez Sarmiento CA, Doncel GF. Use of laptop computers connected to internet through Wi-Fi decreases human sperm motility and increases sperm DNA fragmentation. Fertil Steril. 2012;97(1):39-45.e2.
18. Falahati S, Anvari M, Khalili M. Effects of combined magnetic fields on human sperm parameters. Iran J Radiat Res. 2011;9(3):195-200.
19. Hajiuon B. Effects of cell phone radiation on testosterone levels and testicular changes in rats treated with garlic (Allium sativum L.) hydroalcoholic extract. Prog Biol Sci. 2014;4(1):63-72.
20. Gupta U, Chaudhary R, Goyal P. Post-treatment

effects of Alstonia scholaris extract against radiation-induced biochemical alterations in Swiss albino mice. Iran J Radiat Res. 2010;8(3):169-177.
21. Zahedifar Z, Baharara J. Effect of green tea in decreasing electromagnetic waves damages. Zahedan J Res Med Sci. 2015; in press.
22. Ramadan L, Abd-Allah A, Aly HA, Saad-el-Din A. Testicular toxicity effects of magnetic field exposure and prophylactic role of coenzyme Q10 and L-carnitine in mice. Pharmacol Res. 2002;46(4): 363-370.
23. Arfat Y, Mahmood N, Ahmad M, et al. Effect of date palm pollen on serum testosterone and intra-testicular environment in male albino rats. Afr J Pharm Pharmacol. 2014;8(31):793-800.
24. El-Neweshy MS, El-Maddawy ZK, El-Sayed YS. Therapeutic effects of date palm (Phoenix dactylifera L.) pollen extract on cadmium-induced testicular toxicity. Andrologia. 2013;45(6):369-378.
25. Hassan WA, El-kashlan AM, Ehssan NA. Egyptian date palm pollen ameliorates testicular dysfunction induced by cadmium chloride in adult male rats. J Am Sci. 2012;8(4):659-669.
26. Al-dujaily SS, Al-shahery NJ, Zabbon AA. Effect of Phoenix dactylifera pollen on in vitro sperm activation of infertile men saad. Al-Mustansiriyah J Sci. 2012;23(6):27-34.
27. Elkerm Y, Tawashi R. Date palm pollen as a preventative intervention in radiation- and chemotherapy-induced oral mucositis: a pilot study. Integr Cancer Ther. 2014;13(6):468-472.
28. Gabr GA, Soliman GA, Ganaie MA, Hassan HM. The potential protective activity of date palm (Phoenix dactylifera) pollen and Panax ginseng against cisplatin-induced testicular toxicity in rats. Int J Biol Phar Allied Sci. 2014;3(5):605-623.

Effect of *Phoenix dactylifera* pollen grain on maturation of preantral follicles in NMRI mice

Farzaneh Salek Abdollahi[1], Javad Baharara[2*], Khadijeh NejadShahrokhabadi[3], Farideh Namvar[4], Elaheh Amini[5]

[1]MSC Student, Department of Biology, Faculty of Sciences, Mashhad Branch, Islamic Azad University, Mashhad, Iran
[2]PhD. Research Center for Animal Development Applied Biology, Mashhad Branch, Islamic Azad University, Mashhad, Iran
[3]PhD, Department of Biology, Faculty of Sciences, Islamic Azad University, Mashhad Branch, Mashhad, Iran
[4]Ph.D. Institute of Tropical Forestry and Forest Products (INTROP), University Putra Malaysia, UPM Serdang, Selangor 43400, Malaysia
[5]Department of Animal Biology, Faculty of Biological Sciences, Kharazmi University, Tehran, Iran

ARTICLE INFO

Keywords:
Follicle
Oocyte
In vitro maturation (IVM)
Date palm pollen grain

ABSTRACT

Introduction: Optimizing an ideal culture system that is comparable to follicle environment to obtain mature oocytes is one of the important criteria in in vitro maturation (IVM). *Phoenix dactylifera* L. commonly known as date palm is an important herb in Asia folk medicine that is used to improve fertility in women from ancient time. The aim of this study was to investigate the effect of date palm pollen grain extract on IVM of mouse follicles.
Methods: In this study follicles with 1 or 2 layers of granulosa cells and round oocytes were isolated from 2-3 weeks old female NMRI mice ovaries. Follicles were cultured in IVM media with different concentrations 0, 10, 20, 30, 40 μg/ml of palm pollen grain extract for 12 days. Then, the effect of date palm pollen grain on follicular growth and maturation were analyzed.
Results: There was a significant increase in follicle growth and maturation rate in all treated groups as compared to the control group, but maturation rate was significantly higher in the presence of 20 μg/ml palm pollen grain.
Conclusion: Supplementation of IVM media with date palm pollen grain extract improves the IVM of follicles.

Implication for health policy/practice/research/medical education:
Date palm pollen has antioxidant property and may have a beneficial effect on in vitro maturation (IVM) of follicle and improve survival and growth rates of preantral follicles. Supplementation of IVM media with date palm pollen grain extract may improve IVM of follicles

Introduction

Ovarian follicles are the main structural and functional units of female reproductive system which supply the essential microenvironment for the advantages of oocyte growth and maturation. Preantral follicles are considered as a potential source of oocytes to play an important role in in vitro studies of folliculogenesis and embryo production (1). In vitro maturation (IVM) of immature oocyte in laboratory conditions have been considered as an additional approach in assisted reproductive technology (ART) (2). The in vitro embryo production (IVEP) system involves IVM of the primary oocytes, in vitro fertilization (IVF) of the matured oocytes and in vitro embryo culture (IVC). IVM has been considered as one of the most critical part of this process towards successful IVEP (3). Currently, IVM system has been improved and applied as an effective infertility treatment for women with polycystic ovary syndrome (PCOS) to reduce the rate of ovarian hyper stimulation and to preserve fertility in patients at high risk of fertility-threatening disease or treatment regimens like chemotherapy (4). The combination of these reproductive technologies with cryopreservation is a useful method of fertility preservation for cancer patients before undergoing chemotherapy or radiation therapy (5). Maturation of oocyte depends on 2 essential aspects of cytoplasmic and nuclear maturation. So, the loss of complete maturation

*Corresponding author: Javad Baharara, PhD. Research Center for Animal Development Applied Biology, Mashhad Branch, Islamic Azad University, Mashhad, Iran, Email: baharara@yahoo.com

can reduce the success of oocyte developmental competence. However nuclear and/or cytoplasmic maturation are not supported properly by current culture systems (6). Providing effective culture medium comparable to follicular environment is a critical step toward obtaining mature oocytes (3). The intracellular glutathione (GSH) and reactive oxygen species (ROS) levels are recognized to play important role in oocyte IVM and embryo production. Reduction of intracellular GSH content can cause lower oocytes developmental competence (7). The generation of ROS is an essential cellular process. However, excessive amounts of ROS can change cellular molecules like lipids, proteins and nucleic acids (8). The production of high levels of during in vitro cultures leads to impress fertilization rate, embryo development and the change of clinical pregnancy rates (6). Natural antioxidants are compounds that play an important role in prevention of oxidative stress and associated diseases. Plants are considered as excellent sources of natural antioxidants (9).

Phoenix dactylifera L. generally known as the date palm is one of the important main plants of the Middle East (10). Date (*Phoenix dactylifera*) is a member of the palm family arecaceae or palmae (11). Palm pollen grains contain a wide range of nutritional contents such as: vitamins, minerals, trace elements, carbohydrates, lipids, organic acids, sterols, nucleic acids, free amino acids, enzymes and cofactors (10). The antioxidant activities of date palm pollen (DPP) is mainly due to phenolic components, such as flavonoids, phenolic acids, and phenolic diterpenes (12,13). Usually, the different parts of Phoenix dactylifera are used in traditional medicine for the cure of wide range of disorders like memory disturbances, fever, inflammation, paralysis, loss of consciousness and nervous disorders (14). The ancient Chinese and Egyptians used pollen as a medicinal agent (15). It has been demonstrated that DPP has gonadal stimulating potency and in ancient times was used by Egyptian to improve fertility in women (16).

Materials and Methods

Chemicals

All the reagents were obtained from Sigma-Aldrich (Germany) unless otherwise specified.

Animals

The NMRI mice were purchased from Razi Institute (Mashhad, Iran), and housed under standard conditions of temperature 25°C and 12 hours light: 12 hours dark. They were fed water and pellets ad libitum.

Preparation of extract

Samples of the plant were collected from botanical garden at Bushehr city (South of Iran). Pollen grains were washed with distilled water and then dried. The extract was prepared by mixing 0.1 g of palm pollen within 1 ml of PBS with vigorous shaking and vortexing.

DPPH free radical scavenging activity

The percentage of antioxidant activity of DPP extract was estimated by the scavenging free-radical DPPH as compared with butylated hydroxy anisole (BHA) as a standard compound (3). The different concentration of DPP extract was added to methanol solution of DPPH (250-4000 µg/ml). Then, absorbance was measured at 517 nm after 30 minutes incubation in dark with a micro plate reader. The scavenging activity percentage (%) was determined by using the following formula:

DPPH radical scavenging (%) = (control OD - sample OD/control OD) ×100

Isolation of preantral follicles

Female mice, 2-3 weeks old, were killed by cervical dislocation and ovaries were instantly transferred to culture medium that consisted of α-minimal essential medium (α-MEM, Gibco, UK) supplemented with 10% fetal bovine serum (FBS, Gibco, UK), 100 µg/ml penicillin and 50 µg/ml streptomycin under mineral oil. Preantral follicles from ovaries were mechanically isolated by using 30-gauge needles under a stereomicroscope. Isolated follicles that were preantral follicles with 120-150 µm diameter were chosen and cultured in culture medium of MEM-α supplemented with different concentrations of DPP (0, 10, 20, 30, 40 µg/ml extract) for 12 days. Then, the effect of DPP grain on follicular growth and maturation was analyzed (17).

Culture of preantral follicles

The preantral follicles isolated were cultured in 96-well plates which contained 19×35 µl droplets of α-MEM supplemented with 5% FBS, 100 mIU/ml recombinant follicle stimulating hormone, 1% insulin transferrin selenium mix (ITS; Gibco, UK), 100 µg/ml penicillin and 50 µg/ml streptomycin under mineral oil and was incubated at 37°C, humidified atmosphere of 5% CO2 in air for 12 days (18).

Evaluation of follicle parameters

Measurement of follicle diameter was performed with ocular micrometer at 100 X magnification and Image J imaging system software version 1.43 (National Institutes of Health, Bethesda, MD) every 48 hours during the culture period.

From the day four, we could not measure the exact diameter of the growing follicles because of overgrow of granulosa cells. The survival rate of the follicles was confirmed by evaluation of follicle morphology under an inverted microscope. Follicle survival in culture was considered positive during the time that maintained oocytes were surrounded by granulosa cells attached to the culture dish (1).

Ovulation induction

Ovulation was induced on day 12 of culture, by addition of fresh medium supplemented with 1.5 IU/ml human chorionic gonadotropin (HCG; Organon) to the droplets. The cumulus oocyte complexes (COC) were observed 14-16 hours later under the inverted microscope (5).

Statistical analysis

The data are presented as mean ± standard deviation (SD). Statistical analysis was performed using SPSS version 16. Criteria including survival rate, degeneration, germinal vesicle stage, antrum formation rate and oocyte maturation were analyzed by one-way analysis of variance (ANOVA). $P<.05$ was considered to be statistically significant.

Results

DPPH free radical scavenging activity

The anti-oxidative potential of the DPP grain extract was estimated by using the DPPH free radical scavenging activity assay. As shown in Figure 1, DPP grain extract showed dose dependent activity and also the DPPH scavenging effect was 65.6% at a concentration of 1 mg/ml. As a result, depending on concentration, the DPP grain extract demonstrated a moderate DPPH-scavenging activity as compared to the BHA as a standard compound (Figure 1).

Evaluation of follicle parameters

In the present study, we showed the promoting effect of different concentrations of DPP grain extract on IVM of mice follicles (Figure 2).

The results showed that there was a significant increase in follicle diameter in all treated groups as compared to the control but maturation rate was significantly higher in the presence of 20 µg/ml palm pollen grain ($P<.01$). Survival rate of follicles on day 12 of culture was significantly higher in the presence of 20 µg/ml palm pollen grain compared with the control group ($P<.05$).

As shown in Figure 3, the supplementation of DPP to maturation medium increased the rate of oocyte maturation. The survival rate, maturation rate, antrum formation rate were significantly improved in this group compared to the control group ($P<.05$). All three dosages of DPP improved IVM rate. However, a significant increase in the IVM rate was seen only in the group treated with 20 µg/ml ($P<.05$).

The percentage of arrested oocytes at GV stage showed significant ($P<.05$) difference compared to the control group (Table 1). The percentage of GV stage oocytes in the control group was significantly higher than other treatment groups ($P<.05$). The oocytes treated with 20 µg/ml extract showed the lowest percentage of GV stage compared with control group, 10 and 40 µg/ml extract groups ($P<.05$); however, no significant difference was observed

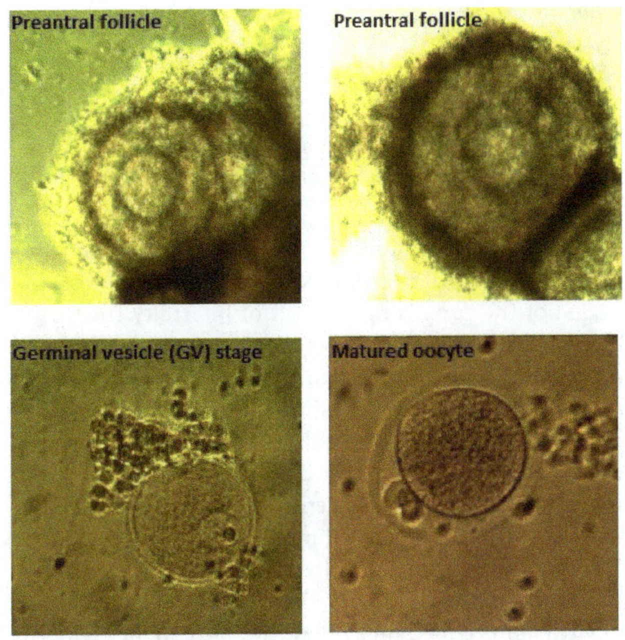

Figure 2. Development of follicles during in vitro culture. Preantral follicles on day 0 and 2, Germinal vesicle (GV), Matured oocyte under exposer with 20 µg/ml DPP.

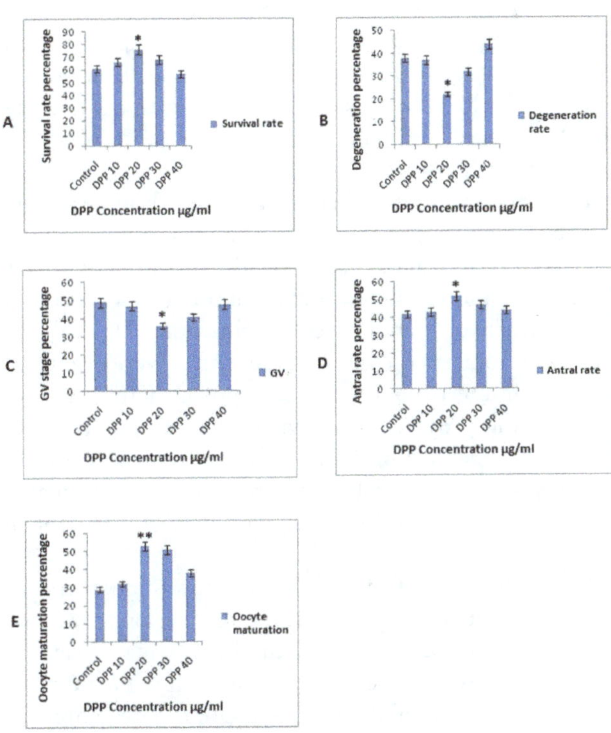

Figure 3. Effect of date palm pollen on follicles parameter. (A) Survival rate, (B) Degeneration, (C) Germinal vesicle stage, (D) Antral rate, (E) Oocyte maturation. (Mean ± SD, $P<.05$ was considered significant).

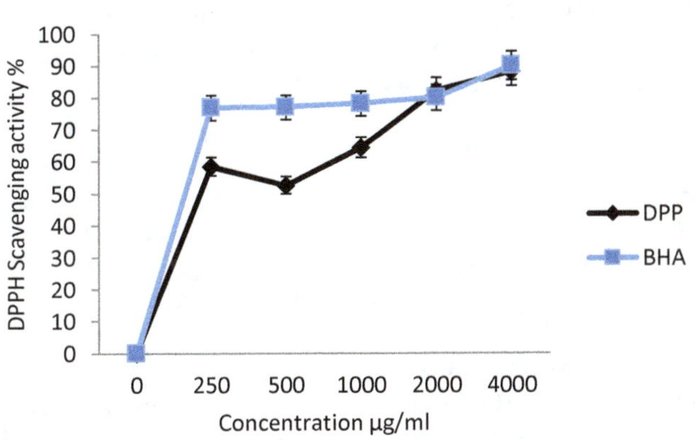

Figure 1. DPPH free radical scavenging activity of date palm pollen extract (sample) and BHA (Mean ± SD).

Table 1. Effect of DPP on IVM of preantral follicle[a]

DPP concentrations µg/ml	Total (%)	Survival rate (%)	Degeneration rate (%)	GV (%)	Antral rate (%)	Oocyte Maturation (%)
Control (DPP 0)	92	61 ± 4.04	38 ± 5.56	49 ± 4.00	42 ± 4.35	29 ± 2.51
DPP 10	81	66 ± 4.50	37 ± 5.03	47 ± 6.65	43 ± 5.29	32 ± 6.02
DPP 20	79	76 ± 6.11	22 ± 5.13	36 ± 4.04	52 ± 3.00	53 ± 4.72
DPP 30	76	68 ± 6.42	32 ± 5.50	41 ± 4.00	47 ± 6.55	51 ± 3.00
DPP 40	87	57 ± 4.16	44 ± 4.00	48 ± 2.51	44 ± 6.42	38 ± 5.85

[a] The data were represented as mean ± SD.

when compared to 30 µg/ml extract ($P > .05$).

Discussion

Recently in vitro culture of preantral follicles plays important role in ART (18). IVM of oocytes has developed as one of the promising method of infertility treatment. Retrieval of immature oocytes without gonadotropin stimulation and culture in maturation media is used in women with ovarian hyper stimulation syndrome (OHSS) (19). IVM has been suggested as an effective strategy for fertility preservation, since it does not need gonadotropin stimulation and is consequently related with serum E2 levels that are in the normal range. As a result, IVM provides an opportunity for serious fertility preservation and also in women suffering from E-sensitive diseases (20,21). In vitro culture mediums of oocytes have higher concentrations of oxygen in comparison to in vivo conditions, which caused an increase of ROS levels. Nowadays natural antioxidants are gaining a great attention which may prevent oxidative damage and related diseases (8). Different culture media have been used to provide optimum conditions for appropriate in vitro oocyte maturation (4). In 2014 Barakat et al (3) evaluated the oocyte maturation and embryo development of sheep and demonstrated that the supplementation of maturation media with low concentration of GTE as an antioxidant can enhance the rate of oocytes maturation and formation of morula and blastula in sheep.

Heidari et al. indicated that fibroblast co-culture improves the growth and viability rate of preantral follicles through development of granulosa cell proliferation (1). The effects of fibroblast co-culture and activin A were evaluated on IVM and fertilization of mouse preantral follicles that elevated the growth and survival rate of preantral follicles (2). The effect of *Papaver rhoeas* L. extract on IVM of sheep oocytes indicated that the rate of oocyte maturation and MII stage increased compared to the control group (8).

Lately, a study revealed that the addition of quercetin in maturation media improved embryos development (22). It has been shown that the natural antioxidants saffron (*Crocus sativus* L.) aqueous extract in culture medium increases the oocyte maturation and embryo development (6). In another study it was demonstrated the antioxidant properties of saffron (*Crocus sativus* L.) aqueous extract and its component like crocin could improve the rate of IVM, IVF and embryo development of mouse oocytes. However, this study showed that saffron aqueous extract had a stronger effect than pure crocin (23). The previous studies documented the antioxidant activity of DPP grain. It was suggested that the supplementation of DPP as an antioxidant enhanced GSH and restored LPO in the testes of Cd-treated rats. In addition, DPP could improve Cd-induced oxidative stress in the testicular tissues (24). The antioxidant potential of DPP was demonstrated by its bioactive components that could protect the oral mucosa by blocking oxidative free radicals, preventing DNA damage, and neutralizing inflammatory reactions (25).

These studies exhibited that the administration of DPP as a source of antioxidant in the maturation medium increased maturation rate of oocytes. In other studies various antioxidants like β-mercaptoethanol (β-ME), cysteine, cysteamine and anthocyanin were applied to develop IVM of oocytes (7). DPP as an antioxidative substance prevented harmful actions of free radicals. Extract of DPP is an herbal mixture that is generally used as a folk remedy for curing male infertility in traditional medicine (16). It was concluded that the supplementation of IVM media with DPP grain extract may improve IVM of follicles.

Conclusions

Finally, the results of the present study demonstrated that DPP has antioxidant property and in proper dose to medium as an antioxidant may have a beneficial effect on IVM of follicle and improve survival and growth rates of preantral follicles. Supplementation of IVM media with DPP grain extract may improve IVM of follicles.

Acknowledgments

The authors would like to thank Research Center of Animal Development Applied Bilogy, Islamic Azad University, Mashhad, Iran for its support.

Authors' contributions

All the authors wrote the manuscript equally.

Conflict of interests

The authors declared no competing interests.

Ethical considerations

Ethical issues (including plagiarism, misconduct, data fabrication, falsification, double publication or submission, redundancy) have been completely observed by the authors.

References

1. Heidari M, Malekshah AK, Parivar K, Khanbabaei R, Rafiei A. Effect of fibroblast co-culture on in vitro maturation and fertilization of mouse preantral follicles. Int J Fertil Steril. 2011;5(1):1-8.
2. Malekshah A, Heidari M, Parivar K, Azami NS. The effects of fibroblast co-culture and activin a on in vitro growth of mouse preantral follicles. Iran Biomed J. 2014;18:49-54.
3. Barakat IA, Al-himaidi AR, Rady AM. Antioxidant effect of green tea leaves extract on in vitro production of sheep embryos. Pak J Zool. 2014;46(1):167-175.
4. Park KE, Kim YY, Ku S-Y, et al. Effects of alginate hydrogels on in vitro maturation outcome of mouse preantral follicles. Tissue Eng Regen Med. 2012;9(3):170-174.
5. Heidari M, Malekshah AK, Azami N, Mirhoseini SM. In-vitro maturation of mouse preantral follicles in two culture media : A comparative study. Ann Biol Res. 2012;3(10):4937-4941.
6. Tavana S, Eimani H, Azarnia M, Shahverdi A, Eftekhari-Yazdi P. Effects of saffron (Crocus sativus L.) aqueous extract on in vitro maturation, fertilization and embryo development of mouse oocytes. Cell J. 2012;13(4):259-264.
7. Kwak S, Hyun S. The effects of resveratrol on oocyte maturation and preimplantation embryo development. J Emb Trans. 2012;27(2):71-80.
8. Rajabi-Toustani R, Motamedi-Mojdehi R, Roostaei-Ali Mehr M, Motamedi-Mojdehi R. Effect of Papaver rhoeas L. extract on in vitro maturation of sheep oocytes. Small Rumin Res 2013;114(1):146-151.
9. Vijaya Kumar Reddy C, Sreeramulu D, Raghunath M. Antioxidant activity of fresh and dry fruits commonly consumed in India. Food Res Int. 2010;43(1):285-288.
10. Baliga MS, Baliga BR, Kandathil SM, Bhat HP, Vayalil PK. A review of the chemistry and pharmacology of the date fruits (Phoenix dactylifera L.). Food Res Int. 2011;44(7):1812-1822.
11. Rahmani A, Aly S, Ali H, Babiker A, Srikar S, Khan A. Therapeutic effects of date fruits (Phoenix dactylifera) in the prevention of diseases via modulation of anti-inflammatory, anti-oxidant and anti-tumour activity. Int J Clin Exp Med. 2014;7(3):483-491.
12. Bahmanpour S, Kavoosi F, Talaei T, Panjehshahin MR. Effects of date palm (Phoenix dactylifera) gemmule extract on morphometric parameters of reproductive tissues, hormones and sperm quality in rat. Anatomical Sciences. 2013;10(3):144-150.
13. Gabr GA, Soliman GA, Ganaie MA, Hassan HM. The potential protective activity of date palm (phoenix dactylifera) pollen and panax ginseng against cisplatin-induced testicular toxicity in rats. International Journal of Biology, Pharmacy and Allied Sciences 2014;3(5):605-623.
14. Abedi A, Parviz M, Karimian SM, Sadeghipour Rodsari HR. The effect of aqueous extract of phoenix dactylifera pollen grain on sexual behavior of male rats. Journal of Jahrom University of Medical Sciences. 2012;2(6):235-242.
15. Hassan HM. Chemical composition and nutritional value of palm pollen grains. Global J Biotechnol Biochem. 2011;6(1):1-7.
16. Elberry A, Mufti ST, Al-Maghrabi J, et al. Anti-inflammatory and antiproliferative activities of date palm pollen (Phoenix dactylifera)on experimentally-induced atypical prostatic hyperplasia in rats. J Inflamm (Lond). 2011;8(1):40.
17. Kim C, Cheon Y, Lee Y, et al. The effect of fibroblast co-culture on in vitro maturation of mouse preantral follicles. Dev Reprod. 2013;17(3):269-274.
18. Nottola SA, Cecconi S, Bianchi S, et al. Ultrastructure of isolated mouse ovarian follicles cultured in vitro. Reprod Biol Endocrinol. 2011;9(3):1-13.
19. Grynberg M, El Hachem H, de Bantel A, Benard J, le Parco S, Fanchin R. In vitro maturation of oocytes: uncommon indications. Fertil Steril. 2013;99(5):1182-1188.
20. Berwanger AL, Finet A, El Hachem H, Le Parco S, Hesters L GM. New trends in female fertility preservation: in vitro maturation of oocytes. Futur Oncol. 2012;8(15):67-73.
21. Maman E1, Meirow D, Brengauz M, Raanani H, Dor J, Hourvitz A. Luteal phase oocyte retrieval and in vitro maturation is an optional procedure for urgent fertility preservation. Fertil Steril. 2011;95(1):64-67.
22. Orlovschi D, Miclea I, Zahan M, Miclea V, Pernes A. Quercetin efficacy on in vitro maturation of porcine oocytes. Scientific Papers Animal Science and Biotechnologies. 2014;47(1):113-115.
23. Mokhber Maleki E, Eimani H, Bigdeli MR, et al. A comparative study of saffron aqueous extract and its active ingredient, crocin on the in vitro maturation, in vitro fertilization, and in vitro culture of mouse oocytes. Taiwan J Obstet Gynecol. 2014;53(1):21-25.
24. El-Neweshy MS, El-Maddawy ZK, El-Sayed YS. Therapeutic effects of date palm (Phoenix dactylifera L.) pollen extract on cadmium-induced testicular toxicity. Andrologia. 2013;45(6):369-378.
25. Elkerm Y, Tawashi R. Date palm pollen as a preventative intervention in radiation- and chemotherapy-induced oral mucositis: A pilot study. Integr Cancer Ther. 2014;13(6):468-472.

Kelussia odoratissima Mozaff. a rich source of essential fatty acids and phthalides

Mehdi Ghasemi[1], Aghafakhr Mirlohi[2*], Mahdi Ayyari[1], Abdolali Shojaeiyan[1]

[1]Department of Horticulture Science, Tarbiat Modares University, Tehran, Iran
[2]Department of Agronomy and Plant Breeding, Isfahan University of Technology, Isfahan, Iran

ARTICLE INFO

Keywords:
Kelussia odoratissima Mozaff.
Essential oil
Fatty acids
(*Z*)-Ligustilide
Omega-3
Omega-6

ABSTRACT

Introduction: The present study was aimed to assess the fatty acids of leaf and essential oil compositions of of aerial parts of *Kelussia odoratissima*.
Methods: The aerial parts of *K. odoratissima* from the three habitats were dried. The essential oils were obtained by hydrodistillation for 3 hours in a Clevenger-type apparatus, then the analysis of the components was carried out using gas chromatography–mass spectrometry (GC-MS). To study the oil yield and fatty acids, the dried leaves were subjected to extraction in hexane by using Soxhlet apparatus. To analyze fatty acids from the oil fractions by GC technique, the oil was subjected to transesterification to obtain the fatty acid methyl esters (FAMEs), which were dissolved in hexane and were subjected to GC analysis.
Results: According to the results, a total of 43 components were detected, the major constitutes of essential oil compositions were (*Z*)-Ligustilide (76.45%), Unknown-A (4.47%), (*E*)-Ligustilide (2.57%), (*Z*)-Butylidene phthalide (2.37%), 5-pentyl cyclohexa-1,3-diene (1.57%) and kessane (0.77%). Sixteen fatty acids were separated from the oil (5% yield per 100 g dry matter). Linoleic acid (25.46%), α-linolenic acid (16.66%), palmitic acid (11.92%), oleic acid (9.33%), stearic acid (4.72%), petroselinic acid (2.53%), arachidonic acid (2.51%) and erucic acid (1.76%) were the major fatty acids.
Conclusion: Generally, *K. odoratissima* is a rich source of essential fatty acids and phthalide derivatives, specially (*Z*)-ligustilide. This study presented valuable information about the phytochemical properties, which can be useful for the future research on the pharmacological effects of *K. odoratissima*.

Implication for health policy/practice/research/medical education:
Kelussia odoratissima with pharmaceutical beneficial compounds such as (*Z*)-Ligustilide, ω-3 and ω-6 can be served as fresh and garnish in the diet. Reducing high blood pressure and cardiovascular diseases by these components has been proved in other researches.

Introduction

Ethnopharmacology is a scientific study on the biological activities of botanical drugs used by local people, which have beneficial, toxic or other direct pharmacological effects (1). Iran has appreciable past regarding folk medicines, especially based on medicinal plants because its flora includes about 8000 plant species and endemic species (2).

Kelussia odoratissima Mozaff. is a wild, perennial and medicinal herb that belongs to the Apiaceae family. This species is found only in Central Zagros Mountains, and so far there has not been reported in other areas of the world (3). The aerial parts harvested and sold in the local markets in the early spring as spice and has been used to cure inflamed ulcers, hypertension, and cardiovascular diseases by the indigenous people (4). The genetic and ecological factors such as precipitation, temperature, plant competition and edaphic conditions, affects the chemical variation of the medicinal plants (5). The results of the study by Shojaei et al showed that the dominant consti-

***Corresponding author**: Aghafakhr Mirlohi, Department of Agronomy and Plant Breeding, Isfahan University of Technology, Isfahan, Iran.
Email: : mirlohi@cc.iut.ac.ir

tutes of essential oil of *K. odoratissima* are phthalides from the Koohrang, Bazoft and Samsami habitats in Iran (6). In the other studies, phthalides such as (*Z*)-Ligustilide, (*E*)-Ligustilide, (*Z*)-Butyldiene phthalide, (*E*)-Butyldiene phthalide and 3-*n*-Butylphthalide have been reported as the major compositions of essential oil (7,8).
Edible oils are biological mixtures of plant origin consisting of ester mixtures derived from glycerol with chain of fatty acids, which play a crucial role in growth and development of the body (9). Fatty acids are usually classified in classes as saturated (SFA), monounsaturated (MUFA) and polyunsaturated (PUFA). On the other hand, the unsaturated fatty acids are classified into a series known as omega, being omega-3, omega-6, omega-9 and Omega-12 as the essential fatty acids (EFAs) (10). In a related study, only the fatty acids of the seeds of *K. odoratissima* were discussed (11).
In Iran, most of the researches on *K. odoratissima* have been focused on the limited and unknown habitats. To the best of our knowledge, there is no report on the fatty acids of aerial parts and the chemical compounds of *K. odoratissima* from the major habitats of Dareh-Sepestan, Landeroun (Isfahan province) and Vastegan (Chaharmahal and Bakhtiari province). The aim of this study was to investigate the essential oil compositions and the fatty acids of aerial parts of *K. odoratissima* using gas chromatography-mass spectrometry (GC-MS) from the above mentioned habitats.

Materials and Methods

Essential oil extraction and analysis

The aerial parts (leaves) of *K. odoratissima* from the habitats of Dareh-Sepestan, Vastegan (Isfahan province) and Landeroun (Chaharmahal and Bakhtiari province), Iran, were dried at room temperature in shade at 25 ± 3°C. The essential oil of samples was obtained by hydrodistillation for 3 hours in a Clevenger-type apparatus according to the method recommended (12). The essential oils were dried over anhydrous Na_2SO_4, and stored at 4°C before analysis. GC analysis was carried out using a Thermoquest gas chromatograph with a flame ionization detector (FID) equipped with a fused silica capillary DB-5 column (30 m × 0.25 mm i.d., 0.25 µm film thickness). Detector (FID) temperature was 280°C and the injector temperature was 250°C. Nitrogen was used as the carrier gas at a flow rate of 1.1 ml/min within a split ratio of 1:100; the oven temperature program was 60°C–250°C at the rate of 5°C min^{-1} and finally held isothermally for 10 minutes. GC–MS analysis was carried out with a Thermoquest–Finnigan gas chromatograph equipped with fused silica capillary DB-5 column (60 m × 0.25 mm i.d., 0.25 µm film thickness) coupled with a TRACE mass spectrometer (Manchester, UK). Helium was used as the carrier gas with an ionization energy of 70 eV, the mass range was 40–460 a.m.u. Ion source, and interface temperatures were 200°C and 250°C, respectively. The oven temperature program was similar as above for the GC. Compositions were identified based on their retention indices (*n*-alkanes), by comparison of their mass spectra with those reported in the literature and stored in NIST, Willey and Adams libraries.

Fatty acid extraction and analysis

The plant sample was collected from the Birahgan habitat in Chaharmal and Bakhtiari province, weighed and dried to remove excess moisture. The oil was extracted for 5 hours using hexane as the extraction solvent. The extract was then evaporated, dried and weighed.
To prepare fatty acid methyl esters (FAMEs), 2% NaOH and 2 mg pentadecanoic acid (C15:0) as an internal standard were added to the 0.11 g oil, which was incubated for 10 minutes in a heated bath and cooled. The methanolic BF_3 (2.18 ml) was then added, and the sample was heated in the bath for 2 to 3 minutes and cooled again. In the following, FAMEs was dissolved in 1.5 ml hexane, and partitioned in 1 ml of saturated sodium chloride and then vigorously shacked. In the final step of dehydration, 1 ml of upper layer was separated and was mixed with 0.5 mg sodium sulfate by centrifuging. The upper layer was injected to GC.
The identification of FAMEs was carried out by GC (UNICAM 4600, SB Analytical, UK) equipped with GC-FID and a BPX-70 fused-silica capillary column (30 m length, 0.25 mm i.d., 0.22 µm film thickness). The operating conditions were as follows: the initial temperature was 50°C, increased by 5°C min^{-1} up to the 160°C; and with a ramp of 20°C min^{-1} reached 180°C and finally 200°C. The injector and detector temperatures were 250 and 250°C, respectively. The column head pressure (Helium) was 20 psi. Each fatty acid was identified in its methyl ester form by comparing its retention time with the internal standard.

Results

Chemical compositions of essential oils

The percentages and retention indices of the compounds in the essential oils of *K. odoratissima* accessions are listed in Table 1. In total, the number of compounds identified and quantified were 38 in Dareh-Sepestan, 42 in Vastegan and 39 in Landeroun accessions, representing 97.90%, 98.13% and 95.65% of the total oil, respectively.
In the essential oil of Dareh-Sepestan accession, (*Z*)-Ligustilide (76.09%), Unknown-A (7.40%), 5-pentyl cyclohexa-1,3-diene (2.21%), (*E*)-Ligustilide (2.16%), (*Z*)-Butylidene phthalide (1.40%), kessane (1.07%) and α-copaene (0.81%) were the main constituents. (Z)-Ligustilide (75.87%), unknown-A (3.93%), (*E*)-Ligustilide (3.20%), (Z)-Butylidene phthalide (2.47%), 5-pentyl cyclohexa-1,3-diene (2.15%), α-copaene (0.93%) and (*Z*)-γ-Bisabolene (0.89%) were the main constituents in the essential oil of Vastegan accession. In the essential oil of Landeroun accession, (Z)-Ligustilide (77.40%), (Z)-Butylidene phthalide (3.25%), unknown-A (2.39%), (*E*)-Ligustilide (2.35%), (Z)-β-Santalol acetate (1.03%), 5-pentyl cyclohexa-1,3-diene (0.89%), 4-Hydroxybenzaldehyde (0.84%) were the main constituents.

Table 1. Chemical composition of essential oils (%) of three accessions of *K. odoratissima*

No.	Component	RI[a]	RI[b]	1[c]	2	3	Mean
1	Propyl benzene	951	951	0.19	0.09	0.13	0.14
2	(*E*)-2-methyl-3-Octen-5-yne	953	958	0.32	0.10	0.06	0.16
3	Limonene	1027	1024	0.17	0.09	0.10	0.12
4	α-Terpinolene	1088	1086	0.28	0.16	0.16	0.20
5	5-Pentyl cyclohexa-1,3-diene	1159	1156	2.21	2.15	0.89	1.75
6	Unknown-A	1277	-	7.40	3.93	2.39	4.57
8	2-Undecanone	1291	1293	-	0.12	-	0.12
9	Menthyl acetate	1294	1294	0.17	-	0.07	0.12
10	p-Vinylguaiacol	1315	1315	0.19	0.46	0.12	0.26
11	α-Cubebene	1351	1351	0.08	0.13	0.08	0.10
12	4-Hydroxybenzaldehyde	1354	1355	0.17	0.39	0.84	0.47
13	α-Copaene	1377	1377	0.81	0.93	0.06	0.60
14	9-Decenyl acetate	1389	1384	0.06	0.14	0.09	0.10
15	(*Z*)-Caryophyllene	1406	1406	0.23	0.18	0.19	0.20
16	(*E*)-Caryophyllene	1421	1421	0.25	0.34	0.22	0.27
17	α-Humulene	1455	1455	0.31	0.42	0.28	0.34
18	α-Acoradiene	1466	1465	0.48	0.34	0.37	0.40
19	10-*epi*-β-acoradiene	1475	1475	0.42	0.61	0.24	0.42
20	Germacrene D	1481	1481	0.31	0.52	0.40	0.41
21	(*Z,E*)-α-Farnesene	1489	1489	0.12	0.17	0.13	0.14
22	(E)-Muurola-4(14),5-diene	1493	1493	0.07	0.19	0.06	0.11
23	β-Himachalene	1499	1499	0.46	0.18	0.35	0.33
24	β-Bisabolene	1505	1505	-	0.21	-	0.21
25	β-Curcumene	1508	1508	0.13	0.23	0.22	0.19
26	(*Z*)-γ-Bisabolene	1513	1514	0.48	0.89	0.31	0.56
27	δ-Cadinene	1522	1522	0.13	0.66	0.68	0.49
28	Kessane	1528	1529	1.07	0.47	0.78	0.77
29	γ-Cuprenene	1531	1532	0.19	0.13	0.24	0.19
30	β-Spathulenol	1579	1577	-	0.14	0.08	0.11
31	3-Butylhexahydro phthalide	1638	1632	0.06	0.06	-	0.06
32	3-*n*-Butylphthalide	1654	1656	0.11	0.38	0.40	0.30
33	(*Z*)-Butylidene phthalide	1676	1677	1.40	2.47	3.25	2.37
34	(*E*)-Butylidene phthalide	1722	1717	0.15	0.42	0.32	0.30
35	(*Z*)-Ligustilide	1759	1741	76.09	75.87	77.40	76.45
36	(*E*)-Ligustilide	1805	1797	2.16	3.20	2.35	2.57
37	(*Z*)-β-Santalol acetate	1823	1818	0.35	0.59	1.03	0.66
38	Neophytadiene	1834	1841	0.05	0.07	0.10	0.07
39	*Z*-Ternine [d]	1848	1845	-	0.06	0.08	0.07
40	*n*-Nonadecane	1894	1900	0.19	0.06	-	0.13
41	Hexadecanoic acid	1958	1959	0.10	0.17	0.27	0.18
43	Phytol	2114	2114	0.06	0.09	0.34	0.16
	Total			97.42	97.81	95.08	

According to the average percentage of chemical compositions, the major constitutes were (*Z*)-Ligustilide, unknown-A, (*E*)-Ligustilide, (*Z*)-Butylidene phthalide, 5-pentyl cyclohexa-1,3-diene and kessane in all the essential oils.

The classification of the identified compounds, based on chemical groups, is shown in Figure 1. The principle compounds in the essential oil of the three accessions of *K. odoratissima* were phthalides (82.12%), followed by 'others' (8.91%), sesquiterpene hydrocarbons (5.96%) and monoterpene hydrocarbons and oxygenated sesquiterpenes were very low in the percentage. Unknown components and hydrocarbons were classified into 'others' group.

Fatty acid composition

The oil yield of the leaf of *K. odoratissima* was 5% (per 100 g dry matter). Table 2 shows the fatty acid compositions of *K. odoratissima* leaf as mg/100 g and percentage. The number of fatty acids identified were fifteen. In the oil, obtained from leaf, Linoleic acid (25.46%), α-linolenic acid

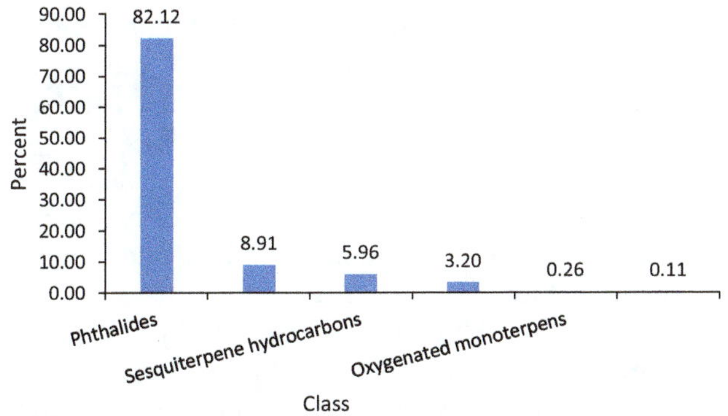

Figure 1. The classification of essential oil compositions of *K. odoratissima*, based on chemical groups.

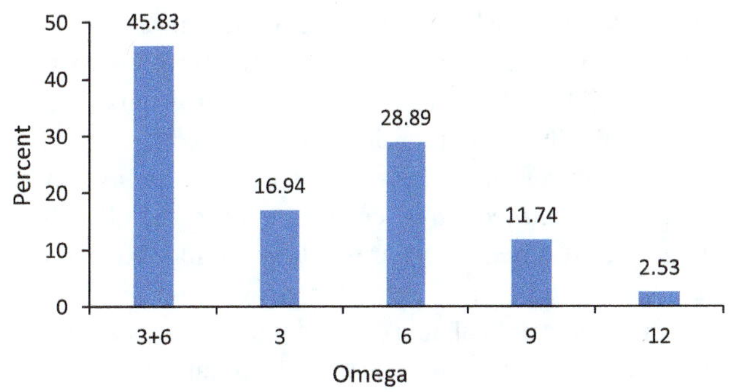

Figure 2. The classification of fatty acids of *K. odoratissima*, based on the omega type.

Table 2. Fatty acid compositions of *K. odoratissima* Mozaff. aerial parts

No.	Fatty acid	mg/100 g	%	Structure
1	Palmitic acid	61.74	11.92	C16:0
2	Palmitoleic acid	3.34	0.64	C16:1n7
3	Heptadecanoic acid	0.18	0.03	C17:0
4	Stearic acid	24.48	4.72	C18:0
5	Petroselinic acid	13.11	2.53	C18:1n12
6	Oleic acid	48.33	9.33	C18:1n9
7	Linoleic acid	131.92	25.46	C18:2n6c
8	Linolelaidic acid	3.13	0.60	C18:2n6t
9	α-Linolenic acid	86.33	16.66	C18:3n3
10	Arachidic acid	5.17	0.10	C20:0
11	Eicosenoic acid	3.38	0.65	C20:1n9
12	Eicosapentaenoic acid	1.45	0.28	C20:5n3
13	Henicosanoic acid	1.64	0.32	C21:0
14	Arachidonic acid	12.99	2.51	C20:4n6
15	Erucic acid	9.14	1.76	C22:1n9

(16.66%), palmitic acid (11.92%), oleic acid (9.33%), stearic acid (4.72%), petroselinic acid (2.53%), arachidonic acid (2.51%) and erucic acid (1.76%) were the major fatty acids. The presence of other fatty acids was very low. Fatty acids were classified in classes as SFA, MUFA and PUFA. The percentage of PUFA, MUFA and SFA was 45.83, 14.91 and 23.17, respectively.

The fatty acids identified from *K. odoratissima* oil were categorized based on the type of omega (Figure 2). Omega-6 had the highest percentage (28.89%). The total of EFAs including omega-3 and omega-6 was 45.83%.

Discussion

Based on our findings, (*Z*)-Ligustilide is the dominant component in the essential oil of *K. odoratissima*, which is in accordance with previous reports (7,8,13). The other components such as (*Z*)-Butylidene phthalides, (*E*)-Ligustilide, Kessane, 3-*n*-Butylphthalide and caryophyllene oxide reported as the main compounds of essential oil of *K. odoratissima* (6). (*Z*)-Ligustilide, (*Z*)-Butylidene phthalide, unknown, 5-Pentyl cyclohexa-1,3-diene, kessane, cuparene, β-cadinene and pulegone have been identified as the main components (14). The second main compound (2.39 to 10.34%) was not fully identified and it has also been reported by the other researchers, with a similar retention index, as an unknown compound (14,15).

Phthalides are rich in the essential oil of *K. odoratissima.* The anti-inflammatory effects of ligustilides from *Ligusticum chuanxiong* and *Angelica sinensis* have been confirmed (16,17). The studies indicate that (*Z*)-ligustilide can facilitate blood circulation, attenuate pain behavior in mice, act to limit ischemic brain damage in rats and exhibit the strongest antioxidant activity (18,19). Some of the studies have also focused on relaxation of smooth muscles in the gastrointestinal, respiratory and circulatory systems and hepatoprotective, immunomodulatory and cardiovascular properties (20). 3-Butylhexahydro phthalide and (*Z*)-Ternine, as known phthalide derivatives are reported for the first time from *K. odoratissima*, but have been reported from *Levisticum officinale* (21).

Petroselinic acid was one of fatty acids in the oil of *K. odoratissima.* The presence of Petroselinic acid (72.35%) in the seeds of *K. odoratissima* was also reported by Saaidi and Omidbaigi (11). It is an uncommon and rare fatty acid that comprises nearly 85% of the total fatty acids of Apiaceae seeds (22). This fatty acid is used to show chemotaxonomical relationships among the genera of the Apiaceae family (23). Petroselinic acid as an unsaturated fatty acid and isomers of oleic acid with a melting point higher than oleic acid can be useful in cosmetics, pharmaceuticals, and perfume and food industries (24).

According to the percentage of standard fatty acids in dietary fats (25,26), the total saturated fatty acids in *K. odoratissima* leaf represent lower value of 23.17% in comparison with the coconut, palm and cottonseed oils, while being higher than the other oils. In comparison with fatty acids in dietary fats, the percentage of MUFAs (14.91%) was more than all the dietary fats, except in coconut and safflower oils. Foods containing MUFAs reduce low-density lipoprotein (LDL) cholesterol, while possibly increasing high-density lipoprotein (HDL) cholesterol (27). PUFAs are also present in much more amounts than coconut, palm, olive and rapeseed oils. PUFAs protect against cardiovascular disease by providing more membrane fluidity than MUFAs, but they are more vulnerable to lipid peroxidation (28). EFAs in *K. odoratissima* leaf have higher value of 45.53% in comparison with the coconut, palm, olive, sunflower and rapeseed oils, while being lower than the cottonseed, soya, corn and safflower oils. Both omega-3 and omega-6 are important components of cell membranes and these needed for growth and repair. The human body is not capable of producing them. The plants and seed oils are very good sources to obtain the essential fatty acids (29,30).

In summary, this study investigated the fatty acid profile of the leaf and the chemical compositions of new three accessions of *K. odoratissima*. Overall, *K. odoratissima* is a rich source of essential fatty acids and phthalide derivatives, especially (*Z*)-ligustilide with the effects of diverse biological activities. This study provided valuable information about the phytochemical properties, which can be useful for the subsequent studies on the pharmacological effects of *K. odoratissima*.

Acknowledgements

We thank Saadat Sarikhani and Hadi Kazemi for help in the oil extraction and identification of fatty acids, respectively.

Authors' contributions

MGh did the experiment and prepared the first draft. All authors contributed in the conception and design of the work, drafting and revising the draft, approval of the final version of the manuscript, and agreed for all aspects of the work.

Conflict of interests

The authors declared no competing interests.

Ethical considerations

Ethical issues (including plagiarism, misconduct, data fabrication, falsification, double publication or submission, redundancy) have been completely observed by the authors.

Funding/Support

This study was granted by Tarbiat Modares University (TMU), Tehran, Iran (grant No. 82.120364).

References

1. Heinrich M. Ethnopharmacology: quo vadis? Challenges for the future. Rev Bras Farmacogn. 2014;24(2):99-102.
2. Sadeghi Z, Kuhestani K, Abdollahi V, Mahmood A. Ethnopharmacological studies of indigenous medicinal plants of Saravan region, Baluchistan, Iran. J Ethnopharmacol. 2014;153(1):111-118.
3. Mozaffarian V. Two new genera of Iranian Umbelliferae. Bot Zhourn. 2003;2:88-94.
4. Ahmadipour B, Hassanpour H, Asadi E, Khajali F, Rafiei F, Khajali F. Kelussia odoratissima Mozzaf–A promising medicinal herb to prevent pulmonary hypertension in broiler chickens reared at high altitude. J Ethnopharmacol. 2015;159:49-54.
5. Ghasemi Pirbalouti, A, Aghaee K, Kashi A, Malekpoor F. Chemical composition of the essential oil of wild and cultivated plant populations of Kelussia odoratissima Mozaff. J Med Plants Res. 2012;6;449-454.
6. Shojaei ZA, Ebrahimi A, Salimi M. Chemical composition of three ecotypes of wild celery (Kelussia odoratissima). J Herbs Spices Med Plants. 2011;17;62-68.
7. Omidbaigi R, Sefidkon F, Saeedi K. Essential oil content and composition of Kelussia odoratissima Mozaff. as an Iranian endemic plant. J Essent Oil Bearing Plants. 2008;11:594-597.
8. Sajjadi SE, Shokoohinia Y, Mehramiri P. Isolation and characterization of steroids, phthalide and essential oil of the fruits of Kelussia odoratissima Mozaff., an endemic mountain celery. Res Pharmaceut Sci. 2013;8:35-41.
9. Eqbql MA, Halimah AS, Abdulah MK, Zalifah MK. Fatty acid composition of four different vegetable oils (red palm olein, corn oil and coconut oil) by gas chromatography. IPCBE. 2011;14;31-34.
10. Ristic V, Ristic G. Role and importance of dietary polyunsaturated fatty acids in the prevention and therapy of atherosclerosis. Med Pregled. 2003;56(1-2):50-53.
11. Saeedi KA, Omidbaigi R. Evaluation of content and composition of fatty acids, total phenolic and essential oil content of Kelussia odoratissima Mozaff. seed. Iranian J Med Aroma Plants. 2009;25(1): 113-119.
12. British Pharmacopoeia. British Pharmacopoeia, vol 2. London: HMSO; 1988:137-138.
13. Raeisi S, Mirjalili MH, Nadjafi F, Hadian J. Variability in the essential oil content and composition in different plant organs of Kelussia odoratissima Mozaff. (Apiaceae) growing wild in Iran. J Essent Oil Res. 2015;27(4):283-288.
14. Raiisi S, Nadjafi F, Hadian J, Kanani MR, Ayyari M. Autecological and phytochemical studies of Kelussia odoratissima Mozaff. an endangered ethnomedicinal plant of Iran. J Biol Active Prod Nat. 2013;3:285-294.
15. Rabbani M, Sajjadi SE, Sadeghi M. Chemical composition of the essential oil from Kelussia odoratissima Mozaff. and the evaluation of its sedative and anxiolytic effects in mice. Clinics. 2011;66:843-848.
16. Huang J, Lu XQ, Zhang C, et al. Anti-inflammatory ligustilides from Ligusticum chuanxiong Hort. Fitoterapia. 2013;91:21-27.
17. Chao WW, Hong YH, Chen ML, Lina BF. Inhibitory effects of Angelica sinensis ethyl acetate extract and major compounds on NF-B trans-activation activity and LPS-induced inflammation. J Ethnopharmacol. 2010;129:244-249.

18. Du J, Yu Y, Ke Y, Wang C, Zhu L, Qian ZM. Ligustilide attenuates pain behavior induced by acetic acid or formalin. J Ethnopharmacol. 2007;112:211–4.
19. Li W, Wu Y, Liu X, et al. Antioxidant properties of cis-Z, Z'-3a. 7a', 7a. 3a'-Dihydroxy-ligustilide on human umbilical vein endothelial cells in vitro. Molecules. 2013;18:20-534.
20. Wedge DE, Klun JA, Tabanca N, et al. Bioactivity-guided fractionation and GC/MS fingerprinting of Angelica sinensis and Angelica archangelica root components for antifungal and mosquito deterrent activity. J Agric Food Chem. 2009;57:464–470.
21. Santos PA, Figueiredo AC, Oliveira MM, et al. Growth and essential oil composition of hairy root cultures of Levisticum officinale WDJ Koch (lovage). Plant Sci. 2005;168:1089-1096.
22. Nguyen QH, Talou T, Cerny M, Evon P, Merah O. Oil and fatty acid accumulation during coriander (Coriandrum sativum L.) fruit ripening under organic cultivation. Crop J. 2015;3(4):366-369.
23. Bagci E. Fatty acids and tocochromanol patterns of some Turkish Apiaceae (Umbelliferae) plants; a chemotaxonomic approach. Acta Botanica Gallica. 2007;154(2):143-151.
24. Coşge B, Kiralan M, Gürbüz B. Characteristics of fatty acids and essential oil from sweet fennel (Foeniculum vulgare Mill. var. dulce) and bitter fennel fruits (F. vulgare Mill. var. vulgare) growing in Turkey. Nat Prod Res. 2008;22(12):1011-1016.
25. Kris-Etherton PM, Harris WS, Appel LJ. Fish Consumption, Fish Oil, Omega-3 Fatty Acids, and Cardiovascular Disease. Circulation. 2002;106(21):2747-2757.
26. Priya Patil D, Chavan NS, Anjali BS. Sonneratia alba J. Smith, A Vital Source of Gamma Linolenic Acid (GLA). Asian J Pharm Clin Res. 2012;5(1):172-175.
27. Gilmore LA, Crouse SF, Carbuhn A, et al. Exercise attenuates the increase in plasma monounsaturated fatty acids and high-density lipoprotein cholesterol but not high-density lipoprotein 2b cholesterol caused by high-oleic ground beef in women. Nut Res. 2013; 33(12):1003-1011.
28. Yehuda S, Rabinovitz S, Carasso RL, Mostofsky DI. The role of polyunsaturated fatty acids in restoring the aging neuronal membrane. Neurobiol Aging. 2002;23(5):843-853.
29. Lunn J, Theobald H. The health effects of dietary unsaturated fatty acids. Nutr Bull. 2006;31:178-224.
30. Stanley JC, Elsom RL, Calder PC, et al. UK Food Standards Agency Workshop Report: the effects of the dietary n-6:n-3 fatty acid ratio on cardiovascular health. Br J Nutr. 2007;98:1305-1310.

Total phenolic compounds and in vitro antioxidant potential of crude methanol extract and the correspond fractions of *Quercus brantii* L. acorn.

Ali Karimi[1], Mohammad-Taghi Moradi[2*]

[1]Faculty of Paramedicine, Shahrekord University of Medical Science, Shahrekord, Iran
[2]PhD student, Medical Plants Research Center, Shahrekord University of Medical Science, Shahrekord, Iran

ARTICLE INFO

Keywords:
Antioxidant
Phenolic compounds
Fraction
Medicinal plants
Quercus brantii Lindl.

ABSTRACT

Introduction: Due to their roles in the maintenance of human health, phytochemicals and antioxidants in plants are raising interest. Phenolic and flavonoids are components with potential to protect against human diseases such as cardiovascular disease and cancers. *Q. brantii* is one of the traditional folk medicinal plants widely used in Iran. In this study, crude methanol extract and four correspond fractions of this plant were used to evaluate the total phenolic, total flavonoids, total flavonol, and antioxidant activities.

Methods: The identification of phenolic, flavonoid, and flavonol components and assay of antioxidant activity were carried out using standard in vitro procedures.

Results: The n-butanol fraction (376.2±7.1) had the highest amount of total phenolic compounds and the n-butanol fraction exhibited the lowest IC50 value (6.5±0.6 μg ml). There was significant relationship between the total phenolic contents and the free radical scavenging property in the four fractions in this study (R= -0.768, P< 0.01).

Conclusion: The results indicate that at least, n-butanol fraction of this plant with high phytoconstituents and less toxicity could be a promising source of medicinally important natural compound.

Implication for health policy/practice/research/medical education:
This study indicates that, at least some fractions of methanolic extract of *Q. brantii* acorn can be used as an accessible source of natural antioxidants. However, further works might be needed to the other extracts of this plant to reveal and evaluate its antioxidant potential.

Introduction

As an available source of innovative active biological compounds, medicinal plants are increasingly analyzed to determine the components on the structural level (1). These new compounds are pivotal for the discovery of new herbal medicines. Some kinds of side effects such as carcinogenesis have been attributed to synthetic antioxidants and thus, there is increasing interest to replace them with naturally occurring antioxidants (2,3). Antioxidant activity is one of the most important biological properties of these natural compounds. As natural antioxidants are capable of promoting food quality and stability and could act as nutraceuticals to end free radical chain reaction in biological systems, an increasing attention has been recently paid to directly evaluating the antioxidant properties of plant extracts as the source of natural antioxidants (4,5).

Many of naturally occurring antioxidants have been found to be free radical or active oxygen scavengers (6) and thus plants have been investigated for their biological activities and antioxidant properties (7-10). Flavonoides which are of the largest group of herbal polyphenols (11) contain tannins (12). Recent reports about antioxidant activity and polyphenol contents of herbals, used for fighting cancer, show that polyphenols, i.e. flavonoids, tannins, and phenolic acids, have antioxidant properties.

Belongs to the family of Fagaceae, Genus Quercus contains 500 species, some of which such as *Quercus brantii L.* are

***Corresponding author**: Mohammad-Taghi Moradi, Medical Plants Research Center, Shahrekord University of Medical Science, Rahmatieh, Shahrekord, Iran. Email: mtmoradi65@gmail.com predominant in central and northern regions of Iran (13). The fruit of Oak tree is called acorn and is placed within a cup called Gland. Vitamins, nutrients, and Carbohydrates have been reported to comprise a large portion (48%-85%) of acorn components. Acron also contains considerable amounts of phenolic, tannin, catechin, epicatechin, and gallocatechin components (13-16).

There are some reports indicating different biological activities of some species of Genus Oak include Iranian Oak with use of the acorn and bark in treatment of some diseases such as chronic dermatological diseases, eczema, and varis (2,7,14,17-19). Additionally, some of the biologically active substances of acorn are utilized in preparing functional foods (20-22). To the best of our knowledge, to date, there has been no reports on the phytochemical analysis and antioxidant potential of different fractions of *Q. brantii* acorn. The main aim of this work was to evaluate phytochemical screening and antioxidant activity of both crude methanol extract and four correspond fractions of *Q. brantii* acorn.

Materials and Methods

Plant collection

The fruits of Oak were gathered from southwest region of Iran. Then, in Herbarium of Medical Plants Research Center of Shahrekord University of Medical Sciences (Iran), genus and species of the plant were identified and confirmed.

Extraction and fractionation of plant material

The fruits were harvested and powdered three times per maceration method. The plant material was dissolved in 70% ethyl alcohol and kept at room temperature for 96 hours. After that, the mixture was filtered and concentrated under nearly vacuum pressure and at 40°C using rotary evaporator. Having crude methanol extract of the plant, four fractions of the crude extract, with different polarity through in-solution isolation and using the difference in various secondary metabolites' polarity, were prepared. To isolate hexane fraction, the extract concentrated, suspended in 70% ethyl alcohol, and mixed with equal volume of normal hexane with sufficient shaking. The remaining plant material, from which the methanol was removed, mixed with distilled water and with chloroform in equal volume, shaked, dried over anhydrous sodium sulfate and used as the chloroform fraction. To prepare butanol fraction, equal volume of butanol was added to the remaining aqueous phase of the material, shaked and concentrated at 40°C and in vacuum condition. The remaining aqueous phase was concentrated, with the similar condition, mentioned above and used as aqueous fraction. The extracts were kept in sterile bottles, under refrigerated conditions, until further use.

Determination of the free-radical scavenging activity

The free-radical scavenging activity was measured by the 2,2 diphenyl-1-picrylhydrazyl (DPPH) method described by Moon and Terao, with some modification (23). Different amounts of each extract and methanol were added to a solution of 0.3 mg/mL methanolic solution of DPPH to make up a total volume of 3.0 mL. After standing for 15 min at room temperature, the absorbance was measured at 517 nm using UV–Vis spectrophotometer (UNICO 2100: USA). High absorbance of the reaction mixture indicated low free radical scavenging activity. Butylated hydroxytoluene (BHT) was used as positive control. Inhibition of free radical by DPPH was calculated as follows: Antiradical activity (%) = $(A_{control} - A_{sample})/A_{control} \times 100$. The IC_{50} value, defined as the amount of antioxidant necessary to decrease the initial DPPH concentration by 50% and was calculated based on linear regression of plots of the percentage antiradical activity against the concentration of the tested compounds (24). The experiment was carried out in triplicate and the results are average values.

Determination of total phenolic content

The total phenolic content of the crude extract and four correspond fractions of *Q. brantii* fruits was determined using Folin-Ciocalteu method (25). Briefly, 0.1 ml of each of the diluted samples was added to 0.5 ml of 10% (v/v) Folin-Ciocalteu reagent. After 3-8 min, 0.4 ml of 7.5% (w/v) sodium carbonate solution was added to the mixture. After being kept in total darkness for 30 min, the absorbance of the reaction mixture was measured at 765 nm using a UV–Vis spectrophotometer (UNICO 2100: USA). Amounts of total phenolic were calculated using a gallic acid calibration curve. The results were expressed as gallic acid equivalents (GAE) g/g of dry plant matter.

Determination of total flavonol content

The total flavonol content was measured following a previously reported method (26). Briefly, 0.5 ml of each diluted plant material was independently mixed with 1.5 ml of methanol, 0.1 ml of 10% (w/v) aluminum chloride, 0.1 ml of 1M potassium acetate, and 2.8 ml of distilled water. After incubation at room temperature for two and a half h absorbance of the reaction mixture was read at 440 nm using a UV–Vis spectrophotometer (UNICO 2100: USA). The results were expressed in mg of rutin equivalents of dry plant matter by comparison with the standard curve, which was made in the same condition. All measurements were done in triplicate and statistical analysis was done by statistical software using one-way analysis of variance (ANOVA) and the post-hoc Tukey's test. All the data are expressed as ± SEM.

Results

DPPH radical scavenging activity

Our results showed that the scavenging effect of the fractions increases as the concentration increases. The four fractions of *Q. brantii* fruit significantly reduced the DPPH. The concentration of each fraction which showed inhibition of higher than 50% were found to be significant ($P<0.05$; Table 1). The n-butanol fraction exhibited the lowest IC_{50} value (6.5±0.6 µg ml) as compared to the other fractions under study. The crude extract, chloroform fraction, and aqueous fraction had IC_{50} values of 15±3, 12.7±1, and 22.4±1.7 µg/ml, respectively, and the n-hexane fraction showed highest value (144.54±5). The results are expressed relative to butylated hydroxytoluene (BHT), a reference standard having IC_{50} of 25.41±1.89 µg/ml. The IC_{50} values of the chloroform fraction, the n-butanol fraction, the crude extract, and the n-hexane fraction were found to be significant ($P<0.05$) while that of the aqueous soluble fraction non-significant ($P>0.05$) as compared with BHT (Table 2).

Total phenolic content

The total phenolic content of the *Q. brantii* extract and the four fractions were expressed as gallic acid equivalent and are presented in Table 2. The results showed total phenolic content of the fractions ranged from 24.4 to 376.2 mg gallic acid equivalent (mgGAE/g). Among the four fractions, the n-butanol (376.2±7.1) and the n-hexane (24.4±3.5) had the highest and the lowest amount of total phenolic compounds, respectively. The total phenolic contents of the crude extract, the chloroform fraction, the n-butanol fraction, and the aqueous fraction were significantly different from that of the n-hexane fraction ($P<0.05$; Table 2). There was good relation between the total phenolic contents and the free radical scavenging property in the four fractions in this study ($R= -0.768$, $P<0.01$).

Total flavonoid and flavonol content

The total flavonoid and flavonol contents of the crude extract and the four fractions of *Q. brantii* fruit were expressed as gallic acid equivalent, as rutin equivalent (mg/g) and are presented in Table 2. The most amount of flavonoid and flavonol (91.6 and 105 mg/mL, respectively) was extracted in chloroform fraction and the lease amount (5.8 and 1.1 mg/mL, respectively) was extracted in aqueous fraction ($P<0.05$).

Discussion

In this study, crude methanol extract and the four correspond fractions of fruit of *Q. brantii* with different polarities were prepared through in-solution isolation and using the difference in different secondary metabolites' polarity. Also, the ability of these plant materials to inhibit

Table 1. DPPH radical-scavenging activity of the crude extract and various fractions of *Quercus brantii* L. acorn.

Sample	Concentration (µg/ml)	Scavenging of DPPH radical activity inhibition (%) (main ± SEM)
Crude extract	25	80.9±0.5
	20	66.4±1.1
	15	49.7±0.9
	10	34.5±0.3
	5	19±1
n-hexane fraction	150	55.3±1.5
	125	47.5±2
	100	40±2/1
	75	37.7±.08
	50	17.4±.3
Chloroform fraction	25	91.5±1.5
	20	80.1±1.4
	15	62.5±0.8
	10	40.2±1.3
	5	22.9±2.4
n-Butanol fraction	10	75±1.5
	7.5	58.2±1.2
	5	47.3±0.3
	2.5	25.8±1.3
	1	8.6±1.2
Remaining aqueous fraction	40	86.8±2.5
	30	66.5±1.9
	20	44.3±0.7
	10	19±0.9
	5	11.8±1.4
BHT	50	90.8±1.5
	40	78.3±1.2
	30	55.5±0.7
	20	40.09±1.7
	10	22±1.06

All results are presented as mean ± standard mean error of three assays. DPPH: 1,1-Diphenyl-2-picrylhydrazyl, BHT; Butylated hydroxytoluene

Table 2. DPPH-radical scavenging activity IC_{50}, total phenolics, flavonoid, and flavonol values of the different fractions of *Quercus brantii* L. acorn.

Sample	DPPH-radical scavenging activity IC_{50}/(µg/ml)	Total phenolics (mg GAE/g)	Flavonoid content (mg/g)	Flavonol content (mg/g)
Crude extract	$15\pm3^{\#a}$	201.6±4	14.7 ± 2.2^{a}	33.6±2
n-hexane fraction	$144.5\pm5^{\#}$	24.4±3.5	16.8 ± 2^{a}	2.4 ± 0.5^{a}
Chloroform fraction	$12.7\pm1^{\#ab}$	222.5±2.5	91.6±1.5	105±4.5
n-Butanol fraction	$6.5\pm0.5^{\#b}$	376.2±7.1	22±2	70.9±55
Remaining aqueous fraction	22.4±1.7	120±3.5	5.8±0.5	1.1 ± 0.4^{a}
P-value*	<0.01	<0.01	<0.01	<0.01

All results are presented as mean ± standard mean error of three assays.

*In terms of analysis of variance; ^{a,b} values with the same letter in each column are not significantly different according to Tukey test ($P< 0.05$); # Significant when compared with the reference standard (BHT, IC_{50} of 25.41±1.89 µg/ml).

Abbreviations: DPPH, 1,1-Diphenyl-2-picrylhydrazyl; IC_{50}, the concentration of a sample at which 50% inhibition of free radical activity is observed; GAE, gallic acid equivalent.

free radicals was assessed using DPPH method.
Among the 4 fractions, the n-butanol (376.2±7.1) and the n-hexane (24.4±3.5) had the highest and the lowest amount of total phenolic compounds, respectively. Based on the scavenging capacity of the free radicals, the n-butanol exhibited the highest antioxidant activity with the highest percent inhibition of the DPPH radical, followed by the chloroform fraction with higher percent inhibition of the DPPH radical compared to that of BHT. Also, the n-hexane fraction contained lower percent inhibition of the DPPH radical compared to BHT and the other fractions, indicating proper relation between the total phenolic contents and the free radical scavenging property, given that as IC_{50} value decreases, the ability to inhibit free radicals increases.
Similar to our study, some authors (27,28) have demonstrated a linear relation between the content of total phenolic compounds and their antioxidant capacity of some plant extracts. Therefore, the antioxidant potential of our plant extracts most probably is due to presence of phenolic components (376.2±7.1). Additionally, as tannins have been reported to be considerable components of phenolics in *Q. brantii* fruit (12), notable antioxidant potential of our fractions could be also due to the tannins. Our results, based on the DPPH method, showed that with increasing the polarity of the extracts, their radical scavenging activity will increase. Similar findings were reported on the rate of antioxidant property of the bark of *Quercus robur* (14). In this study, the crude methanol extract of *Q. brantii* fruit and some of the fractions showed promising antioxidant activity, by inhibiting DPPH, which is related to its total phenolic content. The presence of phenols and flavonoids in the plant, as its major constituents, plays a major role in controlling antioxidants. Phenolic compounds are very important plant constituents because their phenolic groups are responsible for high antioxidant activity and their hydroxyl groups confer scavenging ability.

Conclusion

The results of this study showed that at least some fractions of methanolic extract of *Q. brantii* acorn could be used as easily accessible source of natural antioxidants. However, as some of the fractions show lower activity in DPPH and total phenol content as compared with standard, further works may be taken up to the other extracts of this plant to reveal and evaluate its antioxidant potential.

Acknowledgments

Authors are thankful to the Director of Medical Plants Research Center and to the Deputy of Research of Shahrekord University of Medical Sciences, Shahrekord, Iran for financial support.

Authors' contributions

All authors contributed equally.

Conflict of interests

The authors declare that there are no conflicts of interests.

Ethical considerations

Ethical issues (including plagiarism, misconduct, data fabrication, falsification, double publication or submission, redundancy) have been completely observed by the authors.

Funding/Support

Deputy of Research and Technology of Shahrekord University of Medical Sciences, Shahrekord, Iran.

References

1. Clark AM. Natural products as a resource for new drugs. Pharm Res 1996; 13(8): 1133-44.
2. Karimi A, Moradi MT, Saeedi M, Asgari S, Rafieian-Kopaei M. Antiviral activity of Quercus persica L.: High efficacy and low toxicity. Adv Biomed Res 2013; 2: 36.
3. Znati M, Hichem BJ, Cazaux S, Bouajila J. Chemical composition, biological and cytotoxic activities of plant extracts and compounds isolated from Ferula lutea. Molecules 2014; 19(3): 2733-47.
4. Ito N, Fukushima S, Hagiwara A, Shibata M, Ogiso T. Carcinogenicity of butylated hydroxyanisole in F344 rats. J Natl Cancer Inst 1983; 70(2): 343-52.
5. McClements DJ, Decker EA. Lipid Oxidation in Oil-in-Water Emulsions: Impact of Molecular Environment on Chemical Reactions in Heterogeneous Food Systems. J Food Sci 2000; 65(8): 1270-82.
6. Zheng W, Wang SY. Antioxidant activity and phenolic compounds in selected herbs. J Agric Food Chem 2001; 49(11): 5165-70.
7. Basri D, Fan S. The potential of aqueous and acetone extracts of galls of Quercus infectoria as antibacterial agents. Indian J Pharmacol 2005; 37(1): 26-9.
8. Rafieian-Kopaei M, Baradaran A, Rafieian M. Oxidative stress and the paradoxical effects of antioxidants. J Res Med Sci 2013; 18(7): 629.
9. Rafieian-Kopaei M, Baradaran A, Rafieian M. Plants antioxidants: From laboratory to clinic. J Nephropathol 2013; 2(2): 152-3.
10. Riaz T, Abbasi A, Aziz-Ur-Rehman A, Shahzadi T, Ajaib M, Khan M. Phytochemical screening, free radical scavenging, antioxidant activity and phenolic content of Dodonaea viscosa. J Serb Chem Soc 2012; 77(4): 423-35.
11. Kovacevic N. Basic Pharmakognosy. Belgrade: University of Belgrade–Faculty of Pharmacy; 2000.
12. Rakic S, Petrovic S, Kukic J, Jadranin M, Tešević V, Povrenović D, *et al.* Influence of thermal treatment on phenolic compounds and antioxidant properties of oak acorns from Serbia. Food Chem 2007; 104(2): 830-4.
13. Saffarzadeh A, Vincze L, Csapo J. Determination of the chemical composition of acorn (Quercus branti), Pistacia atlantica and Pistacia Khinjk seeds as non-conventional feedstuffs. Acta Agr Kapos. 1999; 3(3): 59-69.
14. Andrensek S, Simonovska B, Vovk I, Fyhrquist P,

Vuorela H, Vuorela P. Antimicrobial and antioxidative enrichment of oak (Quercus robur) bark by rotation planar extraction using ExtraChrom. Int J Food Microbiol 2004; 92(2): 181-7.
15. Cadahia E, Munoz L, Fernandez de Simon B, Garcia-Vallejo MC. Changes in low molecular weight phenolic compounds in Spanish, French, and American oak woods during natural seasoning and toasting. J Agric Food Chem 2001; 49(4): 1790-8.
16. Popovic BM, Stajner D, Zdero R, Orlovic S, Galic Z. Antioxidant characterization of oak extracts combining spectrophotometric assays and chemometrics. Scientific World Journal. 2013; 2013: 134656.
17. Aslani A, Emami S, Ghannadi A, Ajdari M. Formulation and physicochemical evaluation of an herbal antihemorrohid ointment from Quercus, Black cumin and Fenugreek for the treatment of internal anal hemorrhoids. J Pharm Sci Tabriz Univ Med Sci 2009; 14: 247-57.
18. Kaur G, Hamid H, Ali A, Alam MS, Athar M. Antiinflammatory evaluation of alcoholic extract of galls of Quercus infectoria. J Ethnopharmacol 2004; 90(2-3): 285-92.
19. Khosravi A, Behzadi A. Evaluation of the antibacterial activity of the seed hull of Quercus brantii on some gram negative bacteria. Pak J Med Sci 2006; 22(4): 429-32.
20. Cantos E, Espin JC, Lopez-Bote C, de la Hoz L, Ordonez JA, Tomas-Barberan FA. Phenolic compounds and fatty acids from acorns (Quercus spp.), the main dietary constituent of free-ranged Iberian pigs. J Agric Food Chem 2003; 51(21): 6248-55.
21. Rakić S. Effect of oak acorn extracts on lipide oxidation kinetics. J Agric Sci 2000; 45(2): 139-43.
22. Rakić S, Maletić RO, Perunović MN, Svrzić G. Influence of thermal treatment on tannin content and antioxidation effect of oak acorn Quercus cerris extract. J Agric Sci 2004; 49(1): 97-107.
23. Moon JH, Terao J. Antioxidant Activity of Caffeic Acid and Dihydrocaffeic Acid in Lard and Human Low-Density Lipoprotein. J Agric Food Chem 1998; 46(12): 5062-5.
24. Nahak G, Sahu RK. In vitro antioxidative acitivity of Azadirachta indica and Melia azedarach Leaves by DPPH scavenging assay. Nat Sci 2010; 8(4): 22-8.
25. Folin O, Ciocalteu V. On tyrosine and tryptophane determinations in proteins. J Biol Chem 1927; 73(2): 627-50.
26. Rabiei Z, Rafieian-kopaei M, Heidarian E, Saghaei E, Mokhtari S. Effects of zizyphus jujube extract on memory and learning impairment induced by bilateral electric lesions of the nucleus basalis of meynert in rat. Neurochemical research 2014; 39(2): 353-60.
27. Rahnama S, Rabiei Z, Alibabaei Z, Mokhtari S, Rafieian-kopaei M, Deris F. Anti-amnesic activity of Citrus aurantium flowers extract against scopolamine-induced memory impairments in rats. Neurological Sciences Neurol Sci 2014 Nov 4.
28. Shirzad H, Taji F, Rafieian-Kopaei M. Correlation between antioxidant activity of garlic extracts and WEHI-164 fibrosarcoma tumor growth in BALB/c mice. J Med Food 2011; 14(9): 969-74.

Antifungal effects of *Zataria multiflora* and *Nigella sativa* extracts against *Candida albicans*

Hassan Moghim[1], Simin Taghipoor[1], Najmeh Shahinfard[2], Soleiman Kheiri[3], Ramin Panahi[1]

[1]Medical Plants Research Center, Shahrekord University of Medical Sciences, Shahrekord, Iran
[2]Department of E-learning in Medical Education, Virtual School, Tehran University of Medical Sciences, Tehran, Iran
[3]Social Health Determinants Research Center, Shahrekord University of Medical Sciences, Shahrekord, Iran

ARTICLE INFO

Keywords:
Candida albicans
Zataria multiflora
Nigella sativa

ABSTRACT

Introduction: Candidiasis is a fungal infection caused by *Candida albicans*. Recent studies suggest that the side effects of herbal drugs with significant therapeutic effects are far less than chemical drugs. This study was therefore, conducted to examine antifungal activities of *Zataria multiflora* and *Nigella sativa* extracts on *C. albicans*.
Methods: Powders of *Z. multiflora* and *N. sativa* were macerated with ethanol 70% and evaporated at 38°C by rotary evaporator. The suspension of *C. albicans* was prepared according to McFarland at a concentration of approximately 0.5-2.5 × 10^3 CFU/ml. Testing was performed according to microbroth dilution in 96-well micro-dilution plates. Minimum inhibitory concentration (MIC), MIC50%, MIC90% and minimum fungicidal concentration (MFC) were separately evaluated by counting the fungal colonies for *Z. multiflora* and *N. sativa*.
Results: The measured values of MIC, MIC50%, MIC90% and MFC of *Z. multiflora* on the *C. albicans* were 0.13, 0.38, 0.74 and 1.03 mg/ml, and those of *N. sativa* were 10, 27.7, 52.3 and 72.3 mg/ml, respectively.
Conclusion: The results indicate that both *Zataria multiflora* and *Nigella sativa* extracts are effective against *Candida albicans*, but the former species has the highest antifungal activity. If the clinical trials confirm the results of this study, *Z. multiflora*, as a new antifungal agent by replacing chemical drugs can be used to develop antifungal medicinal herbs.

Implication for health policy/practice/research/medical education:
The results indicate that *Zataria multiflora* and *Nigella sativa* extracts are effective against *Candida albicans*, but the former species has the highest antifungal activity. If the clinical trials confirm the results of this study, *Z. multiflora*, as a new antifungal agent by replacing chemical drugs, can be used to develop antifungal medicinal herbs.

Introduction

Candidiasis is a primary or secondary infection involving a member of the genus *Candida*. Essentially, this disease is an infection caused by *Candida albicans*. The clinical manifestations of the disease are extremely varied, ranging from acute and/or chronic to episodic involvement probably localized to the mouth, throat, skin, scalp, bronchi, lungs, or the gastrointestinal tract or systemic as in septicemia, endocarditis, and meningitis. Since *C. albicans* is an endogenous species, the disease represents an opportunistic infection (1-3).
Thymus vulgaris (*Zataria multiflora*) is a shrub plant in the family Lamiaceae. It is an aromatic and mountain herb which is commonly used as a spice to flavor food (4,5). Recent studies suggest that the side effects of herbal drugs with significant therapeutic effects are far less than chemical drugs (6). Researches have shown that *Z. multiflora* is effective in treating many diseases, particularly in bacterial and fungal infections and parasitic diseases (7).
Nigella sativa is from the order Ranunculales in the family Ranunculaceae. This aromatic plant with tiny and dark seeds is usually used to flavor food such as bread. *Nigella sativa* is a plant from the buttercup family which grows as self-propelled in various parts of Europe and Asia including Iran (8).
In recent years much research has been done on the ef-

***Corresponding author:** Hassan Moghim, Medical Plants Research Center, Shahrekord University of Medical Sciences, Shahrekord, Iran.
Email: Hassan.moghim@yahoo.com

fectiveness of *N. sativa* extract including thymoquinone, thymohydroquinone, dithymoquinone, thymol and carvacrol, nigellicine, nigellimine-N-oxide, nigellidine and alpha-hedrine compounds (6).

Many reports have been published regarding several pharmacological effects of *N. sativa* extract, some of which have been identified through application of modern techniques, including antimicrobial activity of *N. sativa* oil (extract) and other through medicinal compounds such as thymoquinone and thymohydroquinone, on some bacteria including *Staphylococcus aureus* and particularly recently on *Pseudomonas aeruginosa*, Both *Escherichia coli* and *C. albicans*. Thymoquinone have been reported to be effective on *Aspergillus* (7), and some opportunistic fungi which can cause mycotic infection in patients with AIDS and other immunodeficiency syndromes (7). This study was conducted to examine antifungal activities of *Zataria multiflora* and *Nigella sativa* extracts on *C. albicans.*

Materials and Methods

To prepare extracts, *Z. multiflora* and *N. sativa* were purchased from a reputable grocery and after separation of brushwood with an electric mill, they were pulverized. The resulting powder was passed through a No. 10 sieve and then poured into the flasks and mixed with 300 cc of 70% ethanol. The solution was kept for 72 hours in a dry environment. The solution was passed through the filter paper and then transferred into percolation system for extraction. At a temperature of 38°C of the system, the extract was transferred into the incubator with removing alcohol completely. Finally, various concentrations of the extracts were prepared using distilled water and 0.5 ml of dimethyl sulfoxide (9).

Preparation of *C. albicans* suspensions

The standard fungal strain (code No. PTCC5027) used in this study was provided from Scientific Research Center of Iran. *C. albicans* was cultured on dextrose agar medium at 35°C. After 24 hours, some colonies were transferred to 1 ml normal saline to prepare a solution with a concentration of 0.5 McFarland 1.5×10^{6} CFU/ml (neobar slides were used for colony counting). The resulting solution was diluted to a ratio of 1:1000 and suspensions with concentrations of $(0.5\text{-}2.5)\times10^{3}$ CFU/ml were provided (10).

Preparation of *Z. multiflora* and *N. sativa* extracts

Different dilutions were prepared from *Z. multiflora* and *N. sativa* extracts using microbroth dilution according to the method proposed by the National Committee for Clinical Laboratory Standards for yeasts (NCCLSM27-A). Thus, two-fold dilution of the extract was poured into the first well of 96-well plates, and subsequent dilutions were prepared by serial dilution (10,11).

Different concentrations of the extracts prepared were as follows:

Z. multiflora: 0.093, 0.13, 0.185, 0.38, 0.5, 0.74, 1, 1.03, 1.25, 1.5 mg/ml and *N. sativa* : 5, 10, 20, 30, 40, 50, 60 and 70 mg/ml.

100 µl of each dilution of the extract was added separately to the socket of 96-well plates containing 100 ml of Sabouraud broth liquid medium (Sabouraud broth). Then 100 ml of yeast cell suspension in volumes equivalent to 2500 cells/ml was inoculated into all the sockets, except the control plates. The plates were shaker-incubated at 35°C for 48 hours. After incubation, 10 µl of the contents of each socket was cultured on Sabouraud dextrose agar medium and left for 48 hours at 35°C. After this period, minimum inhibitory concentration (MIC) and minimum fungicidal concentration (MFC) (CFU) were separately evaluated based on counting the fungal colonies for *Z. multiflora* and *N. sativa* extracts and compared with the control group (11,12).

Results

Z. multiflora extract

The measured values of MIC, MIC50%, MIC90% and MFC of *Z. multiflora* extract on the *C. albicans* were 0.13, 0.38, 0.74 and 1.03 mg/ml, respectively (Figure 1).

N. sativa extract

The measured values of MIC, MIC50%, MIC90% and MFC of the *N. sativa* were 10, 27.7, 52.3 and 72.3 mg/ml, respectively (Figure 2).

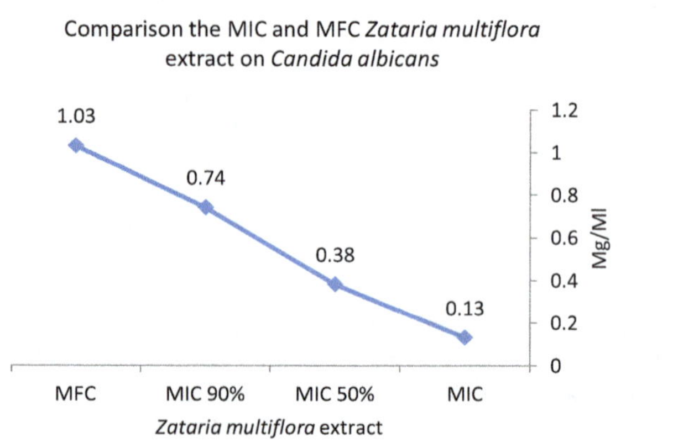

Figure 1. Comparison of the minimum inhibitory concentration (MIC) and minimum fungicidal concentration (MFC) of *Zataria multiflora* extract on *Candida albicans.*

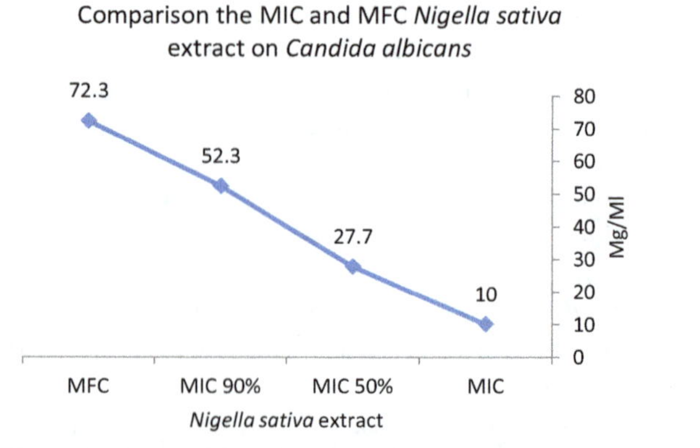

Figure 2. Comparison of the minimum inhibitory concentration and minimum fungicidal concentration of *Nigella sativa* extract on *Candida albicans*

Comparison of inhibitory and fungicidal effects of extracts
The logistic regression test showed that there were significant differences between the inhibitory and fungicidal effects of each of the plants extracts ($P<0.05$). *Z. multiflora* had the highest inhibitory and fungicidal effects on *C. albicans* but *N. sativa* had the lowest antifungal effect (Figure 3). The measured values of MIC, MIC50%, MIC90% and MFC of *Z. multiflora* and *N. sativa* extracts are compared in Table 1.

Discussion

Candidiasis is a primary or secondary infection involving a member of the genus *Candida*. Essentially, this disease is an infection caused by *C. albicans*. The clinical manifestations of the disease are varied, including acute, chronic and episodic involvement which is occasionally localized to the mouth, throat, skin, scalp, bronchi, lungs, or the gastrointestinal tract or systemic as in septicemia, endocarditis, and meningitis. Since *C. albicans* is an endogenous species, the infection is opportunistic (1-3).

Various studies have shown that many species of *Candida* have developed resistance to antifungal drugs. Nowadays traditional medicine and the use of herbal medicines to treat fungal infections are important because herbal medicines have fewer side effects and are less likely to develop drug resistance compared with chemical ones (1-3).

Due to difficulties in treatment of candidiasis, it is necessary to find new antifungal drugs. This increases the spectrum of antifungal drugs and eliminates the drug resistant strains. Herb plants can be beneficial for their therapeutic effects.

Akbari evaluated antifungal activities of *Thymus vulgaris*

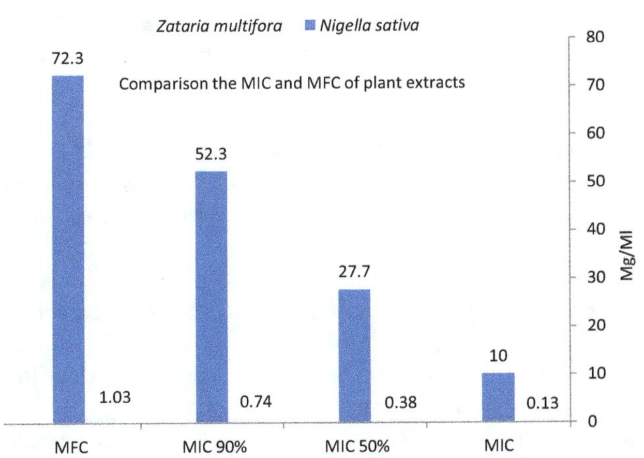

Figure 3. Comparison of minimum inhibitory concentration (MIC), MIC50%, MIC90%, and minimum fungicidal concentration of *Zataria multifora* and *Nigella sativa* extracts on *Candida albicans*.

Table 1. MIC, MIC50%, MIC90% and MFC of *Zataria multifora* and *Nigella sativa* extracts on *Candida albican* (mg/ml)

Plant	MIC	MIC50%	MIC90%	MFC
Zataria multiflora	0.13*	0.38	0.74	1.03
Nigella sativa	10	27.7	52.3	72.3

Abbreviations: MIC, minimum inhibitory concentration; MFC, minimum fungicidal concentration.

L. and *Origanum vulgare* L against fluconazol-resistant susceptible *C. albicans* isolates and found that the essence and extract of both plants were able to inhibit the growth of the isolates susceptible to fluconazole in a predictably concentration-dependent manner. The methanol extracts of *Origanum* had the highest antifungal effect with 0.49 mg/ml MIC (13). In our study, the obtained MIC of Z. *multiflora* extract was 0.13 mg/ml for *C. albicans*, which is greater than the effect on *C. albicans* obtained for this extract in Akbari's study. The contrasting results could be due to the different species of *Z. multiflora*, plant chemical compounds and/or methodologies.

In another study by Fuladi et al (14), the inhibitory effects of clotrimazole cream and herbal vaginal thyme cream were compared and the obtained MIC of *Z. multiflora* methanol and ethanol extracts were estimated to be 0.079 and 0.125 mg/ml, respectively.

Katiraei et al (15) compared the MIC of essential oils of *Z. multiflora*, Geranium and Artemisia with regard to the growth of the *C. albicans* isolates resistant to azole drugs. They showed that the MIC levels of essential oils of the plants were statistically significant from those of azoles. In that study, the obtained MIC of *Z. multiflora* for *C. albicans* was 0.18 mg/ml.

The effect of alcoholic extract of thyme on the growth of *Aspergillus* was investigated and found that the use of plant extracts in food was useful for control of fungal growth without production of toxins in foods (16).

In another study performed by Gandomi Nasr Abadi et al (17), the effect of essential oils of *Z. multiflora* on *Aspergillus flavus* was evaluated . It was found that all concentrations of oils had a significant effect on the growth and sporulation of *A. flavus*. Also, they reported the levels of MIC and MFC 400 and 1000 PPM, respectively. This extract has inhibitory effects on the mold and hence, it is recommended as alternatives to chemical preservatives in the food industry (17).

In a study by AL-Quarashi et al (18) on the antifungal activity of *N. sativa* extract (thymoquinone) against *Aspergillus niger* and amphotericin b was investigated. It was found that the oil extract of *N. sativa* affected the growth of *A. niger* by 100% and could inhibit the growth of *A. niger* by 93.8%. The antifungal activity of *N. sativa* could be attributed to the thymoquinone.

To the best of our knowledge, No study has yet been conducted to assess the MIC and minimum bactericidal concentration of *N. sativa* on *C. albicans*. Further studies will be needed to investigate antifungal activities of *N. sativa*.

In our study, the obtained values of MIC, MIC50%, MIC90% and MFC of *Z. multiflora* extract on the *C. albicans* were respectively 0.13, 0.38, 0.74 and 1.03 mg/ml, which are consistent with other studies. Therefore *Z. multiflora* extract has antifungal effect against *C. albicans* and can be used as an antifungal agent to treat fungal infections such as candidiasis.

In the present study, the obtained values of MIC, MIC50%, MIC90% and MFC of *N. sativa* were 10, 27.7, 52.3 and 72.3 mg/ml, respectively. Both *Z. multiflora* and *N. sativa* extracts are able to inhibit the growth of *C. albicans*, but the former species has a greater impact on fungal infections. The major constituents of *Z. multiflora* are carvacrol, thymol, and phenolic compounds with antifungal activities (5). In recent years much research has been done on the effectiveness of *N. sativa* extract including thymoquinone, thymohydroquinone, dithymoquinone, thymol and carvacrol compounds. It has been shown that the antifungal activity of *N. sativa* could be attributed to thymol and carvacrol contents (6).

Conclusion

In this study, antifungal effects of *Z. multiflora* and *N. sativa* extracts were determined for *C. albicans*. It was shown that, an increase in the concentration of plant extracts caused fungal growth inhibition. Antifungal drugs are expensive with side effects and harmful for patients which frequently lead to drug resistance. As herbal medicines have fewer side effects and are less likely to develop drug resistance compared with chemical ones, they could be useful for treatment.

The results of the current study show that *Z. multiflora* extract plays a significant role in preventing of *C. albicans* growth. If the clinical trials confirm the results of this study *Z. multiflora*, as a new antifungal agent by replacing chemical drugs can be used to develop antifungal medicinal herbs.

Acknowledgements

This paper was derived from MD thesis of Ramin Panahi. The authors gratefully thank the Medical Plants Research Center staff for their assistance.

Authors' contributions

HM prepared the proposal and the manuscript draft as well as conducting the study. All authors contributed to the conception of the work, revising the draft, approval of the final version of the manuscript, and agreed for all aspects of the work.

Conflict of interests

The authors declare no competing interests.

Ethical considerations

Ethical issues (including plagiarism, misconduct, data fabrication, falsification, double publication or submission, redundancy) have been completely observed by the authors.

Funding/Support

The research was funded by Deputy of Shahrekord University of Medical Sciences, Iran (code number: 290-75-01-1389).

References

1. Moghim H, Taghipour S, Shahinfard N, Kheiri S, Heydari S, Rafieian S. Antifungal effects of Allium ascalonicum, Marticaria chamomilla and Stachys lavandulifolia extracts on Candida albicans. J HerbMed Pharmacol. 2014;3(1):9-14.
2. Moghim H. Role of cellular immunity in prevention of Candidiasis in Leukemia and Lymphomatic patients using flowcytometry method. J Shahrekord Univ Med Sci. 2001;3(3):42-48.
3. Moghim H. Detection of CH50 and role of C3, C4 complement in patients with Candidiasis. J Shahrekord Univ Med Sci. 2000;2(1):62-65.
4. Hematkhah F. Medicinal Plants. 2nd ed. Iran: Asreketab Publisher; 2004: 48-118.
5. Velag G. Medicinalplans. 2nd ed. Iran: Ghoghnoos publisher; 2007:80-87.
6. Saad B, Azaizeh H, Said O. Tradition and perspectives of Arab herbal medicine: a review. Evid Based Complement Alternat Med. 2005;2:475-479.
7. Samsam SH. Breedingand propagation of medicinal plants. Iran: Mani Publisher; 2005:125-7.
8. Shabooee E. Medicinal Plants and Fruits. Iran: Barbod Publisher; 2001.
9. Sharafati R, Sherafati F, Rafieian-Kopaei M. Biological characterization of Iranian walnut (Juglans regia) leaves. Turk J Biol. 2011;35:635-639.
10. Willinger B, Apfalter P, Hirschl AM, Makristathis A, Rotter M, Seibold M. Susceptibility testing of Candida species: comparison of NCCLS microdilution method with Fungitest. Diagn Microbiol Infect Dis. 2000;38(1):11-15.
11. Moghim H, Taghipour S, Shahinfard N, Kheiri S, Khabbazil H. Comparative study on the antifungal activity of hydroalcoholic extract of Iranian Propolis and Royal jelly against Rhizopus oryzae. J HerbMed Pharmacol. 2015;4(3):89-92.
12. Razzaghparast A, Shams Ghahfarokhi M, Yadegari MH, Razzaghi Abyaneh M. Antifungal effects of Allium cepa and some azoles in intact forms and in combinations to each other against pathogenic yeasts. Kowsar Med J. 2008;13(2):103-113.
13. Akbari S. Antifungal activity of Thymus vulgaris L. and Origanum vulgare L. against fluconazol-resistant and susceptible Candida albicans isolates. J Med Plants. 2007;6(1):53-62.
14. Fuladi Z, Afshari P, Gharibi T, Dabbagh MA. The comparison oF Zataria multiflora boiss (Avishan Shirazi) and Clotrimazol vaginal cream in the treatment of candidiasis vaginitis. Iranian South Medical of Journal. 2009;12(3):214-224.
15. Katiraei F, Eydi S, Bahonar Ar, Zarinfar H, Khosravi A. Comparision of MICS of some Iranian herbal essences against azole resistance and azole susceptible of Candida albicans. Journal of Medicinal Plants. 2008;7(27):37-44.
16. Javanmard M, Ramazan Y. Application of edible coatings incorporated Avishan-E Shirazi (Zalaria multiflora) alcoholic extract for inhibition of Aspergillus flavus growth on the pistachio kernel. J Med Plants. 2009;8(30):61-65.
17. Gandomi Nasr Abadi H, Misaghi A, Akhoundzadeh Basti A, Khosravi AR. Effects of Zataria multiflora Boiss essential oil on Aspergillus flavus. Journal of Medicinal Plants. 2008;7(27):45-51.
18. AL-Quarashi AR, Akhtar N, Al-Jabre S, AL-Akloby O, Randhawa MA. Anti-fungal activity of Thymoquinone and Amphotericin B against Aspergillus niger. Scientific Journal of King Faisal University. 2007;8(1):143-8.

Effect of *Crocus sativus* Stigma (saffron) alone or in combination with chloroquine on chloroquine sensitive strain of *Plasmodium berghei* in mice

Nader Pestechian[1], Somayeh Abedi-Madiseh[1], Mustafa Ghanadian[2,3*], Mehdi Nateghpour[4]

[1]Department of Medical Mycoparasitology, School of Medicine, Isfahan University of Medical Sciences, Isfahan, Iran
[2]Pharmaceutical Sciences Research Center, Isfahan University of Medical Sciences, Isfahan, Iran
[3]Pharmacognosy Department, Isfahan Faculty of Pharmacy, Isfahan University of Medical Sciences, Isfahan, Iran
[4]Department of Medical Parasitology and Mycology, School of Public Health, Tehran University of Medical Sciences, Tehran, Iran

ARTICLE INFO

Keywords:
Crocus sativus
Saffron
Plasmodium berghei
Combination therapy
Chlor

ABSTRACT

Introduction: In malaria treatment protocols, treatment failure or drug resistance of synthesized drugs like alkaloids related to quinine, and aminoquinolines are the main problems now. Therefore, discovering efficient drugs or combination therapy of blood schizonticidal drugs with different mechanisms or different targets in the parasite is a crucial effort to solve this problem. In this study, the effectiveness of *Crocus sativus* Stigma (saffron) individually and in combination with chloroquine, was considered against chloroquine-sensitive strain of *Plasmodium berghei*.
Methods: At the first stage, using 4 day suppressive Peter's test in mice, ED_{50} and survival times of saffron methanol extract, and its aqueous and ethyl acetate fractions and chloroquine on *P. berghei* were calculated. Then, based on the toxicity and survival time results, combination therapy was conducted with the best saffron fraction and chloroquine against the parasite.
Results: The saffron extract, aqueous and ethyl acetate fractions resulted in suppression of parasitemia with ED_{50} values of 587.0±78.7, 323.7±37.2, and 508.7±35.6 mg/kg, respectively. Combination of ethyl acetate fraction with chloroquine, potentiated the antimalarial property and the survived percent of the treated mice on days 7, 14, and 28 significantly more than chloroquine or ethyl acetate fraction alone.
Conclusion: Saffron and its fractions individually can be effective in reducing the parasitemia in mice. The outcome of combination of ethyl acetate fraction with chloroquine on the mice showed synergistic effect on the chloroquine-sensitive strain of parasite.

Implication for health policy/practice/research/medical education:
Saffron and its fractions are effective in reducing the parasitemia in mice. The combination of ethyl acetate fraction with chloroquine has synergistic effect on the chloroquine-sensitive strain of parasite. Hence, the combination therapy might be useful in the treatment of malaria.

Introduction

In the mid of 19th century, it was supposed that malaria would be eradicated but now the disease is reached to an epidemic problem in the tropical regions in Africa and south of Asia. It is due to the several factors including increasing the drug resistance of malarial parasites, and limitation of use of insecticides because of toxicological problems and consequent failure in controlling anopheline mosquitoes. Malaria is caused by *Plasmodium falciparum*, *P. vivax, P. malariae* or *P. ovale*. Among them *P. falciparum* is reported to have more morbidity because of resistance of plasmodiums to chloroquine or other drugs. *P. vivax* is usually sensitive to treatment and *P. malariae* and *P. ovale* are uncommon (1). Current anti malarial drugs include quinine an alkaloid extracted from the bark of cinchona tree which is frequently used in the prevention and treatment of malaria. Quinimax, quinidine and mefloquine are other alkaloids related to quinine in the treatment or pre-

***Corresponding author**: Mustafa Ghanadian, Department of Pharmacognosy, School of Pharmacy, Isfahan University of Medical Sciences, Isfahan, Iran.
Email: ghannadian@gmail.com

vention of malaria (2). Chloroquine, and amodiaquine are another widely used antimalarial drugs with 4-aminoquinolone structure but, drug-resistant was rapidly decreased their effectiveness (2,3). Primaquine is 8-aminoquinolone for treatment of different types of malaria infection with blocking the oxidative metabolism in plasmodia (2). Artemisinin and artesunate are sesquiterpene lactones with a chemically rare peroxide bridge linkage effective against multidrug resistant *P. falciparum* (4).

Despite the administration of drugs, increasing the risks of treatment failure because of developing resistance is the main problem, now. Therefore, discovering new and efficient drugs or combination therapy of 2 or more blood schizonticidal drugs with different mechanisms and different targets in the parasite is a crucial effort to solve this problem (5). Saffron is a spice derived from the styles and stigmas of the flower of *Crocus sativus* L., commonly known as the "za'ferân" in Persian. It is grown from Spain in the west to India in the east but southeastern provinces in Iran including Khorasan region produce approximately most of the world production (6). The stigmas are mostly used as food spice and colorant. There are also some reports on the effectiveness of saffron for the treatment of malaria (*Tab-e- se-yek* in Persian) in the Islamic medical manuscripts (7). Saffron contains carotenoids, including zeaxanthin, lycopene, and α- and β-carotenes (8). Crocin is a carotenoid that may comprise up to 10% of dried saffron. Picrocrocin and safranal has insecticidal and pesticidal properties and may comprise to more than 4% of saffron's mass (8). In a recent research crocin derived from saffron and safranal semi-synthetic derivatives showed in vitro anti-malarial properties (9). Therefore, saffron was selected alone or in combination with chloroquine in this study for evaluation of its anti-malarial properties in *P. berghei* infected mice as an experimental in vivo model.

Materials and Methods

Plant material

Saffron, the dried stigmas of the *Crocus sativus* flowers, was obtained from Global international saffron company, Torbat-e-Heydarieh, Khorasan, Iran and identified at the Pharmacognosy Department, School of Pharmacy, Isfahan University of Medical Sciences. The plant material was milled into a fine powder (100 g) and then macerated with ethanol (600 mL × 3), at room temperature for three days. The extract was evaporated in a vacuum system at 40°C (Rotary evaporator, Heidolph Co. Germany) to a dark red residue which was subjected to liquid/liquid partitioning between water and ethyl acetate. Aqueous and ethyl acetate fractions were evaporated to remove solvent and kept in refrigerator in -20°C before use.

Animals

Male albino sourian mice, weighing between 23 to 27 g supplied from Pasteur Institute of Iran, were randomly assigned to treatment and control groups with 7 mice in each group. The mice were kept at room temperature in accordance with the internationally accepted principles for laboratory animal use and care, and were given ad libitum access to food and water.

Parasites

Chloroquine-sensitive *P. berghei* NICD strain from Haffkine Institute of India was used in the study. Two weeks previous to the tests the parasites (stored in nitrogen liquid) were rethawed and maintained by blood passage in saurian mice, intra-peritoneal. The donor mice with 10% parasitaemia were then sacrificed and blood was collected and diluted with normal saline into heparinized falcon tubes (5×10^6/mL infected erythrocytes). Treatment mice were inoculated with 10^6 parasitized erythrocytes in 0.2 ml dilution, intra peritoneal.

Antimalarial in vivo assay

The anti-malarial study requires in vitro methods or in vivo test models. The most common in vivo test utilize *P. berghei* in a 4 day suppressive test in mice (Peter's test). Different dose levels (350, 700, and 1000 mg/kg) of saffron total extract, aqueous and ethyl acetate fractions and chloroquine (20 mg/kg) were administered to groups of 5 mice in each group in addition to 5 mice uninfected mice as negative control and 5 infected but treated with physiological saline + 2% tween 80 as placebo were prepared. Two hours after parasite inoculations in day zero, plant extracts and chloroquine were injected into the infected mice and repeated once daily for 4 consecutive days. On fifth day a thin blood smear of the tail blood of each of the mice was prepared on microscope slides, fixed with absolute methanol, and stained with 10% Giemsa stain in distilled water. Percentage of parasitaemia suppression was determined by counting parasites against 200 erythrocytes on days 5, 7, 14 and 28 for Peter's test using the following formula (10).

$$\%\text{suppression} = \frac{\text{Mean parasitemia of placebo} - \text{mean parasitemia of treated group}}{\text{Mean parasitemia of placebo}}$$

If any animals died before the end of the fourth day, the death was considered for the extract toxicity (1). Combination therapy was then conducted with three treatment groups 1, 2 and 3 treated with best fraction of saffron extract, chloroquine (20 mg/kg) and a combination of these two, in addition to negative control (nor infected , nor receiving any of the agents) and placebo. Interaction was evaluated as additive, synergism or antagonism, respectively. The treated mice were followed up in both screening and combination method for 28 days after injection (on days 5, 7, 14, and 28), and survival time of the mice was recorded in each test group (10-12).

Ethics

All the animals were handled in accordance with the internationally accepted principles and guides for the care and use of laboratory animals in 2010 (11), and the Ethics Committee of Isfahan University of Medical Sciences.

Statistical analysis

The ED_{50} value (drug concentration causing 50% of maximum suppression) of the samples were calculated based on semi-log graphs. Values are given as mean ± standard error of mean (SEM). Statistical analysis was performed using Student's *t* test and/or one-way analysis of variance (ANOVA) as appropriate and Bonferroni post hoc test to identify the differences between treated groups and control.

Results

General mean ± SD for all study samples for age and weight on day zero was 4 weeks old and 27.1 ± 3.4 g, respectively. There were no statistically significant differences between groups in terms of basic characteristics.

The data were analyzed with 2 factors related to the parasitemia suppression and survival time.

In between group analysis, there was a significant difference between the mean of placebo and total extract and ethyl acetate fraction at concentrations of 700 and 1050 mg/kg on day 4 (24 hours after the last dose), $P < 0.001$. Aqueous extract in all the concentrations (350, and 1050 mg/kg) showed parasitemia suppression significantly more than placebo ($P < 0.001$; Figure 1).

The saffron extract, aqueous and ethyl acetate fractions resulted in suppression of parasitemia with ED_{50} values of 587.0 ± 78.7, 323.7 ± 37.2, and 508.7 ± 35.6 mg/kg, respectively. It means that aqueous fraction with lower ED_{50} is more effective in decreasing the parasitemia than ethyl acetate and total extract. However, none of the observed activities of the extracts and fractions was comparable to that of chloroquine ($P < 0.05$).

The mice were followed up for 28 days and ANOVA results showed that mean survival time of the treated mice with chloroquine 20 mg/kg (23.6 days) and ethyl acetate 700 mg/kg (17.8 days) were significantly ($P < 0.05$) more than placebo (10.8 days) while total extract and aqueous fraction treated groups did not show significant differences with placebo. It means that ethyl acetate fraction (700 mg/kg) has longer survival time than other saffron derived treated groups.

Considering the toxicity of total extract, ethyl acetate and aqueous fraction in various concentrations, aqueous fraction (1050 mg/kg) showed more toxicity with two mice died and ethyl acetate fraction (700 mg/kg) exhibited less toxicity with no death in mice under test before the end of the fourth day.

Combination therapy was then conducted with three treatment groups 1, 2 and 3 treated with ethyl acetate fraction of saffron extract (700 mg/kg), chloroquine (20 mg/kg) and a combination of these 2, in addition to negative control and placebo (Figure 2).

There was a significant difference between the parasitemia suppression of ethyl acetate fraction, chloroquine and combination of these 2 with placebo on day 4 ($P < 0.001$) but there was no statistically significant difference between combination group and chloroquine alone ($P > 0.05$).

ANOVA results showed that survived percent of the treated mice with chloroquine + ethyl acetate fraction on days 7, 14, and 28 were significantly ($P < 0.05$) more than chloroquine or ethyl acetate fraction alone. It means that survival time interaction between ethyl acetate fraction and chloroquine against the *P. berghei* showed a synergism pattern (Table 1).

Discussion

The saffron total extract, aqueous and ethyl acetate fractions significantly resulted in suppression of parasitemia in mice infected with *P. berghei*. However, their effectiveness against *P. berghei* parasitemia was not comparable with chloroquine. Combination therapy of chloroquine (20 mg/kg) with saffron ethyl acetate fraction (700 mg/kg) significantly prolonged survival time against the *P. berghei* parasitemia in comparison with chloroquine or ethyl acetate fraction alone.

Investigation on the antimalarial effects of medicinal herbs alone or in combination with current antimalarial drugs opened a new field of research against plasmodium infections.

Motevalli Haghi et al (12) examined the effectiveness of *Peganum harmala* on *P. berghei.* with considerable effect in 100 mg/kg dosage. Nahrevanian and colleagues reported antimalarial activity of *Artemisia khorassanica* and *Artemisia sieberi* against *P. berghei* in mice (13,14). Different parts of plants of the Simaroubaceae family are used traditionally in the treatment of malaria. These plants contain quassinoid alkaloids like simaroubolide compound that are responsible for this activity (15). Stem bark of Alstonia

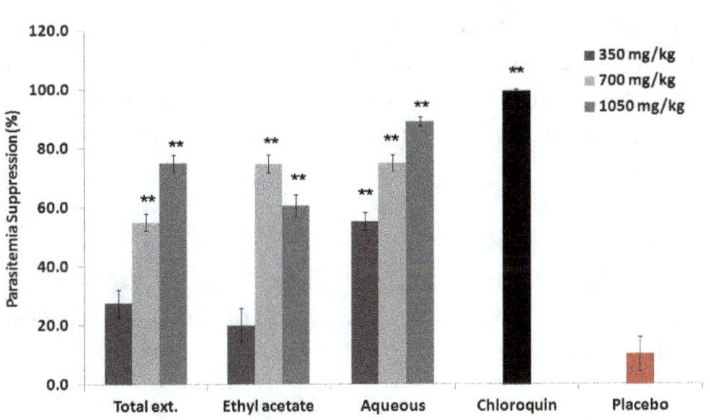

Figure 1. Parasitemia suppression (mean ± SEM) of infected mice treated with crude extract, ethyl acetate and aqueous fractions of saffron on day 4 (1 day after cessation of treatment) in Peter's antimalarial test.

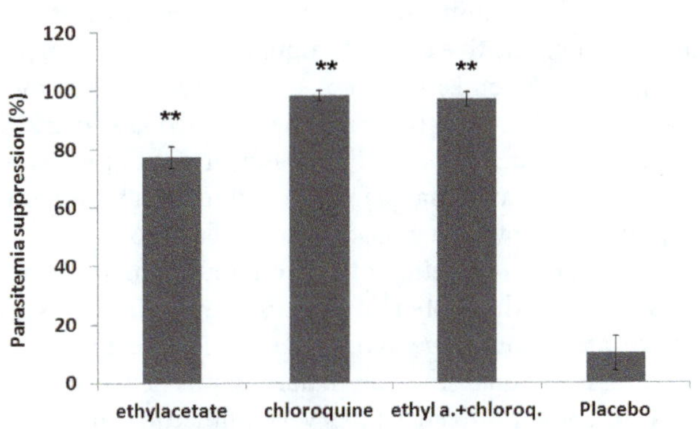

Figure 2. Parasitemia suppression (mean ± SEM) of infected mice treated with ethyl acetate fraction of saffron (700 mg/kg), chloroquine (20 mg/kg), ethyl acetate fraction (700 mg) + chloroquine (20 mg) and placebo on day 4 (1 day after cessation of treatment) in Peter's antimalarial test.

Table 1. Mean survival time (days) after injection (%) of infected mice treated with ethyl acetate fraction of saffron (700 mg/kg), chloroquine (20 mg/kg), ethyl acetate fraction (700 mg) + chloroquine (20 mg) and placebo

	Lived from 100%			
Group	**Ethyl acetate fraction**	**Chloroquine**	**Ethyl acetate + chloroquine**	**Placebo**
in day 7th	77.6	79.6	100.0	75.5
in day 14th	74.5	75.5	99.0	68.4
in day 28th	61.2	73.5	91.8	36.7

(Apocynaceae) exhibits antipyretic and antimalaria properties and has been used in the past for malarial treatment (16). The roots of *Cryptolepis sanguinolenta* from Asclepiadaceae family have been used in Africa as antimalarial drug. Cryptolepine and isocryptolepine are identified from these plants as responsible indoloquinoline alkaloids for this effect (17). The barks of Cinchona species a rich source of quinine and other quinolidine alkaloids were used for treatment of malaria fever from times long ago (18). The African antimalarial medicinal plants genus *Ancistrocladus* and *Triphyophyllum peltatum* contain naphthyl isoquiniline alkaloids like Yaoundamine and Habropetaline alkaloids with considerable in vitro antimalarial activity with good selectivity indices (19,20). Stem bark of *Pogonopus tubulosus* a tree from South America used traditionally in Bolivia against malaria and contains tubulosine indoline alkaloid with potent antimalarial activity in mice (21). *Glycyrrhiza glabra* a plant native to Iran contains licochalcone A and 18β-glycyrrhetinic acid with promised in vitro activities against *P. falciparum* (22,23). However, in comparison with previous reports on medicinal plants with antimalaria activity, it is the first report of *Crocus sativa* to be effective against *P. berghei*. This research was in agreement with another report recently published on 2 bioactive compounds isolated from *Crocus sativa* including crocin and safranal and their semi-synthetic derivatives with potent antimalarial activity in vitro against *P. falciparum* chloroquine sensitive strain with IC_{50} less than 20 μg/mL (9).

Ethyl acetate fraction of *Crocus sativus* stigma in combination with chloroquine exhibited a synergic pattern against chloroquine sensitive *P. berghei*. In comparison with other antimalarial plants, *Otostegia persica* combinational therapy with chloroquine revealed potentiating against the chloroquine sensitive and chloroquine resistant *P. berghei* strains (24). Artemisinin from *Artemisia anova* and mefloquine combination treatment has showed also marked synergism against *P. berghei* (25). But, *Artemisia aucheri*, an effective antimalarial plant, in combination with chloroquine has shown an antagonistic pattern (26).

The mechanism of action of saffron and its main bioactives crocin with carotenoid structure and safranal as an unsaturated monoterpenoid against malaria is not clear. In a cross-sectional study on malaria status between plasma carotenoids with structures very similar to crucin and indicators of disease severity like parasitemia, and antioxidant status with malaria, carotenoid concentrations were lower in the patients than in the control subjects (27). This study suggested that subjects with acute malaria have suppressed plasma concentrations of antioxidants, and that higher plasma carotenoids are associated with more and rapid clearance of malaria parasitemia (28,29). There are some reports also on immune modulation properties of *Crocus sativus* stigma (30). So, saffron as a rich source of crucin with carotenoid structure might act as a biological antioxidant supplement useful for reducing the parasitemia through alteration of oxidative stress and immune modulation especially in combination with malaria standard drugs. This study showed for the first time that saffron and its fractions has antimalarial activity as well as combination of its ethyl acetate fraction with chloroquine, which has a synergistic effect on chloroquine sensitive *P. berghei*. However, the exact mechanism of action of saffron, its fractions and its main bioactive like crocin and safranal in reducing blood parasite count is not clear and more studies are recommended in this regard.

Acknowledgments

The authors are grateful to the Pharmaceutical Sciences Research Center, Isfahan University of Medical Sciences, Isfahan, Iran and Department of Medical Parasitology and Mycology, School of Public Health, Tehran University of Medical Sciences (TUMS), Tehran, Iran for their help.

Authors' contributions

All contributed to the conception of the work, conducting the study, revising the draft, approval of the final version of the manuscript, and agreed for all aspects of the work. All the authors wrote the manuscript equally.

Conflict of interests

The authors declared no competing interests.

Ethical considerations

Ethical issues (including plagiarism, misconduct, data fabrication, falsification, double publication or submission, redundancy) have been completely observed by the authors.

Funding/Support

This work was financially supported by the Vice-Chancellor of Research, Isfahan University of Medical Sciences, Isfahan, Iran (gant No. 189128).

References

1. Evans WC. Trease and Evans Pharmacognosy. 15th ed. Edinburg: WB Saunders; 2002:407-413.
2. World Health Organization. Guidelines for the

treatment of malaria. Geneva: World Health Organization; 2010:164-165.
3. Famin O, Ginsburg H. Differential effects of 4-aminoquinoline-containing antimalarial drugs on hemoglobin digestion in Plasmodium falciparum-infected erythrocytes. Biochem Pharmacol. 2002;63:393-398.
4. White NJ. Qinghaosu (artemisinin): the price of success. Science. 2008;320:330-334.
5. White NJ. Antimalarial drug resistance. J Clin Invest. 2004;113:1084-1092.
6. Ghorbani M. The efficiency of saffron's marketing channel in Iran. World Appl Sci J. 2008;4:523-527.
7. Majlesi MB. Bihār al-Anwār. Trans by Kamarey MB. vol 14. Tehran: Entesharat-e Eslamieh; 2006.
8. Moghaddasi MS. Saffron chemicals and medicine usage. J Med Plants Res. 2010;4:427-430.
9. De Monte C, Bizzarri B, Gidaro MC, et al. Bioactive compounds of Crocus sativus L. and their semi-synthetic derivatives as promising anti-Helicobacter pylori, anti-malarial and anti-leishmanial agents. J Enzyme Inhib Med Chem. 2015. doi:10.3109/14756366.2014.1001755.
10. Peters W. The chemotherapy of rodent malaria. XXII. The value of drug resistant strains of Plasmodium berghei in screening for blood schizonticidal activity. Ann Trop Med Parasitol. 1975;69:155-171.
11. McGrath JC, Drummond GB, McLachlan EM, Kilkenny C, Wainwright CL. Guidelines for reporting experiments involving animals: the ARRIVE guidelines. Br J Pharmacol. 2010;160:1573-1576.
12. Motevalli Haghi A, Nateghpour M, Edrissian GH, Souri E, Satvat MT. Evaluation of the effectiveness of ethanolic extract of Peganum harmala L. against Plasmodium berghei in comparison with chloroquine in saurian mice using in vivo test. Public Health Res. 2004;2:1-2.
13. Nahrevanian H, Kazemi M, Naszm H, Amini M. In vivo antimalarial effects of Iranian flora Artemisia khorassanica against Plasmodium berghei and pharmacochemistry of its natural components. Iran J Parasitol. 2010;5:6-19.
14. Nahrevanian H, Sheykhkanlooye Milan B, Kazemi M, Hajhosseini R, Soleymani Mashhadi S, Nahrevanian SH. Antimalarial effects of Iranian flora Artemisia sieberi on Plasmodium berghei in vivo in mice and phytochemistry analysis of its herbal extracts. Malar Res Treat. 2012. doi:10.1155/2012/727032.
15. Muhammad I, Samoylenko V. Antimalarial quassinoids: past, present and future. Expert Opin Drug Discov. 2007;8:1065-1084.
16. Adotey JPK, Adukpo GE, Opoku Boahen Y, Armah FA. A review of the ethnobotany and pharmacological importance of Alstonia boonei De Wild (Apocynaceae). ISRN Pharmacol. 2012;2012:587160.
17. Grellier P, Ramiaramanana L, Millerioux V, et al. Antimalarial activity of cryptolepine and isocryptolepine, alkaloids isolated from Cryptolepis sanguinolenta. Phytother Res. 1996;10:317-321.
18. Andrade-Neto VF, Brandão MGL, Stehmann JR, Oliveira LA, Krettli AU. Antimalarial activity of Cinchona-like plants used to treat fever and malaria in Brazil. J Ethnopharmacol. 2003;87:253-256.
19. Karn A, Mewada A, Sharon M, Sharon M. Antimalarial Activity of Yaoundamine a Naphthyl Iso-quinoline Alkaloid, Extracted from Stem of Ancistrocladus heyneanus. Annals Biol Sci. 2014;2:40-44.
20. Bringmann G, Messer K, Schwöbel B, Brun R, Assi LA. Habropetaline A, an antimalarial naphthylisoquinoline alkaloid from Triphyophyllum peltatum. Phytochemistry. 2003;62:345-349.
21. Frederich M, Tits M, Angenot L. Potential antimalarial activity of indole alkaloids. Trans R Soc Trop Med Hyg. 2008;102:11-19.
22. Asl MN, Hosseinzadeh H. Review of pharmacological effects of Glycyrrhiza sp. and its bioactive compounds. Phytother Res. 2008;22:709-724.
23. Chen M, Theander TG, Christensen SB, Hviid L, Zhai L, Kharazmi A . Licochalcone A. A new antimalarial agent, inhibits in vitro growth of the human malaria parasite Plasmodium falciparum and protects mice from P. yoelii infection. Antimicrob Agents Chemother. 1994;38:1470-1475.
24. Nateghpour M, Farivar L, Souri E, Hajjaran H, Mohebali M, Haghi AM. The Effect of Otostegia persica in Combination with Chloroquine on Chloroquine-Sensitive and Chloroquine-Resistant Strains of Plasmodium berghei Using In-vivo Fixed Ratios Method. Iran J Pharm Res. 2012;11:583-588.
25. Chawira AN, Warhurst DC, Robinson BL, Peters W. The effect of combinations of qing-haosu (artemisinin) with standard antimalarial drugs in the suppressive treatment of malaria in mice. Trans R Soc Trop Med Hyg. 1987;81:554-558.
26. Khodadadi M, Nateghpour M, Souri E, et al. Evaluation of effectiveness of ethanolic extract of artemisia aucheri, individually and in combination with chloroquine, on chloroquine-sensitive strain of plasmodium berghei in sourian mice. Iran J Public Health. 2013;42:883-888.
27. Das BS, Thurnham DI, Das DB. Plasma alpha-tocopherol, retinol, and carotenoids in children with falciparum malaria. Am J Clin Nutr. 1996;64:94-100.
28. Metzger A, Mukasa G, Shankar AH, Ndeezi G, Melikian G, Semba RD. Antioxidant status and acute malaria in children in Kampala, Uganda. Am J Trop Med Hyg. 2001;65:115-119.
29. Nussenblatt V, Semba RD. Micronutrient malnutrition and the pathogenesis of malarial anemia. Acta Tropica. 2002;82:321-337.
30. Escribano J, Díaz-Guerra MJ, Riese HH, et al. In vitro activation of macrophages by a novel proteoglycan isolated from corms of Crocus sativus L. Cancer Lett. 1999;144:107-114.

GABA mediated response of aqueous, ethanol and ethyl acetate extracts of *Dicranopteris linearis* leaf in Swiss Albino mice

Mohammad Mustakim Billah[1*], Kashfia Nawrin[1], Kh Tanvir Ahmed[2], Mohammed Sahek Ullah Jabed[1], Md. Nasidul Islam[3], Md. Main Uddin[4]

[1]Department of Pharmaceutical Sciences, North South University, Bangladesh
[2]Mylan School of Pharmacy, Duquesne University, USA
[3]Department of Pharmacy, East West University, Bangladesh
[4]Department of Clinical Pharmacy and Pharmacology, University of Dhaka, Bangladesh

ARTICLE INFO

Keywords:
Dicranopteris linearis
Maze test
Hole cross
Open field
Head dipping

ABSTRACT

Introduction: The objective of the study was to assess the potential of the leaf of *Dicranopteris linearis* in altering the CNS functions with three different extracts; aqueous, ethanol and ethyl acetate.
Methods: To evaluate and compare the activities Morris maze, elevated plus maze (EPM), open field, hole cross and head dip tests were performed and many behavioral parameters were observed. The forced swim in Morris water maze analyzed the depression of rodents in terms of inability to self-rescue. Alongside, hole cross and open field tests assessed the inhibition of locomotor activities. Moreover, EPM test screened the anxiolytic potential while the head dipping hole board test supported the previous experiments by evaluating both sedative, depressive and anxiolytic potentials of the extracts.
Results: The results showed that the ethanol extract significantly suppressed CNS activity by reducing number of locomotor activities and increasing the stability phase (in EPM and Morris maze) supporting mild sedation, depression and anxiolysis. Furthermore, the ethyl acetate extract also possessed moderate to high potential in reducing locomotor activities depending on gradient doses. Results were compared with control group and found statistically significant.
Conclusion: As this plant mimic the activity of a gamma-aminobutyric acid (GABA) agonist, it can be concluded that the plant may have GABA mediated involvement in central nervous system. However, the responsible compounds for these activities are yet to be investigated and this may potentiate a new source of drug development.

Implication for health policy/practice/research/medical education:
Dicranopteris linearis mimics the activity of a gamma-aminobutyric acid (GABA) agonist and the plant may have GABA mediated involvement in central nervous system. This may potentiate a new source of drug development. The research work can be a lead for fellow researchers to investigate in depth pharmacology of the compounds present in this plant leaf extract.

Introduction

Dicranopteris linearis is a medicinal plant used by tribes in different localities of Bangladesh for various ailments. The plant belongs to Gleicheniaceae family and is characterized as forking fern by its segmented leaves in linear shape, up to 7 centimeters long and a few millimeters wide. The undersides are hairy and sometimes waxy. The young leaf juice has also been reported to be used by the Garo tribes of Haluaghat (Mymensingh) for cough, allergic symptoms and respiratory troubles (1). Many other pharmacological responses including analgesic, antipyretic, anti-inflammatory (2), antibacterial, antioxidant (3), hepatoprotective (4), gastroprotective (5) and cytotoxic (6) activities have been reported in scientific literatures and other potential activities are under investigation. However, no CNS activity has been reported in literatures

***Corresponding author:** Mohammad Mustakim Billah; Department of Pharmaceutical Sciences, North South University, Bangladesh.
Email: mustakimbillah@hotmail.com

and no comparison study on different extracts was found. Thus, the aim of this study was to investigate the CNS activity of the leaf of this plant, to support the scientific basis of its medicinal use and to find most potent extract by comparison. To assess the potentials, three different solvents were selected to extract the maximum potent compounds depending on the polarity of the solvents. The study was designed accordingly to compare the activity of these three extracts.

Materials and methods

Collection and preparation of leaf samples

The plant leaves were collected from the district of Mymensingh of Bangladesh in June, 2014 (Accession Number: DACB 42009). The leaves were processed by washing, drying and crushing into powder. The powdered material was soaked for 7 days in water (DLAQ), ethanol (DLET) and ethyl acetate (DLEA) solvents in separate closed vessels intended to extract the pharmacological active components. The solution was then filtered and condensed through a rotary evaporator to get the viscous extracts.

Drugs and Chemicals

Diazepam, ethanol and ethyl acetate obtained for the experiments were of analytical grades.

Grouping of animals

Swiss albino mice were used for all the experiments. Animals were obtained from the university animal house and selected based on their age (2.5 months), weight (25-30 gm) and capability of free movement. For each experiment, mice were divided into eight groups (n = 5) for different treatments; control (dH2O), standard (diazepam 1 mg/kg), DLAQ (200 mg/kg), DLAQ (400 mg/kg), DLET (200 mg/kg), DLET (400 mg/kg), DLEA (200 mg/kg) and DLEA (400 mg/kg) as per body weight. For handling and treating animals, institute adopted animal research standards were followed (7).

Morris maze test

The test was performed according to the method established by Morris (8) and as described by Alikatte et al (9) with slight modifications. A round bowl measuring 70 cm diameter and 14 cm height was filled with water where there was only one crystal clear glass stand at water level intended to make it almost completely invisible. The glass stand was subjected to avoid forced swim. The animals were trialed for their response in forced swimming the day before the experiment for 5 minutes and the mice able to rescue themselves were selected for the experiment. On day of experiment, 30 minutes after oral gavages of control, standard diazepam and test samples the mice were placed in the water away from the stand and were observed for the time being they find the place to rescue themselves from the induced stress. Five minutes were considered as the withdrawal time. The drug induced depressed groups were compared to the control group which served as the model of natural behavior.

Elevated plus maze test

Elevated plus maze (EPM) test is a well-established method to analyze the anxiolytic potential of samples. A cross sectional four armed (two closed and two open) apparatus was used for this assessment. One hour after drugs and samples treatment of respective groups the animals were placed in the centre of maze to observe and record their tendency to entry in the open or closed arms and their duration spent in those arms. The 5 minutes observation of this parameter identifies their behavioral changes (10).

Hole cross test

A specially designed rectangular shaped (30×20×20 cm) apparatus having a mid-partition with an integrated hole (3 cm diameter) which divided the box into two equal compartments was used for this test. Animals were placed in the apparatus 20 minutes after treatment of drugs and samples and observed for the number of hole crossed and number of rearing by them for next 10 minutes (11).

Open field test

The open field apparatus was designed as a square floor divided into several small squares colored alternatively black and white. Like the hole cross tests, 20 minutes after oral treatments animals were placed in the apparatus and observed accordingly for next 10 minutes for their behavior of distance travelled (number of square crossing) and number of rearing (12).

Head dipping test

This method was described by Clark et al (13). A specially designed square board containing uniformly distanced 4X4 holes and having in-between walkways for the animals was used for this experiment. The animals after being treated with standard and samples were placed in the board where they were observed for 20 minutes for their activity of dipping the head into the hole (14).

Statistical analysis

Statistical analysis for animal experiments was carried out using one-way analysis of variance (ANOVA) followed by Dunnett's multiple comparison tests using SPSS 20 for windows. The results obtained were compared with the vehicle control group. P values < 0.05, 0.01 and 0.001 were considered to be statistically significant.

Results

Morris maze test

The results showed that the ethanol extract in higher dose significantly increased (P<0.01) the time for the animals to find the rescue object which was reluctance of the animal and the indication for depressive pattern

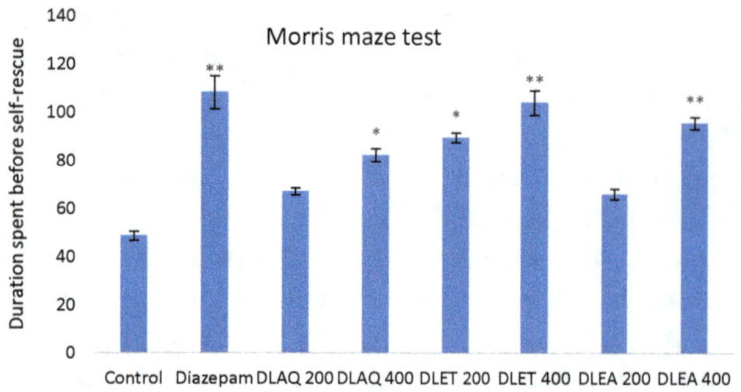

Figure 1. Effect of different extracts of *D. linearis* on duration spent before self-rescuing (swimming time in seconds) in Morris maze test. Data are presented as the mean ± SEM (n = 5). $^{**}P < 0.01$, $^{*}P < 0.05$

of behavior (Figure 1). In comparison, the control group showed a rapid recognition of the rescue object (glass stand). Ethyl acetate extract also increased the duration compared to the standard ($P < 0.01$).

Elevated plus maze test

Figure 2 compared the parameters of number of entry in open arm and duration spent in open arm exhibited by the extracts to control group. This indicates the development of confidence level. The result showed firm activity of the standard to increase both the parameters as an indication of anxiolytic activity. Only ethyl acetate and ethanol extract exerts their potential to mimic the standard. The result was statistically significant.

Hole cross test

Two parameters (number of hole crossing and rearing) regarding the pattern of depressive behavior was studied and the result found standard ($P < 0.001$), DLET 200, DLET 400 ($P < 0.001$) and DLEA 400 significantly reduced the locomotor activities which was the indication of depressive behavior (Figure 3).

Open field test

Like hole cross test, open field test also produced similar results observing the depressive parameters of distance travelling and rearing (Figure 4). Both parameters exhibit that DLET 400 suppressed the CNS functions compared to the standard ($P < 0.001$). However, DLET 200 and DLEA 400 also showed moderate activity in reducing locomotor function.

Head dipping test

Like all the above experiments DLET 400 mimics the activity of standard in reducing the CNS functions significantly in head dip test. The number of head dip into the holes were significantly reduced compared to control and was statistically significant at $P < 0.01$ (Figure 5).

Discussion

The use of three different solvents in extraction procedure rationalized for the presence of maximum potent compounds. Water served to extract the polar compound, ethanol for slightly polar to nonpolar compounds while ethyl acetate obtained the nonpolar compounds. Both sedative, depressive and anxiolytic potentials were assessed by the performed experiments.

Morris water maze test is widely used method for evaluating the memory retention behavior of experimental animal (15). However some literature suggests that the forced swimming in Morris maze can also assess the depression in rodents (16). Thus method was slightly modified and designed accordingly to evaluate depression in mice. Mice with natural behavior tends to reach the rescue object quickly than that of the mildly sedated or depressed mice.

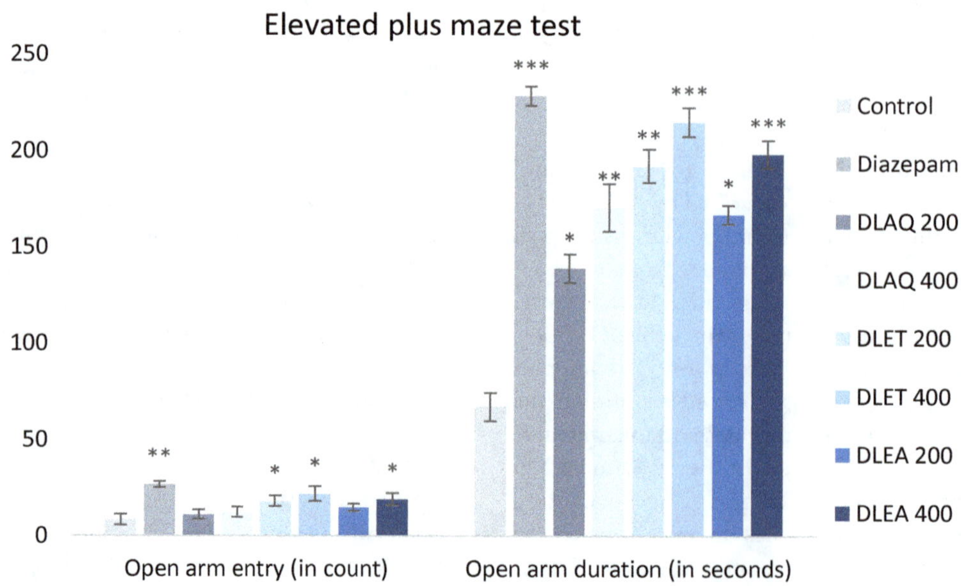

Figure 2. Effect of different extracts of *D. linearis* on number of open arm entry and duration spent in seconds at open arm in elevated maze apparatus. Data are presented as the mean ± SEM (n = 5). $^{***}P < 0.001$, $^{**}P < 0.01$, $^{*}P < 0.05$

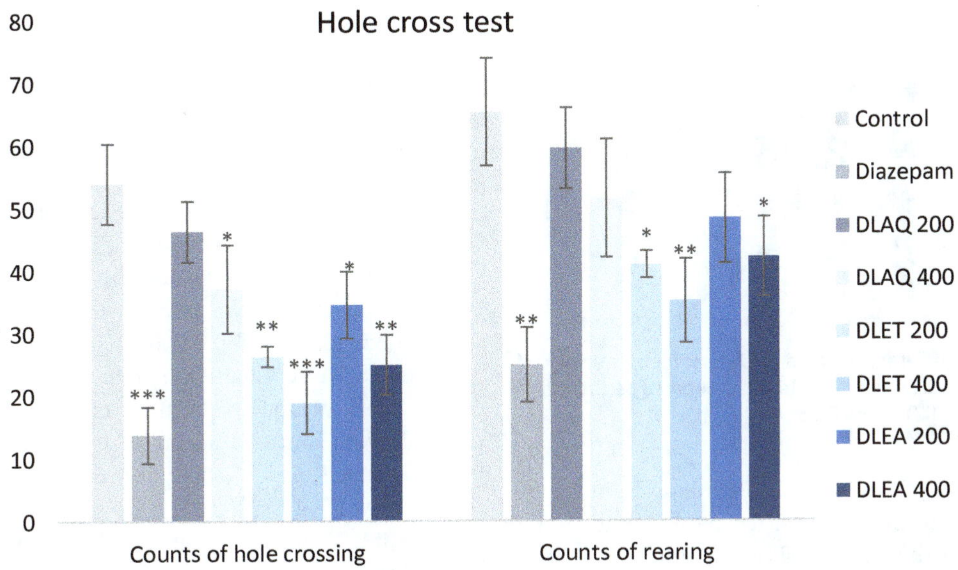

Figure 3. Effect of different extracts of *D. linearis* on number of hole crossed and number of rearing in hole cross apparatus. Data are presented as the mean ± SEM (n = 5). ***$P < 0.001$, **$P < 0.01$, *$P < 0.05$.

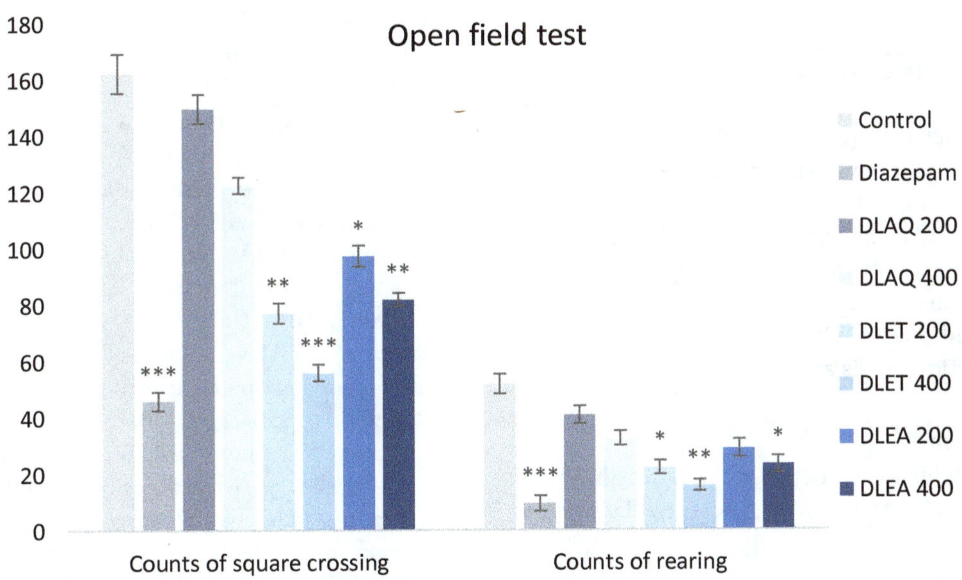

Figure 4. Effect of different extracts of *D. linearis* on number of square crossed (distance travelled) and number of rearing in open field. Data are presented as the mean ± SEM (n = 5). ***$P < 0.001$, **$P < 0.01$, *$P < 0.05$.

Therefore, increase in swimming time indicates mild sedation or depression for the experimental subject. The ethanol extract significantly increased the swimming time compared with standard suggesting mild sedation or hypnosis whereas ethyl acetate extract at higher dose also increased swimming time proposing a mild depression by inhibiting neurotransmission.

EPM test screened the anxiolytic potential by observing different parameters (17). The frequency of open arm entry and time spent in open arm of maze apparatus are the measures to assess emotional aspects and psychomotor performance of the rodents. The effect of the extract was possibly due to the action on gamma-aminobutyric acid (GABA) benzodiazepine receptor complex, stimulation of glucocorticoid production and release in the adrenal cortex (18). Alongside, Head dipping test on a hole board also suggests the measure of anxiolytic as well as sedative properties being assessed (19). Head dipping is considered as the sign of exploratory behavior. The ethanol and ethyl acetate extracts confirmed both the anxiolytic and depressive properties via responding to these tests.

Hole cross and open field tests examine the Inhibitory activities of locomotor functions of mice (20,21). The ethanol extract found to reduce the exploratory activities of mice. Since GABA is the major inhibitory neurotransmitter of the central nervous system (22) and

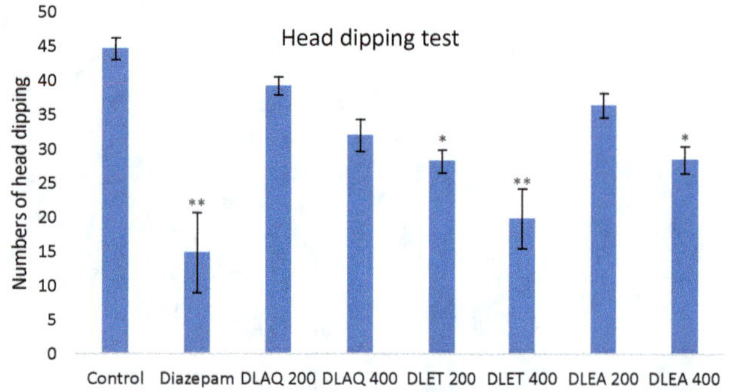

Figure 5. Effect of different extracts of *D. linearis* on number of head dip in hole board appartus. Data are presented as the mean ± SEM (n = 5). ***P* < 0.01, **P* < 0.05.

most of the anxiolytic as well as CNS depressant drugs like diazepam act through GABA receptor (23), it can be hypothesized that the extracts showing similar activities acted similarly by membrane hyperpolarization to potentiate GABAergic inhibition. This was led by either decrease in the firing rate of critical neurons in the brain or by direct activation of GABA receptor (24).

Conclusion

The ethanol leaf extract of *Dicranopteris linearis* possess significant neuropharmacological potential. Alongside the ethyl acetate extract also produced moderate to significant activities. Behavioral alteration in regard of depression was observed through the different experiments. Therefore it can be concluded that the plant leaf is a good source for new drug development. However, the sample is yet to be investigated for the responsible compounds. Moreover, it can be declared that the use of this plant in medicinal purpose has scientific basis and is safe and nontoxic.

Acknowledgements

Authors are grateful to the department of North South University for the permission to use their laboratory facilities.

Authors' contributions

This work was carried out in collaboration between all authors. MMB and KN performed the neuropharmacological tests and prepared the manuscript. KTA designed the methodology and coordinated the whole project. MSU Jabed prepared the plant extract and assisted in tests. MNI designed and made the apparatuses and assisted in tests. MMU conducted the statistical analysis of data and assisted in tests.

Conflict of interests

Authors declare no conflict of interests.

Ethical considerations

All ethical issues regarding animal and lab works were fully considered.

References

1. Sarker SK, Hossain AB. Pteridophytes of greater Mymensingh district of Bangladesh used as vegetables and medicines. Bangladesh J Plant Taxon. 2009;16(1):47-56.
2. Zakaria ZA, Abdul Ghani ZD, Nor RN, Gopalan HK, Sulaiman MR, Abdullah FC. Antinociceptive and anti-inflammatory activities of Dicranopteris linearis leaves chloroform extract in experimental animals. Yakugaku Zasshi. 2006;126(11):1197-1203.
3. Ismail NA, Shamsahal-Din NS, Mamat SS, et al. Effect of aqueous extract of Dicranopteris linearis leaves against paracetamol and carbon tetrachloride-induced liver toxicity in rats. Pak J Pharm Sci. 2014;27(4):831-835.
4. Lai HY, Lim YY, Tan SP. Antioxidative, tyrosinase inhibiting and antibacterial activities of leaf extract from medicinal ferns. Biosci Biotechnol Biochem. 2009;73(6):1362-1366.
5. Hussaini J, Othman NA, Abdulla MA, Majid NA, Faroq HM, Ismail S. Gastroprotective effects of Dicranopteris linearis leaf extract against ethanol-induced gastric mucosal injury in rats. Sci Res Essays. 2012;7(18):1761-1767.
6. Zakaria ZA, Mohamed AM, Jamil NS, et al. In vitro cytotoxic and antioxidant properties of the aqueous, chloroform and methanol extracts of Dicranopteris linearis leaves. Afr J Biotechnol. 2011;10(2):273-282.
7. Zimmermann M. Ethical guidelines for investigations of experimental pain in conscious animals. Pain. 1983;16:109-110.
8. Morris RG. Development of a water maze procedure for studying spatial learning in the rat. J Neurosci Methods. 1984;11:47-60.
9. Alikatte KL, Akondi BR, Yerragunta VG, Veerareddy PR, Palle S. Antiamnesic activity of Syzygium cumini against scopolamine induced spatial memory impairments in rats. Brain Dev. 2012;34:844-851.
10. Braida D, Capurro V, Zani A, et al. Potential anxiolytic- and antidepressant-like effects of salvinorin A, the main active ingredient of Salvia divinorum, in rodents. Br J Pharmacol. 2009;157:844-853.
11. Khatoon MM, Khatun MH, Islam ME, Parvin MS. Analgesic, antibacterial and central nervous system depressant activities of Albizia procera leaves. Asian Pac J Trop Biomed. 2014;4(4):279-284.
12. Shams-Ud-Doha K, Mahmud ZA, Bachar SC, Qais N. Antinociceptive, anti-inflammatory, antimicrobial and central nervous system depressant activities of ethanolic extract of leaves and roots of Gomphostemma parviflorum var. parviflorum wall. Pharmacognosy Res. 2013;5(4):233-240.
13. Clark G, Koester AG, Pearson DW. Exploratory behavior in chronic disulfoton poisoning in mice. Psychopharmacologia. 1971;20(2):169–171.

14. File SE, Wardill AG. Validity of head dipping as a measure of exploration in a modified hole board. Psychopharmacologia. 1975;44(1):53-59.
15. Zongyang L, Yamin L, Liwei W, et al. Memory-enhancing effects of the crude extract of polygala tenuifolia on aged mice. Evid Based Complement Alternat Med. 2014;2014:392324.
16. Sun MK, Alkon DL. Induced depressive behavior impairs learning and memory in rats. Neuroscience. 2004;129(1):129-139.
17. Walf AA, Frye CA. The use of the elevated plus maze as an assay of anxiety-related behavior in rodents. Nat Protoc. 2007;2:322-228.
18. Nishikava H, Hata T, Funakami Y. A role for corticotropin-releasing factor in repeated cold stress-induced anxiety-like behavior during forced swimming and elevated plus-maze test in mice. Biol Pharm Bull. 2004;27(3):352-356.
19. Takeda H, Tsuji M, Matsumiya T. Changes in head-dipping behavior in the hole-board test reflect the anxiogenic and/or anxiolytic state in mice. Eur J Pharmacol. 1998;350(1):21-29.
20. Takagi K, Watanabe M, Saito H. Studies of the spontaneous movement of animals by the hole cross test; effect of 2-dimethyl-aminoethanol and its acyl esters on the central nervous system. Jpn J Pharmacol. 1971;21(6):797-810.
21. Tatem KS, Quinn JL, Phadke A, Yu Q, Gordish-Dressman H, Nagaraju K. Behavioral and locomotor measurements using an open field activity monitoring system for skeletal muscle diseases. J Vis Exp. 2014;(91):51785.
22. Martin D. The role of GABAA receptors in mediating the effects of alcohol in the central nervous system. J Psychiatry Neurosci. 2003;28(4):263-274.
23. Billah MM, Hasan MR, Nawrin K, Mohiuddin, Habib MR. Evaluation of analgesic and sedative-anxiolytic potential of paderia foetida leaf extract. Am J Biomed Sci. 2015;7(2):98-104.
24. Kolawole OT, Makinde JM, Olajide OA. Central nervous depressant activity of Russelia equisetiformis. Niger J Physiol Sci. 2007;22(1-2):59-63.

Effect of *Aloe vera* on some indicators of cell damage after a period of aerobic exercise in male athletes

Amir-Hosein Barati[1], Faezeh Fazeli[1], Mehdi Lotfipour[2*]

[1]School of Physical Education and Sport Science, Shahid Rajaee Teacher Training University, Tehran, Iran
[2]Department of Sport Physiology, School of Physical Education and Sport Science, Shahid Rajaee Teacher Training University, Tehran, Iran

ARTICLE INFO

Keywords:
Aloe vera
Index of cellular damage
Antioxidant
Boys
Athletic

ABSTRACT

Introduction: *Aloe vera* is a medicinal plant with antioxidant activity. The purpose of this study was to determine the effect of *Aloe vera* on some indicators of cell damage after a period of aerobic exercise in male athletes of 15-18 years old.
Methods: In this clinical trial study, 20 male students with average weight of 64.85 ± 51 and height of 172.05 ± 6.4 were randomly assigned to 2 groups of *Aloe vera* supplement (n = 10) and placebo (n = 10). Then aerobic training was conducted for 4 weeks. The supplemented group took 3 capsules, each capsule contains 2 g of dried *Aloe vera* and placebo group took 3 capsules/day containing dextran after every meal. To determine the index of cell injury markers creatine kinase (CK), lactate dehydrogenase (LDH) and reactive protein C (CRP) were determined and blood samples were collected 24 hours before and after each test. The data were analyzed using ANOVA and independent t test. Significance level was considered as $P \leq .05$.
Results: The use of *Aloe vera* during aerobic exercise significantly reduced LDH ($P = .006$) in the supplement group (15% reduction) compared to placebo group and CRP with 11% reduction in the supplement group compared to placebo ($P = .008$). There was no significant reduction in CK.
Conclusion: The findings of this study showed that *Aloe vera* reduces cell damage and inflammation indicators. This result may reflect the role of *Aloe vera* as anti-inflammatory and antioxidant agent.

Implication for health policy/practice/research/medical education:
Aloe vera can be taken to alleviate the capacity of the antioxidant defense system and might improve athlete's performance.

Introduction

Using of herbs as medicines and food supplements allocated special situation to improve overall health and treat illnesses (1,2). The skill levels of athletes have been developed in various disciplines. Each factor that can make little chance for developing the success has special importance that among them, dietary supplements have most important situation (3,4).

High levels of free radicals and depletion of antioxidants can lead to cellular dysfunction and oxidative damage to membrane lipids and other organelles (4,5). Reactive oxygen species (ROS) are produced in prolongs and intense exercises that may cause cell damage (4). It seems that using the antioxidant supplements can decrease the oxidative stress of exercises (4,6,7). The antioxidant supplements that are introduced to the athletes are mainly synthetic chemical compounds. But today, attention has been paid to the herbal supplements with antioxidant activity (1,4,8,9). Basically, natural supplements have less harms than artificial supplements and against artificial supplements. *Aloe vera* is rich in vitamin C and E with antioxidant activity and enhances the resistance of the body against free radicals (1,8). *Aloe vera* works by inhibiting the production of interleukin (IL) 6 and 8 and decreasing leukocyte adhesion (10,11). It also increases the level of interleukin 10 and reduces the levels of tumor necrosis factor-alpha (TNF α), inhabiting the inflammatory reactions (10,12,13). This study was designed to determine the effect of *Aloe vera* on some indicators of cell damage after a period of aerobic exercise in male athletes of 15-18 years old. The factors evaluated were lactate dehydrogenase (LDH), creatine kinase (CK),

***Corresponding author**: Mehdi Lotfipour, Department of Sport Physiology, School of Physical Education and Sport Science, Shahid Rajaee Teacher Training University, Tehran, Iran. Email: rudkhunehbarfi@yahoo.com and reactive protein C (CRP).

Materials and Methods

This study was a quasi-experimental trial. The population included male athletes of 15 to18 years old from Imam Ali Industrial and Physical Education School of Shahrekord, Iran. Twenty volunteers were divided into 2 groups of *Aloe vera* supplementation (n = 10) and placebo (n = 10) groups. The criteria for entering the research included having general physical and mental health and being athlete. The criteria of eliminating the research were cardiovascular disease, surgery, hormonal disorders, smoking and any intervention affecting on the experimental results. Before the intervention, in order to homogenize 2 groups, the age, height, weight and body mass index (BMI) were matched among them (Table 1). All participants were given written information about research and after studying their parents' consents were gotten.

This research was conducted by a sport physiologist the subjects did not have any history of cardiovascular diseases, high blood pressure, diabetes, kidney and liver diseases affecting the measured variables. Subjects became familiar with the manner of exercise, for decreasing some of the confounding and bias factors which might affect the results. The subjects were asked to avoid the use of anti-inflammatory drugs during the exercises. Students' Cooper tests were done to confirm that they were athletes. All subjects were healthy and did not have any clear diseases. Blood specimens of subjects were collected in 4 steps as follows: 24 hours before Cooper test (first step), 24 hours after Cooper test (second step), 24 hours before second Cooper test (third step), and 24 hours after Cooper test (forth step). Two groups participated in the exercise protocol. The intensity of the exercise was increasing once during 4 weeks from simple to hard. Each group had 12 sections for 1 hour and 2 groups had 15 minutes exercise for warming up, 35 minutes for running with 65%-75% of maximum of heartbeats and 10 minutes for cooling off. Also relating to the intense of exercise, this work was done by determining the subjects' heartbeats before exercising, during it and after doing activity in each section. The weight of the athletes was measured by scale with 0.1 kg accuracy. BMI was obtained by weight (kg) divided to square of height (m). Each of bloodletting was done at 16:00 PM in the supine situation for determining the amount of creatine kinase, lactate dehydrogenase and CRP. It is worth noting that the level of CRP was measured by CJKC method of ELISA kits (Pars Making test). The blood samples were centrifuge for 5 minutes in 4000 rpm and the serum were separated. The obtained data were presented as frequency, mean and standard deviation for each variable (Table 1). Kolmogorov-Smirnov test was used to determine the homogeneity of the data. Independent *t* test was used for comparing the variables of two groups and IFN Boone to separate mean comparison. The statistical calculation was done by SPSS version 16 and the $P \leq .05$.was considered significant.

Results

The demographic characteristics of the subjects including the age, height, weight and BMI are summarized in Table 1. There were no differences for the above-mentioned variables between 2 groups.

The results of repeated measure analysis of variance (ANOVA) for comparison internal of group variables in different steps of exercises are presented in Table 2.

The real effects of exercise on the amount of creatine kinase are shown in the second row of Table 2. This variable shows that creatine kinase in the group which got *Aloe vera* was 63% less than that of control group. The real effects of exercises on the amount of CRP in *Aloe vera* group was 64% less than the variance in control group.

To compare the indicators of cell damage in Aloe vera and placebo groups independent *t* test was done and the results are shown in Table 3.

Regarding the results of Table 3, independent *t* test showed that was significant ($P \leq .05$). So, the using of *Aloe vera* caused to decrease the level of CRP.

Discussion

The goal of doing this research was determining the effect of using the *Aloe vera* on cellular damages indices after a course of aerobic exercise among male athletes of 15-18 years old. The obtained results of research showed that there were no significant differences in the amount of LDH and CRP after doing the exercise protocol. But there was not any significant difference in the amount of CK among groups. The obtained results are in agreement with the results of others (14,15). In these researches antioxidant supplement caused significant decrease in CK in supplemented groups which represents a reduction of oxidative stress during exercise in athletes. But, in

Table 1. Homogeneity of the demographic characteristics of the subjects before the exercise

Variables	Supplementation group	Placebo group	*P* value
Age (y)	17 ± 0.65	17 ± 0.94	1
Weight (kg)	64.80 ± 5.26	64.90 ± 9.75	.97
Height (cm)	173.3 ± 5.05	171.06 ± 6.80	.53
BMI (kg/m^2)	21.73 ± 1.84	22.22 ± 3.12	.67

Abbreviation: BMI, body mass index.

Table 2. Comparison of the effects of inter-group LDH, CK and CRP variables in different steps following the use of *Aloe vera*

Statistic test	Freedom rate	F coefficient	*P* value
LDH	3	6.086	.001
CK	3	4.012	.01
CRP	3	3.05	.03

Abbreviations: CK, creatine kinase; LDH, lactate dehydrogenase; CRP, reactive protein C.

Table 3. Comparison of LDH, CK and CRP in supplement and placebo groups

Variable	Steps	Subjects		*P* value[a]
		Supplement group M ± SD	Placebo group M ± SD	
LDH	Before the Cooper test	357.60 ± 40.61	376.10 ± 44.77	.34
	After the Cooper test	394.90 ± 80.48	380.20 ± 32.88	.59
	After one month, before the Copper test	427.60 ± 94.64	599.80 ± 14.53	.006[b]
	After the second Cooper test	495.70 ± 59.138	624.70 ± 59.138	.01[b]
CK	Before the Cooper test	258.70 ± 125.626	190.60 ± 46.126	.1
	After the Cooper test	279.90 ± 152.581	205 ± 57.941	.2
	After one month, before the Copper test	326.80 ± 157.64	340 ± 121.112	.8
	After the second Cooper test	439.80 ± 160.785	453.60 ± 88.781	.8
CRP	Before the Cooper test	3.90 ± 0.99	4.60 ± 0.84	.17
	After the Cooper test	4.20 ± 1.13	4.90 ± 1.19	.19
	After one month, before the Copper test	5 ± 1.15	6.50 ± 1.08	.008[b]
	After the second Cooper test	5.80 ± 0.91	6.90 ± 1.101	.02[b]

Abbreviations: CK, creatine kinase; LDH, lactate dehydrogenase; CRP, reactive protein C.
[a] The results of Independent t test.
[b] Statistically significant.

this research there were not any significant effects on CK. In 2 studies, antioxidant supplements decreased the muscles damage during the endurance exercise courses (4,10). There were not significant changes in CK among supplemented and placebo groups.
Intense exercise courses such as aerobics or endurance marathon are important factors in the production of free radicals and also production of destructive factors in membrane. The Cooper test which was used in this research showed that cellular damage indexes such as LDH, CK and CRP increased after 24 hours that in comparison between supplemented and placebo groups was significant. The results showed decrease in LDH and CRP which are in agreement with the results of others (1,4,6,11). In a study the cellular inflammation index in *Aloe vara* group significantly reduced in comparison to placebo group. As seen, there are different results about the effects of *Aloe vera* in cellular indexes of damages and aerobic exercises in researches.
The number of participants and duration of supplementation to achieve corollary results are important issues. The results of some researches are different following using of *Aloe vera* supplement.
The level of the readiness and the kind of exercise programs were so effective on the results of it. In this research all the subjects were male athletes 15-18 years old and the exercise was aerobic exercise with certain intense that all subjects in 2 groups did for 4 weeks in 3 courses. *Aloe vera* effect on CRP was not effective on male athletes 15-18 years old after 1 course.
In short, the results of statistical analysis of present research showed that using *Aloe vera* has positive effect on the antioxidant defense system and also causes a decrease in the free radical during the endurance. So the sport can be considered as a profit in intense exercise.

Authors' contributions
All the authors wrote the manuscript equally.

Conflict of interests
The authors declared no competing interests.

Ethical considerations
Ethical issues (including plagiarism, misconduct, data fabrication, falsification, double publication or submission, redundancy) have been completely observed by the authors. This trial's protocol and procedures were approved by Ethics Committee of Hamadan University of Medical Sciences, Iran. Then, this trial was registered at http://www.irct.ir website. The registration number of this trial is IRCT2015040521614N1.

Funding/Support
This project was financially supported by corresponding author.

References

1. Yazdani D, Rezaee MB, Kianbakht S, Khosravani S. An overview of the various aspects of medicinal Aloe vera. Journal of Medicinal Plants. 2006;19(5):521-527.
2. Avijgan M. Aloe vera gel as an effective and cheap option for treatment in chronic bed sores. J Gilan Univ Med Sci. 2004;13:45-51.
3. Sosa S, Morelli CF, Tubaro A, Cairoli P, Speranza G, Manitto P. Anti-inflammatory activity of Maytenus senegalensis root extracts and of maytenoic acid. Phytomedicine. 2007;14(2-3):109-114.
4. Azizi, M, Razmjo S, Rajabi H, Hedayati M, Sharifi K. Effect of antioxidant supplementation on oxidative pressure and muscle damage following a period of

heavy training in female adolescent swimmers. Iran Food Science and Nutrition Journal. 2010;5(19):1-12.

5. Sampedro MC, Artola RL, Murature M, et al. Mannan from Aloe saponaria inhibits tumoral cell activation and proliferation. Int Immunopharmacol. 2004;4(3):411-418.
6. Tanaka M, Misawa E, Ito Y, et al. Identification of five phytosterols from Aloe Vera gel as antidiabetic compounds. Biol Pharmacol Bull. 2006;29(7):1418-1422.
7. Langmead L, Makins RJ, Rampton DS. Antiinflammatory effects of Aloe vera gel in human colorectal mucosa in vitro. Aliment Pharmacol Therapeut. 2004;19(5):521-527.
8. Letita M, Timothy J. Antioxidant activity in medical plants associated with the symptoms of diabetes mellitus used by the indigenous people of the North American bored forest. Ethnopharmacol. 2002;82:197-205.
9. Diams I, Julia K, Thomas R. A depose tissue inflammation and Cardiovascular disease. Rev Assoc Med Brase. 2010;56:116-210.
10. Mosayebi G, Ghazavi A, Aghili B, Mirshafie A. Immunomodulating activity of Aloe Vera in animal model of multiple sclerosis. J Arak Unive Med Sci. 2009;12(3):98-104
11. Muller MJ, Hollyoak MA, Moaveni Z, Brown TL, Herndon DN, Heggers JP. Retardation of wound healing by silver sulfadiazine is reversed by Aloe vera and nystatin. Burns. 2003;29(8):834-836.
12. Raja Sekaran S, Sivagnanam K, Subramanian S. Anti oxidant effect of Aloe vera gel extract in streptozotocin induce diabetes in rats. Pharmacol Reports. 2005;57(1):90–96.
13. Wang ZW, Zhou JM, Huang ZS, et al. Aloe polysaccharides mediated radioprotective effect through the inhibition of apoptosis. J Rad Res. 2004;45(3):447-54.
14. Can A, Akev N, Ozsoy N, et al. Effect of Aloe Vera leaf gel and pulp extracts on the liver in type-II diabetic rat models. Biol Pharm Bull. 2004;27(5):694-698.
15. Bryer SC, Goldfarb AH. Effect of high dose vitamin C supplementation on muscle soreness, damage, function, and oxidative stress to eccentric exercise. Int J Sport Nutr Exerc Metab. 2006;16(3):270-280.

Identification and comparison of the yield and composition of essential oil constituents of four Eucalyptus species adapted to the climatic conditions of Khorramabad

Reza Karamian[1,2], Ali Mohammadian[1,2], Esfandiar Hassanimoghadam[1,2], Lila Alizadeh[1], Nargess Abdali[1,3], Mahtab Keshvari[4], Seyed Masih Hosseini[5], Kolsoum Beyranvand[1*]

[1]Razi Herbal Medicines Research Center, Lorestan University of Medical Sciences, Korramabad, Iran
[2]Agriculture and Natural Resources Research Center, Korramabad, Iran
[3]Student Research Committee, Lorestan University of Medical Sciences, Khorramabad, Iran
[4]Isfahan Cardiovascular Research Center, Cardiovascular Research Institute, Isfahan University of medical Sciences, Isfahan, Iran
[5]Medical Plants Research Center, Shahrekord University of Medical Sciences, Shahrekord, Iran

ARTICLE INFO

Keywords:
Eucalyptus
Essential oil
GC-MS

ABSTRACT

Introduction: Eucalyptus has more than 400 species, while only a few species of this genus have been imported in Iran. In this study we aimed to investigate chemical compounds of the essential oils of Eucalyptus species adapted in Lorestan climate.
Methods: In this study, the fresh young leaves of four different Eucalyptus species including *E. suggrandis*, *E. globulus* subsp. *bicostata*, *E. nitens* and *E. globulus* subsp. *maidenii* were collected in spring (the middle of May) in khorramabad, Iran. The powder of air-dried leaves of different species of Eucalyptus was subjected to hydro-distillation using a Clevenger-type apparatus. The chemical compositions of different essential oils were detected using gas chromatography (GC) and gas chromatography coupled with mass spectrometry (GC/MS) and determination of their retention time (RT), retention index (RI) and Mass Spectra. The obtained data were analyzed using SPSS software.
Results: The results of this study indicated that there was significant difference (P<0.01) among the yield and chemical compounds of the essential oils of studied species. The results showed that the yield of essential oil extracted from *E. suggrandis*, *E. globulus bicostata*, *E. nitens* and *E. globulus maidenii* were 1.12%, 1.34%, 2.57% and 5.38%, respectively.
Conclusion: The essential oil constituents of four Eucalyptus species plant were different in among of some compounds. *E. globulus maidenii* had most content of essential oil and 1.8-Cineole compound so it is necessary to identify quality and quantity characteristics of compounds available in this plant.

Implication for health policy/practice/research/medical education:
E. globulus maidenii has most content of essential oil and 1.8-Cineole compound so it is necessary to identify quality and quantity characteristics of compounds available in this plant.

Introduction

Developed countries tend to use medicinal plants and natural compounds in pharmaceutical, cosmetics and food industries and the public welcome to use these plants need applied research. Damages resulting from the use of chemical drugs despite their significant therapeutic effects in many diseases have been reported. Because of synthetic compounds that there are in chemical drugs, adverse side effects may occur in patients and consumers treated with these drugs. So developed countries gradually eliminated all chemicals in food, pharmaceutical, cosmetic and health products and such industries have been transferred to developing countries. Some developed countries such as America, Germany, France, Belgium and the UK have shown significant advancements in the field of medicinal plants so the herbal medicines can be

*__Corresponding author__: Kolsoum Beyranvand,
Email: Genefanavarq@gmail.com

sold several times higher than chemical ones by these countries. Climate variability and unique ecological conditions of Iran, especially in Zagros region areas such as Lorestan has led to more diversity and richness of plant species, especially in the case of medicinal plants. In the research performed to identify the chemical composition of the extract of *Nardostachys jatamansi* in Iran, a total of 29 components were identified using GC/MS analysis (1). According to the researches carried out in Lorestan, there are approximately 1670 plant species of which 250 species are known to have medicinal properties (2). One of the species with medicinal properties is Eucalyptus that is imported in Iran. Even though there are more than 400 species of Eucalyptus in the world, only a few species were imported in Iran and have been planted in areas with mild winters, such as the north and south of Iran (3). According to the performed researches during ten years in Khorramabad, 7 species of Eucalyptus were compared in terms of survival and adaptation (4). Beside of drug usage, Eucalyptus is used to drain the everglades, prevent soil erosion and produce timber and green space. The main chemical components of Eucalyptus, which have many applications in medicine and other industries are Eucalyptol and 1, 8-cineol. In this study we aimed to investigate chemical compounds of the essential oils of Eucalyptus species adapted in Lorestan climate.

Materials and Methods

Plant collection and extraction of essential oils

Fresh young leaves of four different Eucalyptus species including *E. suggrandis*, *E. globulus* subsp. *bicostata*, *E. nitens* and *E. globulus* subsp. *maidenii* were collected in spring (the middle of May) in Khorramabad, Iran. The leaves were spread on the cloth and dried during 7 days in the laboratory. Air-dried leaves of different species of Eucalyptus (100 g) were powdered and subjected to hydro-distillation using a Clevenger-type apparatus. The oils were separated from water and dried over anhydrous sodium sulfate and kept in sealed vials at low temperature before analysis.

Identification of essential oil constituents

The essential oils extracted from leaves of different Eucalyptus were subjected to gas chromatography (GC) and gas chromatography coupled with mass spectrometry (GC/MS). After injection of oils, using Retention Rime (RT), Retention Index (RI) and Mass spectra of components and their comparison with those of standard ones or by computer matching against the library spectra, the compositions of the oils were studied qualitatively and quantitatively (5).

Statistical analysis

To ensure normal distribution of obtained data, the Kolmogorov-Smirnov test was used. The significance of differences among the yield and components of samples were determined by analysis of variance (ANOVA), using the Duncan test of SPSS. Differences were considered significant at the $P<0.01$ level.

Results

Compositions of essential oils obtained from different Eucalyptus species

In total, 37 compounds in the essential oil of *E. nitens*, 27 compounds in the essential oil of *E. globulus bicostata*, 31 compounds in the essential oil of *E. globulus maidenii* and 38 compounds in the essential oil of *E. suggrandis* were identified.

Compositions of essential oil of E. nitens

Of the 36 components identified in the essential oil of *E. nitens*, 1, 8-cineol (46.67%) was the main constituent. α-pinene (14.56) was in the second place and the other constituents were Aromadendrene (9.02), Viridiflorol (5.65) and β-pinene (4.51). All compounds that were identified in the essential oil of *E. nitens* are recorded in Table 1.

Table 1. The composition of essential oil extracted from *E. nitens*

	Chemical composition	Compound (%)	Retention time	Katz index
1	α- Pinene	14.56	11.64	935
2	β-Pinene	4.51	13.61	975
3	Myrcene	0.35	14.32	988
4	1.8-Cineole	46.67	16.77	1038
5	Gamma-terpinene	0.34	17.90	1061
6	Terpinolene	0.32	19.25	1087
7	Methybuthyl2-methylbutanoate(3)	0.22	20.11	1104
8	Trans-Pinocarveol	1.15	21.88	1140
9	Pinocarvone	0.35	22.85	1160
10	Terpinene-4-ol	0.54	23.69	1170
11	α-Terpineol	0.94	24.45	1192
12	Myrtenol	0.20	24.65	1196
13	Trans-p-Mentha-1(17).8-dien-2- ol	0.32	26.13	1228
14	Geranial	0.27	26.64	1239
15	Delta-Elemene	0.40	31.05	1336
16	Isoledene	0.23	32.62	1371
17	Geranyl acetate	0.20	33.08	1382
18	α-Ggurjunene	0.56	34.27	1409
19	Trans-Caryophllene	0.39	34.68	1419
20	β-Copaene	0.39	35.93	1432
21	Aromadendrene	9.02	35.93	1449
22	Alloaromadendrene	1.68	36.60	1465
23	α-Gurjunene	0.33	36.92	1473
24	Naphthalene,1,2,3,5,6,7,...	0.59	37.59	1489
25	Viridiflorene	0.60	38.03	1500
26	Gamma-Cadinene	0.15	38.60	1514
27	Delta-Cadinene	0.38	38.96	1523
28	Epiglobulol	0.82	40.54	1564
29	Globulol	0.63	40.78	1570
30	Veridiflorol	5.65	41/81	1596
31	1H-Cycloprop(e)azulenn-4-ol	1.34	42.05	1602
32	Leptospermone(iso)	0.65	42.76	1622
33	Eremoligenol	0.62	43.04	1629
34	(gamma)Eudesmol	0.62	43.04	1629
35	2-Naphthalenemathanol, 1, 2, 3, 4,...	0.32	43.60	1645
36	β-Eudesmol	1.79	44.16	1660
	-	99.01	-	-

Compositions of essential oil of E. globulus bicostata
Twenty-seven compounds were identified in the essential oil of *E. globulus bicostata* of these, 1, 8-cineol as the major component with the 70.15% was significantly higher than the other compounds. Aromadendrene with 6.92%, Viridiflorol with 4.49% and α-pinene with 3.65% were the other main constituents. All compounds that were identified in the essential oil of *E. globulus bicostata* are presented in Table 2.

Compositions of essential oil of E. globulus maidenii
As presented in Table 3, 31 compounds were identified in the oil of *E. globulus maidenii,* of which 1, 8-cineol detected as the main constituent with 60.29%. The other major components were α-pinene, α-terpineol and β-eudesmol with 15.05%, 6.11% and 3.88%, respectively.

Compositions of essential oil of E. suggrandis
38 compounds were identified in the oil obtained from *E. suggrandis.* 1, 8 –cineol, α-pinene, Trans-pinocarveol, β-Eudesmol and Pinocarvone were the major detected constituents with 30.94%, 18.52%, 14.89%, 6.87% and 4.96%, respectively. All compounds that were identified in the essential oil of *E. suggrandis* are presented in Table 4.

Table 2. The composition of essential oil extracted from *E. globulus bicostata*

	Chemical composition	Compound (%)	Retention time	Katz index
1	α- Pinene	3.65	11.35	929
2	β-Pinene	0.38	13.34	970
3	1.8-Cineole	70.15	16.80	1039
4	Gamma-terpinene	0.24	17.77	1058
5	Trans-Pinocarveol	1.3.	21.77	1138
6	Pinocarvone	0.71	22.79	1159
7	α-Terpineol	2.54	24.43	1192
8	Trans-carveol	0.18	25.63	1217
9	Trans-p-Mentha-1(17).8-dien-2-ol	0.55	26.10	1227
10	Thymol	2.48	29.22	1294
11	α-Terpinylacetate	0.27	31.60	1348
12	Isoledene	0.20	32.60	1371
13	α-Gurjunene	0.62	34.23	1408
14	Trans-Caryophyllene	0.13	34.61	1417
15	β-Copaene	0.36	35.16	1431
16	Aromadendrene	6.92	35.72	1444
17	Alloaromadendrene	0.22	36.84	1471
18	Propanoic acid,2,2-dimethyl-2-phenylethyl	0.40	37.51	1487
19	Ledene	0.93	37.85	1495
20	Gamma-Cadinene	0.13	38.55	1513
21	Cycloisolongifol-5-ol(trans)	0.16	38.76	1518
22	Delta-Cadinene	0.16	38.90	1522
23	Epiglobulol	0.68	40.43	1561
24	Viridiflorol	4.49	41.54	1589
25	1H-Indene	0.44	42.12	1604
26	β-Eudesmol	0.66	42.87	1625
27	α-Cadinol	0.24	43.99	1656
	-	99.24		

Table 3. The composition of essential oil extracted from *E. globulus maidenii*

	Chemical composition	Compound (%)	Retention time	Katz index
1	α- Pinene	15.05	11.60	934
2	β-Pinene	0.78	13.39	971
3	Myrcene	0.58	14.21	988
4	α-phellandrene	0.47	14.83	1000
5	1.8-Cineole	60.29	16.77	1038
6	(z-β) Ocimene	0.17	17.34	1050
7	Gamma-terpinene	0.38	17.80	1059
8	Terpinolene	0.16	19.17	1086
9	Linalool	0.16	19.81	1098
10	Isopenntyl 2-methylbutanoate (3)	0.09	20.06	1103
11	Trans-Pinocarveol	0.68	21.71	1137
12	Pinocarvone	0.21	22.75	1157
13	Delta-Terpineol	0.31	23.11	1165
14	Terpinene-4- ol	0.62	23.62	1176
15	α- Terpineol	6.11	24.70	1197
16	1,7-Octadien-3-one,2-methyl-6-methylene	0.29	26.08	1227
17	α-Copaene	0.30	32.72	1373
18	Geranial acetate	0.11	30.00	1380
19	α- Gurjunene	0.60	34.20	1407
20	Trans-Caryophyllene	0.24	34.60	1417
21	Aromadendrene	3.32	34.75	1440
22	Aristolene	0.39	37.48	1486
23	Viridiflorene	0.87	37.81	1494
24	Delta- Cadinene	0.5	38.87	1521
25	Epiglobulol	0.31	40.32	1558
26	(-)-Globulol	0.73	41.33	1584
27	Viridiflorol	0.26	41.61	1591
28	Guaiol	0.25	41.80	1596
29	Gamma- Eudesmol	1.53	43.20	1634
30	Hinesol	0.19	43.43	1640
31	β-Eudesmol	3.88	43.13	1659
	-	99.82	-	-

Discussion

The results of this study indicated that the yield of obtained essential oil was varied in case of some species of Eucalyptus in the studied area. Based on the comparison of the averages of the yield of oil by Duncan test, *E. globulus maidenii* had the highest oil yields (5.38%) and *E. suggrandis* showed the lowest oil yields with approximately 1.12% (Figure 1). 7 similar compounds identified in the extracted oils from different species of Eucalyptus that were studied in this study (Table 5). As presented in Table 5, three compounds including 1, 8-cineol, α-pinene and β-pinene had the highest amount in terms of composition between different species.

Conclusion

Based on the results of this study, it can be concluded that the development of culturing of *E. globulus* in Khorramabad weather conditions and exploitation of its leaves to obtain essential oil in large extent is recommendable economically (more than 5% essential oil and 1, 8-cineol up to 66.72%). Therefore, with regard to the specific application and required compound, developing

Table 4. The composition of essential oil extracted from *E. Suggrandis*

	Chemical composition	Compound (%)	Retention time	Katz index
1	α- Pinene	18.52	11.87	940
2	Camphenne	0.41	12.24	947
3	β-Pinene	0.68	13.52	974
4	1.8-Cineole	30.94	16.77	1038
5	Gamma-terpinene	0.64	17.97	1062
6	Metha-Cymenene	0.27	19.30	1088
7	Methybuthy12-methylbutanoate(3)	0.10	20.12	1105
8	-Campholenalα	0.51	21.07	1124
9	Trans-Pinocarveol	14.89	22.87	1160
10	Pinocarvone	4.96	23.46	1172
11	Terpinene-4-ol	0.33	23.94	1182
12	-Terpineolα	1.57	24.73	1198
13	Myrtenol	0.46	24.97	1203
14	Trans-Carveol	0.26	25.87	1222
15	Trans-p-Mentha-1(17).8-dien-2-ol	0.38	26.31	1232
16	2,3-Butanedioldiacetate	0.05	27.07	1248
17	Carvacrol	0.22	29.39	1298
18	Delta-Elemene	0.62	30.65	1326
19	-Copaeneα	0.21	32.81	1375
20	-Elemeneβ	0.15	33.52	1392
21	α- Gurjunene	0.30	34.29	1410
22	Trans-Caryophyllene	0.85	34.80	1422
23	1H-Cycloprop(a)naphthalene	0.08	35.06	1428
24	β -Gurjunene	0.11	35.23	1432
25	Aromadendrene	2.21	35.75	1445
26	Alloaromadendrene	0.83	36.52	1463
27	Germacrene-D	0.30	37.28	1482
28	-Selinneneβ	0.45	37.55	1488
29	Bicyclogermacrene	1.96	38.11	1502
30	Gamma-Cadinene	0.15	38.63	1515
31	Delta- Cadinene	0.38	39.00	1524
32	Epiglobulol	0.41	0.52	1563
33	Globulol	0.42	40.78	1570
34	Viridiflorol	3.67	41.77	1595
35	1H-Cycloprop(e)azulenn-4-ol	1.25	42.04	1602
36	1H-Cycloprop(e)azulenn-1A-2-3,...	0.43	42.67	1619
37	-Naphthalenemethanol, 1,2,3,4,...	2.10	43.48	1642
38	β-Eudesmol	6.87	44.57	1671
	-	98.94		

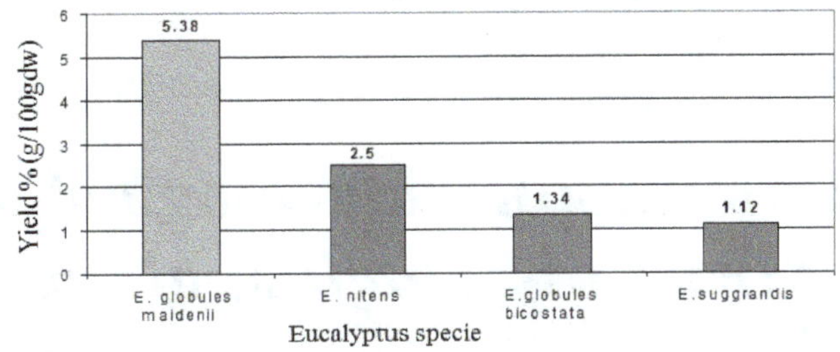

Figure 1. The yield of extracted essential oils from different four species of Eucalyptus

Table 5. The same compounds in the extracted oil of different four Eucalyptus species

	Nitens	*Suggrandis*	*Globulus bicostata*	*Globulus* maidenii 12130
α-Pinene	14.56	18.52	3.65	15.05
–Pineneβ	4.51	0.68	0.38	0.78
1, 8- Cineole	46.67	30.94	70.15	60.29
Gammaterpinen	0.34	0.64	0.24	0.38
Pinocarvone	0.35	4.96	0.71	0.21
Epigloubluol	0.82	0.41	0.68	0.31
-Eudesmolβ	1.79	6.87	0.66	3.88

and planting of mentioned species can be suggested.

Authors' contributions

All contributed to the study. RK, AM, EH, LA, NA, MK, KB acquired data and prepared the drafting. MK revised it critically for important intellectual content and submitted it. KB prepared the main drafting.

Conflict of interests

The authors declared no competing interests.

Ethical considerations

Ethical issues (including plagiarism, misconduct, data fabrication, falsification, double publication or submission, redundancy) have been completely observed by the authors.

Funding/Support

This research was financially supported by Razi herbal medicines research center, Lorestan University of medical science, Korramabad, Iran.

References

1. Ghassemi-Dehkordi N, Sajjadi E, Shafiei-Koojani H, Keshvari M, Hoseini SM. Identification of chemical compounds of Nardostachys Jatamansi essence available in Iran. J HerbMed Pharmacol 2014; 3(2): 83-6.
2. Karamian R. Final report of Investigation on Adaptability and performance of industrial eucalypt Provenances at Khorram Abad in Lorestan province; 2011. p 19. [In Persian]
3. Mohammadian A. Final report of investigation in habitat and distribution of different species of Thymus Genus in Iran. Research Institute of Forests & Rangelands; 2010. p. 109. [In Persian]
4. Assareh MH, Sardabi H. Eucalyptus, description, lustration and propagation by advanced technologies. Research Institute of Forests & Rangelands; 2007. [In Persian]
5. Adams RP. Identification of Essential Oil Components by Gas Chromatography/Mass Spectroscopy. Carol Stream, USA: Allured Publishing Corp; 1959. p. 456.

28

Immunopharmacological screening of aqueous root extract of *Santalum album*

Amit Gupta[1*], Sushama R Chaphalkar[2]

[1]Department of Immunology, Vidya Pratishthan's School of Biotechnology, Baramati, District Pune, Maharashtra India
[2]Director, Vidya Pratishthan's School of Biotechnology, Baramati, District Pune, Maharashtra India

ARTICLE INFO

Keywords:
Santalum album
Hepatitis B vaccine
NDV
Aqueous extract

ABSTRACT

Introduction: In order to scrutinize the anti-microbial and anti-inflammatory agents, many research groups have focused their works on the field of immunopharmacology. Thus, the current study aimed to evaluate the immunopharmacological activity of aqueous root extract of *Santalum album* against Hepatitis B surface antigen (HBsAg) and Newcastle disease virus (NDV) on human peripheral blood mononuclear cells (PBMCs).
Methods: Variable doses of aqueous root extract of Santalum album (0.5-30 mg/ml, 50 µl) were prepared using phosphate buffered saline (PBS) and tested for proliferation assay, nitric oxide production and CD14 monocyte surface marker using flow cytometry.
Results: Aqueous root extract of *Santalum album* inhibited proliferation, nitric oxide production and CD14 monocyte surface marker at higher doses.
Conclusion: Aqueous root extract of *Santalum album* possesses both anti-inflammatory as well as antiviral activities and might be used for these purposes.

Implication for health policy/practice/research/medical education:
Santalum album has anti-inflammatory and antiviral activities and might be used for these purposes.

Introduction

Medicinal plants have been continuously used for thousands of years to treat various disorders and to prevent a number of animal and human diseases (bacteria, viruses, fungi, etc.) (1,2). The knowledge of various medicinal plant properties has been transmitted all over the world. It has been reported that the active constituent is responsible for immunopharmacological properties of medicinal plants so that some of them are continuously used throughout the world for different purposes (3,4).
There are a large number of medicinal plant products, potentially able to control various diseases and also used for specific case of disease treatment (1). For the last twenty years, lot of work was done on many medicinal plant products with description of their chemical constituents in the form of primary and secondary metabolites (2,3). These metabolites could be isolated using various types of qualitative and quantitative based assays, leading to understand the mechanism and correlation between these metabolites and disease model studies (5). Thus, the present work was focused on *Santalum album*, as one of medicinal plants, with emphasis on its antimicrobial properties in human peripheral blood mononuclear cells (PBMCs).
Newcastle disease virus (NDV, single-stranded RNA virus) belongs to the family Paramyxoviridae and genus *Aulavirus* with helical capsid symmetry. Till now, NDV disease still burdens for the poultry industry with several consequences including an increase in mortality rates (5). The only control method for NDV disease is through vaccination but it does not provide hundred percent protection. Thus there is a need to search for those medicinal plants to control the burden of NDV disease.
One of the medicinal plant, *Santalum album* (commonly known as chandan) in the family *Santalaceae*, is usually found in India, china, Indonesia and Philippines (6,7). *Santalum album*, is a widely plant commonly found in India especially parts of Karnataka and adjoining districts of Maharashtra, Tamil Nadu and Andhra Pradesh in India.

***Corresponding author:** Amit Gupta; Vidya Pratishthan's School of Biotechnology, Baramati, District Pune, Maharashtra India.
Email: amitgupta@vsbt.res.in

Actually, this plant is being exploited for various purposes especially sandalwood oil is obtained mostly by steam distillation of its root and heartwood (8,9) with a number of medicinal uses e.g. treatment of many other ailments like diarrhea along with bleeding, intrinsic hemorrhage, inflamed hemorrhoids (piles), eye infections, inflammation of the umbilicus, hiccoughs initial phase of pox, and urticaria (10,11). The current study was focused on the immunopharmacological activity of *Santalum album* on human PBMCs against Hepatitis B surface antigen (HBsAg) and NDV.

Materials and methods

Assemblage and composition of plant material

The fresh roots of *Santalum albumin* were collected from the garden of Vidya Pratishthan's in the morning, between January and February 2015 in Baramati region, District Pune, Maharashtra, India. Afterwards, the fresh roots were washed in tap water and then with distilled water to remove dust and finally dried in a shady area. The plant roots were macerated with liquid nitrogen to prepare a fine powder. This powder was used for subsequent immunopharmacological assays.

Phytochemical screening and extraction

Different qualitative and quantitative based assays were carried out in order to determine the presence of secondary metabolites. Qualitative based assays revealed aqueous root extracts of *Santalum album* and the presence of Saponin (foam test); terpenoids (acetic anhydride test) and flavonoids (alkaline reagent test).

Collection of NDV samples

NDV Samples of suspected birds were collected under the programme of Biovillage scheme, Vidya Pratishthan's School of Biotechnology.

Specific pathogen free chicken eggs were purchased from Venkys India Ltd. The allantoic cavity route of embryonated (9-11 day old) chicken eggs was used for isolation and propagation of NDV from field samples (5). These eggs were observed in dark (using candle) at regular intervals and bigger sized embryos (air cell and area without blood vessels) selected for inoculation. After disinfection of egg shells with spirit, 0.2 ml of supernatant was inoculated at 45° angle into embryonated chicken eggs. Embryo motility was observed every 10 hours by candling. After the death of embryos, amnio-allantoic fluid was harvested and checked for presence of virus. This was determined through haemagglutination test (128 HA titre value).

PBMC proliferation assay and nitric oxide production using HBsAg and NDV

EDTA anti-coagulant human blood samples were collected from Mangal Pathology Laboratory, Maharashtra, India and scrutinized at the VSBT, Baramati, Maharashtra, India, between January to February 2015.

PBMCs were separated by means of density gradient centrifugation and cultured with variable doses of aqueous root extracts (0.5-30 mg/ml, 50 μl) of *Santalum album* along with or without HBsAg (20 μg/ml, 10 μl) and NDV (1:80 dilution, 10 μl). Incubate 96-well plates for 48 hours at 37°C. HBsAg and NDV used as standard for these studies. Centrifuging the plates was done at 2500 rpm for 10 minutes at 4°C with collecting the supernatant for the estimation of nitric oxide production through Griess reagent. Afterwards, fresh complete medium was added into the 96-well plates. Again, incubating the plates for another 4 hours along with (3-(4,5-Dimethylthiazol-2-yl)-2,5-diphenyltetrazolium-bromide; 5 mg/ml, 10 μl) continued. After incubation, the plates were suddenly centrifuged with discarding the supernatant, collecting the pellet and finally dispersing in dimethyl sulphoxide (DMSO) solution. The optical density was measured at 570 nm (12,13). After preincubation of PBMC (10^5 cells/ml) with or without HBsAg and NDV for 48 hours the supernatant (as mentioned above) was collected for estimation of nitric oxide production. Briefly, 50 μl of untreated and treated PBMC cell culture medium along with HBsAg/NDV was assorted with 50 μl of Griess reagent (1% sulfanilamide and 0.1% naphthyl ethylenediamine dihydrochloride [NED] in 2.5% phosphoric acid). For this experiment, Roswell Park Memorial Institute medium (RPMI) containing 10% fetal bovine serum was used as a blank followed by incubation of 96-well plates at room temperature for 10-15 minutes. After incubation, absorbance at 540 nm was measured in a microplate reader (14,15).

Estimation of CD14 monocyte surface marker by flow cytometry

In another set of experiments, human PBMCs were cultured with serial dilutions of aqueous root extracts of *Santalum album* along with or without HBsAg (20 μg/ml, 10 μl)/NDV (1:80 dilution, 10 μl) for 48 hours in 96-well plates. After incubation, samples of the PBMCs treated with or without HBsAg/NDV were collected and stained with CD14 FITC (3 μl) monoclonal antibody. The samples were then incubated, lysed and washed with phosphate buffered saline (PBS). Finally, the samples were prepared for flow cytometric analysis. The resulting stained cell pellet was resuspended in 2000 μl of PBS and run on a FACS Calibur flow cytometer (16,17).

Statistical analysis

All values were mentioned as mean ± SE. Data was represented by one-way analysis of variance (ANOVA) test (Bonferroni multiple comparison test).

Results

PBMC proliferation assay

The effect of variable doses of aqueous root extract of *Santalum album* on PBMC proliferation assay with or without HBsAg and NDV using MTT is shown in Figure 1. The

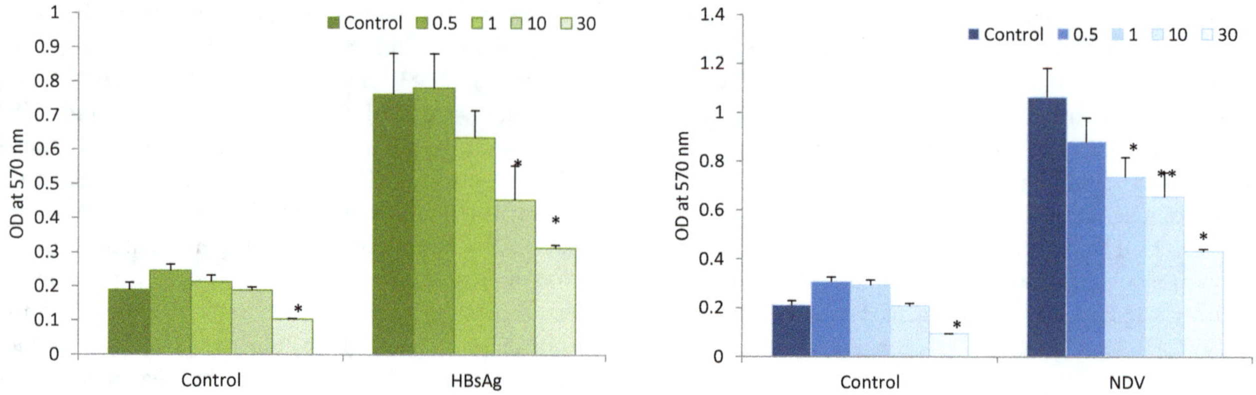

Figure 1. Effect of variable doses of aqueous root extract of *Santalum album* on HBsAg and NDV in human PBMC. PBMC were cultured with or without optimized dose of HBsAg and NDV along with variable doses of aqueous root extract (0.5, 1, 10 and 30 mg/ml, 50 µl) or NDV/HBsAg alone. After 3 days, proliferation was measured by MTT assay. The results are presented as Mean ± S.E. *$P < 0.05$, **$P < 0.01$, ***$P < 0.001$ as compared to control.

aqueous extract showed a dose-dependent decrease in the proliferation assay with or without HBsAg/NDV as compared to control. Also, there was a significant enhancement of PBMC proliferation as compared to control.

Nitric oxide estimation

The observed effect of variable doses of aqueous root extract in the cell culture medium of PBMC along with or without HBsAg/NDV is shown in Figure 2. The aqueous root extract showed a significant decrease in nitric oxide production at higher doses with or without HBsAg/NDV as compared to control. There was a significant enhancement of nitric oxide production as compared to control.

CD14 monocyte surface marker

The effect of aqueous root extract of CD14 monocyte surface marker on PBMC with or without HBsAg/NDV is shown in Figure 3. There was a significant decrease in CD14 monocyte surface marker at higher doses as compared to control.

Discussion

The prime objective of our study was to investigate the aqueous root extract of *Santalum album* for in vitro proliferation, nitric oxide production and CD14 monocyte surface marker on human PBMC using HBsAg and NDV, in order to validate the potential use of this aqueous root extract as a tool in screening for anti-inflammatory and anti-microbial effects on the immune system.

As per the literature survey, there are a number of immunopharmacological studies related to medicinal plants which have already been done using non specific antigens on humoral and cell mediated immune response (18). These studies are a matter of great interest for many immunopharmacologists. For instance, one of the medicinal plant namely, *Santalum album* shows anti-inflammatory (reduction in HBsAg) as well as anti-microbial (inhibitory effect of NDV) activities at higher doses as compared to

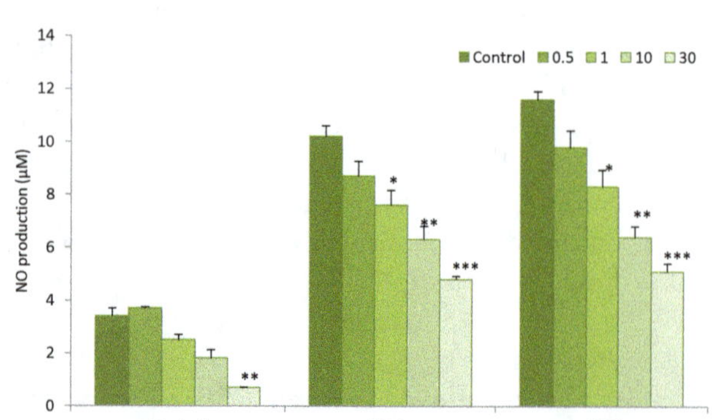

Figure 2. Estimation of nitric oxide production (NO) from human PBMC. The supernatant nitrite concentration was determined by Griess reagent after 48 h culture of cells in presence of with or without HBsAg and NDV along with variable doses of aqueous root extract (0.5, 1, 10 and 30 mg/ml, 50 µl) or NDV/HBsAg alone. Values are expressed as Means ± S.E. The difference between the control and treated groups is determined by One-way ANOVA test (Bonferroni multiple comparison test). *$P < 0.05$; **$P < 0.01$; ***$P < 0.001$.

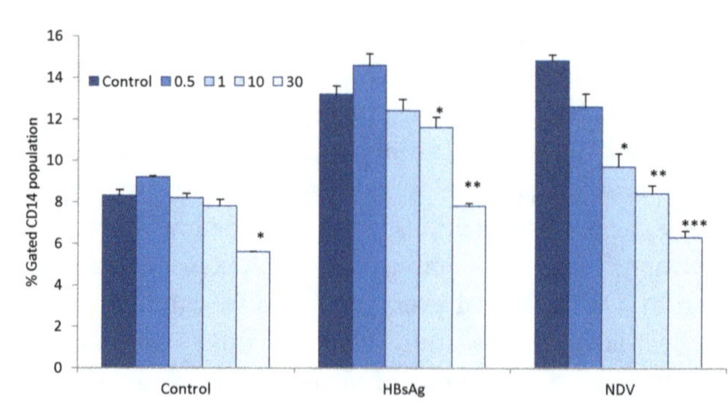

Figure 3. Flow cytometric analysis of aqueous root extract extracted from *Santalum album* on CD14 monocyte surface marker. PBMC were treated with variable doses of aqueous root extract (0.5, 1, 10 and 30 mg/ml, 50 µl) along with or without NDV/HBsAg and then lysed and wash the cells with PBS and analyzed through flow cytometer (FACS, Calibur) using forward and side scatter gating applied for data acquisition of 10000 events of cell populations representing different phenotypes analyzed using cell quest software.

control and standard HBsAg/NDV.

One of the parameters interconnected with our immune system i.e. nitric oxide production, provides reliable information whether the aqueous root extract shows inhibitory or stimulatory effect with respect to PBMC proliferation assay and CD14 monocyte surface marker. The criteria for selecting this parameter i.e. nitric oxide (as a fundamental signaling agent), regulates various immunopharmacological functions and serves as a potent mediator of inflammation, bacteria or viral disease burden and cytotoxicity (14,15). The findings of the preliminary phytochemical investigations of the aqueous root extract of *Santalum album* and the results of anti-inflammatory activity against HBsAg are shown in the respective figures with anti-viral activity against NDV. The results indicate that aqueous root extraction of *Santalum album* shows a dosage-dependent relationship.

The capacity to elicit a decline in T cell immunity can be shown by the CD14 monocyte surface marker. This is determined through flow cytometry and generally used for measuring the properties of the cell suspended in a stream of fluid when passing through one, two or three lasers. It is also used for measuring the immunophenotyping i.e. detection of cell surface molecules such as cluster of differentiation (CD), cell cycle analysis, cell viability, total protein, enzyme activity, gene expression etc. (16,17). The results indicate that aqueous root extract could significantly reduce the CD14 count in human PBMC exposed to HBsAg and NDV. The results of our immunopharmacological studies on human PBMC after exposing with HBsAg and NDV suggest that the aqueous root extract shows anti-inflammatory as well as anti-viral effect on human PBMC.

Conclusion

This study suggests that the aqueous root extract of *Santalum album* significantly inhibits the production of proliferation assay, nitric oxide production and CD14 monocyte surface marker when using HBsAg and NDV. Further investigations of the aqueous root extract should be done through in vivo assessment for immunopharmacological studies in mice models with identification of the major active components responsible for anti-microbial and anti-inflammatory activities.

Acknowledgements

We would also like to thanks Dr. H. Pawar Veterinary Doctor for collection of NDV samples under the project of Biovillage-Sustainable development through Biotechnology.

Authors' contributions

This work was carried out in collaboration between AG and SRC. AG anchored the field study, collected the data and prepared the manuscript. AG and SRC managed the literature searches and produced the initial draft. Both the authors read and approved the final manuscript.

Conflict of interests

None to be declared.

Ethical considerations

All these studies were conducted under surveillance of animal diseases in Baramati taluka which is ethically approved from IBSC committee, Savitri Phule University Pune, India.

Funding/Support

Both the authors are highly thankful to our organization i.e. Vidya Pratishthan's and these studies were conducted for the collection of NDV samples under the project of Biovillage- Sustainable development through Biotechnology.

References

1. Eddouks M, Chattopadhyay D, Feo VD, Cho WC. Medicinal plants in the prevention and treatment of chronic diseases. Evid Based Complement Alternat Med. 2012;458274:1-2.
2. Gupta A, Khamkar PR, Chaphalkar SR. Review on medicinal plants to target and inhibit the epidermal growth factor receptor signaling in cancer and tissue repair therapy. International Journal of Advances in Pharmacy, Biology and Chemistry. 2014;3(1):210-213.
3. Gupta A, Khamkar PR, Chaphalkar SR. Applications and uses of active ingredients from medicinal plants. Indian Journal of Novel Drug Delivery. 2014;6(2): 106–111.
4. Maciel MA, Pinto AC, Veiga VF Jr, Grynberg NF, Echevarria A. Medicinal plants: the need for multidisciplinary scientific studies. Quim Nova. 2002;25(3):429-438.
5. Gupta A, Jagtap RB, Chaphalkar SR. Anti-viral activity of Azadirachta indica leaves against Newcastle disease virus: a study by in vitro and in vivo immunological approach. International Journal of Current Trends in Pharmaceutical Research. 2014;2(6):494-501.
6. Misra BB, Dey S. Biological Activities of east Indian sandalwood tree, Santalum album. Peer J Pre-Prints. 2013;1:e96.
7. Brocke C, Eh M, Finke A. Recent developments in the chemistry of sandalwood odorants. Chem Biodivers. 2008;5:1000-1010.
8. Burdock GA, Carabin IG. Safety assessment of sandalwood oil (Santalum album L.). Food Chem Toxicol. 2008;46:421-432.
9. Benencia F, Courreges MC. Antiviral Activity of Sandalwood oil against Herpes Simplex Viruses 1 & 2. Phytomedicine. 1999;6(2):119-123.
10. Varadaraj P, Shankaranaryana KH. Antibacterial activity of Sandal bark Tannins against Staphylococcus aureus. Van Vigyan 1986;24(3&4):120-121.
11. Scartezzini P, Speroni E. Review on some plants of Indian traditional medicine with antioxidant activity.

J Ethnopharmacol. 2000;71(1-2):23-43.
12. Gupta A, Khamkar PR, Chaphalkar SR. In vitro anti-inflammatory activities of root aqueous extract of Mesua ferrea in human whole blood and peripheral blood mononuclear cells using flow cytometry. International Journal of Pharmacy and Life Sciences. 2014;5(10):3903-3909.
13. Gupta A, Chaphalkar SR. Exploring the immunogenicity potential of plant viruses used as vaccine antigen: Tobacco plant. Journal of International Research in Medical and Pharmaceutical Sciences. 2015;5(4):118-127.
14. Chung HS, Kang M, Cho C, et al. Inhibition of nitric oxide and tumor necrosis factor-alpha by moutan cortex in activated mouse peritoneal macrophages. Biol Pharm Bull. 2007;30:912-916.
15. Gupta A, Khamkar PR, Chaphalkar SR. Inhibition of nitric oxide production and proinflammatory cytokines by aqueous extract of Terminalia arjuna in human peripheral blood mononuclear cells. International Journal of Pharmaceutical and Biological Science Archive. 2014;2(8):29-33.
16. Gupta A, Khamkar PR, Chaphalkar SR. Immunomodulatory and anti-inflammatory activity of aqueous extract of leaf, stem and root of Ficus religiosa on human whole blood and peripheral blood mononuclear cells. International Journal of Medicine and Pharmaceutical Research. 2014;2(4):732-739.
17. Gupta A, Chaphalkar SR. Immunopharmacological activity of Zingiber officinale on human peripheral blood mononuclear cells. Asian Journal of Medical and Pharmaceutical Researches. 2015;5(2):13-17.
18. Gupta A, Khajuria A, Singh J, et al. Immunomodulatory activity of biopolymeric fraction RLJ-NE-205 from Picrorhiza kurroa. Int Immunopharmacol. 2006;6(10):1543-1549.

29

Comparative study on the antifungal activity of hydroalcoholic extract of Iranian Propolis and *Royal jelly* against *Rhizopus oryzae*

Hassan Moghim[1*], Simin Taghipoor[1], Najmeh Shahinfard[1], Soleiman kheiri[2], Hamideh Khabbazi[1]

[1]Medical Plants Research Center, Shahrekord University of Medical Sciences, Shahrekord, Iran
[2]Social Health Determinants Research Center, Shahrekord University of Medical Sciences, Shahrekord, Iran

ARTICLE INFO

Keywords:
Propolis
Royal jelly
Candida albicans
Rhizopus oryzae

ABSTRACT

Introduction: Mucormycosis is an opportunistic fungal infection. *Rhizopus oryzae* is major cause of mucormycosis in humans. This disease is the most common form of the acute fungal infection with rapid progress. Iranian Propolis extract and *Royal jelly* are honey bee products which have been used by human over the past centuries in traditional medicine. In this study the effects of Iranian Propolis and *Royal jelly* were investigated against *Rhizopus oryzae* and *Candida albicans*.
Methods: The used method in this study was microdilution. To perform it, the prepared dilutions of *Royal jelly* and alcoholic extract of Iranian Propolis were added to tubes containing Sabouraud dextrose broth culture media except to control group and then *Rhizopus oryzae* suspension was added to all microtubes. In the next stage, microtubes were maintained in incubator at 25°C for 48 hours and then 10 ml of the content of each microtube was transferred to Sabouraud dextrose agar media. The minimum inhibitory concentration (MIC) and minimum fungicidal concentration (MFC) of the agents were calculated.
Results: In this study, the MIC and MFC of Iranian Propolis alcoholic extract on Rhizopus oryzae were respectively 0.1 and 0.25 mg/ml and the MFC of *Royal jelly* on *Rhizopus oryzae* were respectively 100 ± 34 and 133 ± 46 mg/ml.
Conclusion: The results indicate that Propolis might be used as an ideal combination for the treatment of fungal infections like *Rhizopus oryzae*. However, clinical studies are needed to confirm the effects of these drugs.

Implication for health policy/practice/research/medical education:
Propolis might be used as an ideal combination for the treatment of fungal infections, if clinical studies confirm the effects of these drugs.

Introduction

Mucormycosis is an opportunistic fungal infection caused by fungi in the order of mucorales and can cause acute fungal infection. These fungi have a wide geographical spread. *Rhizopus oryzae* is major cause of mucormycosis in humans. This disease is the most common form of the infection with rapid process (1-4). Therefore, with regard to the increasing incidence of fungal diseases and problems that exist with the use of classical medications and also due to incidence of some drug resistances, there is a need to introduce new drugs with fewer side effects. So, more extensive researches should be performed in this regard (5).

Today, much attention has been paid to the use of therapies with natural and biological materials. *Royal jelly* and Propolis, the bee products, have been used in traditional medicine by humans over the past centuries (6,7). *Royal jelly* is one of bee products that is produced by incomplete digestion in the stomach of workers of honey bees. This material is secreted from hypopharynx and mandibular

***Corresponding author**: Hassan Moghim, Medical Plants Research Center, Shahrekord University of Medical Sciences, Shahrekord, Iran. Email: hassan.moghim@yahoo.com glands for feeding the queen bee (6,7).

Propolis is a plant resin around the hive and is produced by honey bees. This resin is used to block the gaps and disinfect the hive to strength the walls and body of the hive (8).

Several beneficial properties of this compound can be considered for human being. The extract of the Propolis contains flavonoids, tannins, steroids, alcohol and alkaloid. Overall, Propolis has antimicrobial effect with different spectrum and therefore, it might be considered as a potent candidate for treatment of several clinical scenarios (9).

The chemical composition of Propolis is very complex and more than 300 different compounds are identified in Propolis samples depending on the location and time of collection and the plants of the region. There are naturally 50% gum (including flavonoids and phenolic acids), 30% wax, 10% volatile oils, 5% pollen and 5% various organic compounds in composition of Propolis (6,10-12).

In recent years, several reports have been published about the specific antimicrobial characteristics of natural products to treat bacterial infections that Propolis is one of the considerable cases. Studies have also shown antibacterial activity of *Royal jelly* against bacteria and fungi (13-17).

On the other hand, the irregular use of antifungal drugs, has caused drug resistance against them and they also can have many side effects on human health. Thus, investigations to find natural antimicrobial drugs have increased in order to prevent side effects of drugs (18). Although several reports have been published on anti-inflammatory, antitumor, antiallergic (19), and antihypertesive agents (20,21), few information is available on the antimicrobial property of Propolis. Hence, the present study was conducted to investigate the antimicrobial property of Iranian Propolis and *Royal jelly* against *Rhizopus oryzae* and *Candida albicans.*

Materials and Methods

Rhizopus oryzae with 5176 (SBC327.47) code was provided from Iranian Research Organization for Science and Technology (Tehran). First, *Rhizopus oryzae* was cultured on dextrose agar medium at 25°C. After 24 hours, for preparation of suspension of the *Rhizopus oryzae* fungus, some normal saline was poured onto the fungus colonies surface so that the medium was completely covered and then media were shaken to suspend the spores in it. Then, the supernatant was collected in a sterile tube with screw cap and an uniform similar suspension was prepared by vigorous shaking to separate hydrophobic spores from each other (3,5,22).

Extraction

A total of 500 g of Iranian Propolis raw material was purchased from a reputable grocery and to prepare extract, raw material was crushed. The obtained powder was mixed with 80% ethyl alcohol in the ratio of 1:1 and powder was transferred into percolator and the extract was prepared by the percolation method according to instruction no. 10 of German pharmacopeia. The obtained extract was distillated by the rotary vacuum evaporation until alcohol was removed completely. Also *Royal jelly* that was purchased and maintained in special vial was used in next stages to perform examinations (23,24). The needed dilutions of *Royal jelly* and Propolis extract were prepared in distilled water and ethanol (70%), respectively. Then using the micro dilution method, different dilutions were prepared based on the method recommended by National Clinical Laboratories Standards Committee. Two fold dilutions of extract was poured into first microtube and next dilutions were prepared serially (22).

The concentrations of *Royal jelly* and Propolis extracts were prepared as follows:

Royal jelly: 20, 25, 30, 35, 40, 45, 50, 55, 60, 65, 70, 75, 80, 90, 100, 110, 120, 130, 140, 150, 160, 180, 200, 220, 240 mg/ml.

Iranian Propolis extract: 0.015, 0.023, 0.0312, 0.046, 0.0625, 0.0937, 0.1, 0.187, 0.25, 0.375, 0.5, 0.75, 1, 1.5, 2 mg/ml.

To study the effects of Iranian Propolis extract and *Royal jelly* on *Rhizopus oryzae*, 1.5 cc microtubes were used. Then, 500 µl of prepared dilutions of Iranian Propolis and *Royal jelly* were added to tubes containing 500 µl of sabouraud dextrose broth culture media except to control group and then 50 µl of *Rhizopus oryzae* was added to all microtubes. In the next stage, microtubes were maintained in incubator at 25°C for 48 hours and then 10 ml of the content of each microtube was transferred to sabouraud dextrose agar culture media and again maintained at 25°C for 48 hours and finally the minimum fungicidal concentration (MFC) was determined for *Rhizopus oryzae* (3,24).

Effects of *Royal jelly* and Iranian Propolis extract on *Rhizopus oryzae* were compared, minimum inhibitory concentration (MIC) and MFC of them were determined and finally the results of MIC and MFC of *Royal jelly* and Iranian Propolis on *Rhizopus oryzae* were analyzed.

Results

Results of Iranian Propolis

Table 1 shows the MIC and MFC values of alcoholic extract of Iranian Propolis tested on *Rhizopus oryzae* for 3 times. In every experiment MIC and MFC values of alcoholic extract of Iranian Propolis on *Rhizopus oryzae* were respectively obtained 0.1 and 0.25 mg/ml.

The mean of MIC and MFC of alcoholic extract of Iranian Propolis on *Rhizopus oryzae* were respectively 0.1 and 0.25 mg/ml (Table 1).

Results of *Royal jelly*

Table 2 represents the values of MIC and MFC of *Royal jelly* on *Rhizopus oryzae* in 3 times of test that in the first trial MIC and MFC values of *Royal jelly* were respectively 60 and 80 mg/ml, in the second test 120 and 160 mg/ml respectively and in the third test 120 and 160 mg/ml, respectively.

Table 1. MIC and MFC values (mg/ml) of Iranian propolis on *Rhizopus oryzae*

Experiments	MIC	MFC
First test	0.1	0.25
Second test	0.1	0.25
Third test	0.1	0.25
Mean	0.1	0.25

Abbreviation: MIC, minimum inhibitory concentration; MFC, minimum fungicidal concentration.

Table 2. MIC and MFC values (mg/ml) of *Royal jelly* on *Rhizopus oryzae*

Experiments	MIC	MFC
First test	60	80
Second test	120	160
Third test	120	160
Mean ± SD	100 ± 34	133 ± 46

Abbreviation: MIC, minimum inhibitory concentration; MFC, minimum fungicidal concentration.

The mean of MIC and MFC of *Royal jelly* on *Rhizopus oryzae* were respectively 100±34 and 133±46 mg/ml (Table 2).

The MFC of samples containing ethanol extract of Iranian Propolis was 0.25 mg/ml and were 133 mg/ml in samples containing *Royal jelly* on *Rhizopus oryzae*.

Discussion

Royal jelly and Propolis are of honey bee products and has been used in traditional medicine by humans over the past centuries (6,7). In a study Jamali and colleagues (9) have suggested that the physical character of Propolis generally has been used by honey bees to protect their hive, but several beneficial properties of this compound could be considered for human being. Their findings concerning the chemical analysis of the Propolis exhibited the presence of flavonoid, tannin, steroid, alcohol and alkaloid in extracts. Overall, Propolis has antimicrobial effect with different spectrum and therefore, it might be considered a potent candidate for treatment of several clinical scenarios.

The main chemical compounds present in Propolis are silver, mercury, copper, iron, calcium, silis, flavonoids, and phenolic compounds. Propolis contains some volatile oils, terpenes and bee wax, too (9,10).

Ownagh and colleagues (25) expressed that the ethanol extract of Propolis has an inhibitory effect on all tested fungi and the MIC of Propolis was 62.5-500 µg/ml for dermatophytes (*Microsporum canis, Microsporum gypseum, Microsporum nanum, Trichophyton rubrum, Trichophyton* mentagrophytes, *Epidermophyton floccosum*) and 62.5-125 µg/ml for nondermatophytes (*Candida albicans, Aspergillus niger*, and saccharomyces). Twenty-six compounds were identified by gas chromatography-mass spectrometry analysis. The chemical composition of ethanol extract of Propolis included considerable amount of flavonoids (25).

In another study the antifungal activity of alcoholic extract of Propolis was examined and its impact on experimental *Candida* keratitis showed that 1000 µg/ml concentrations of Propolis could completely treat *Candida albicans* keratitis (18). The inhibitory effect of alcoholic extract of Propolis against *Candida albicans* was also examined. Half of the fermented strains were affected by inhibitory effect of 0.25 g/dl concentration of Propolis extract and minimum fungicidal concentration of extract was determined 0.25 g/dl in more than 50% of the isolates (5). In another study the minimum inhibitory concentration of Propolis *on Candida rugosa*, Aspergillus niger and *Rhizopus oryzae* fungi was found to be 2.5 mg/ml (26). In our study, the mean of MIC and MFC of *Royal jelly* on *Rhizopus oryzae* were respectively 100±34 and 133±46 mg/ml that are in agreement with the results of other studies. The means of MIC, and MFC of Iranian Propolis alcoholic extract on *Rhizopus oryzae* were 0.1 and 0.25 mg/m, respectively. These results are in consistent with the results of previous studies which worked on other fungi. Therefore Iranian Propolis extract has antifungal effect on *Rhizopus oryzae* and might be used as an antifungal agent for treatment of fungal infections.

Conclusion

The results of this study show that alcoholic extract of Iranian Propolis has higher effect compared to *Royall jelly* in agreement with the results of other studies. So Propolis might be used as an antifungal agent for treatment of fungal infections like *Rhizopus oryzae*. If clinical studies also confirm the effects of these drugs, they might be used to treat fungal infections.

Acknowledgements

This paper was derived from the MD theses of the Hamideh Khabbazi. The authors gratefully thank the Medical Plants Research Center and Deputy of Shahrekord University of Medical Sciences, Iran, for funding the research (code number of 1096).

Authors' contributions

All the authors wrote the manuscript equally.

Conflict of interests

The authors declared no competing interests.

Ethical considerations

Ethical issues (including plagiarism, misconduct, data fabrication, falsification, double publication or submission, redundancy) have been completely observed by the authors.

Funding/Support

This research was financially supported by Shahrekord University of Medical Sciences, Shahrekord, Iran.

References

1. Moghim H. Detection of CH50 and role of C3, C4 complement in patients with Candidiasis. J Shahrekord Univ Med Sci. 2000;2(1):61-5.
2. Moghim H. Role of cellular immunity in prevention of Candidiasis in leukemic and lymphomatic patients using flowcytometry method. J Shahrekord Univ Med Sci 2001;3(3):42-8.
3. Moghim H, Taghipoor S, Shahinfard N, et al. Antifungal effects of Allium ascalonicum, Marticaria chamomilla and Stachys lavandulifolia extracts on Candida albicans. J Herbmed Pharmacol. 2014;3(1):9-14.
4. Rippon JW. Candidiasis and the pathogenic yeasts. 3rd ed. Philadelphia: Saunders Company Medical Mycology; 1988:532-538.
5. Diba K, Mousavi B, Mahmoudi M, Hashemi J. In-vitro anti-fungal activity of Propolis alcoholic extract on Candida spp and Aspergillus spp. Tehran Univ Med J. 2010;68(2):80-86.
6. Ownagh A, Tukmechi A, Adibhesam M, Ebrahimzadeh S. Comparative study on the effect of ethanol extract of propolis collected from west azarbaijan apiaries against dermatophytes and non-dermatophytes fungi. Urmia Med J. 2010; 21(3):206-214.
7. Shirzad H, Sedaghat A, Ghasemi S, Shirzad M. Effect of Royal Jelly on Sterile Wound Healing in Balb/C Mice. Armaghan Danesh Journal. 2009;15(1):39-46.
8. Greenaway W, Scaysbook T, Whatley FR. The composition and plant origins of propolis. Bee Worked. 1990;71(3):107-118.
9. Jamali F, Baserisalehi Mand B. Antimicrobial activity and chemical screening of propolis Extracts. Am J Life Sci. 2014;2(2):72-75.
10. Milena P, Rosa D, Hassan TA, Iva T, Hristo N, Vassya B. Omani propolis: Chemical profiling, antibacterial activity and new propolis plant sources. Chem Cent J. 2013;7:158.
11. Kirk SM, Callister SM, Lim LC, Schell RF. Rapid susceptibility testing of Candida albicsns by flow cytometry. J Clin Microbiol. 1997;35(2):358-363.
12. Khalil ML. Biological activity of bee propolis in health and disease. Asian Pac J Cancer Prev. 2006;7(1):22-31.
13. Zia M, Mannani R, Mahmoodi M, Bayat M, Mohaghegh F. The effect of alcoholic extract of Propolis obtained from Iran bee hives on the growth of Trichophyton mentagrophytis, Trichophyton rubrum and Trichophyton verrucosom. J Isfahan Med School. 2009;27(95):232-240.
14. Fontana R, Mendes MA, de Souza BM, et al. Jelleines: a family of antimicrobial peptides from the royal jelly of honeybees (Apis mellifera). Peptides. 2004;25(6):919-928.
15. Melliou E, Chinou I. Chemistry and bioactivity of royal jelly from Greece. J Agric Food Chem. 2005;53(23):8987-8992.
16. Kamakura M, Mitani N, Fukuda T, Fukushima M. Antifatigue effect of fresh Royal jelly in mice. J Nutr Sci Vitaminol. 2001;47(6):394-401.
17. Fujiwara S, Imaj J, Fujiwara M, Yaeshima T, Kawashima T, Kobayashi K. A potent antibacterial protein in royal jelly. Purification and determination of the primary structure of royalisin. J Biol Chem. 1990;265(19):11333-11337.
18. Ahangari A, Ownagh A, Tehrani A, Tukmechi A. The effects of ethanol extract of Propolis (EEP) on the experimentally induced Candida keratitis in rabbits. Tehran Univ Med J. 2011;69(1):22-28.
19. Forcing S, Bankova J. Propolis: is there a potential for the development of new drug. J Ethnopharmacaol. 2011;133(2):253-260.
20. Vassya S, Solangel D, Cast R, Mari C. Propolis: recent advances in chemistry and plant origin. Apidologie. 2000;31(1):3-15.
21. Yaghoubi S, Ghorbani GR, Soleimanian Zad R. Antimicrobial activity of Iranian propolis and its chemical composition. DARU. 2007;15(1):45-48.
22. Willinger B, Apfalter P, Hirschl AM, Makristathis A, Rotter M, Seibold M. Susceptibility testing of Candida species: comparison of NCCLS microdilution method with Fungitest. Diagn Microbiol Infect Dis. 2000;38(1):11-15.
23. Kujumgiev A, Tsvetkoval L, Serkedjieva Y, Bankova V, Christov R, Popov S. Antibacterial, antifungal and antiviral activity of propolis of different geographic origin. J Ethnopharmacol. 1999;64(3):235-240.
24. Razzaghparast A, Shams Ghahfarokhi M, Yadegari MH, Razzaghi Abyaneh M. Antifungal effects of Allium cepa and some azoles in intact forms and in combinations to each other against pathogenic yeasts. Kowsar Med J. 2008;13(2):103-113.
25. Ownagh A, Adibhesami M. Treatment of Candidia albicans cutaneous infection by ethanol extract of Propolis in an experimental model. Med J Tabriz Univ Med Sci. 2013;35(2):6-11.
26. Erkmen O, Ozcan MM. Antimicrobial effects of Turkish Propolis, pollen, and laurel on spoilage and pathogenic food-related microorganisms. J Med Food. 2008;11(3):587-592.

The relaxant effect of *Ferula assafoetida* on smooth muscles and the possible mechanisms

Mohammad Reza Khazdair[1], Mohammad Hossein Boskabady[2*]

[1]Pharmaciutical Research Center and Department of Physiology School of Medicine, Mashhad University of Medical Sciences, Mashhad, Iran
[2]Neurogenic Inflammation Research Centre and Department of Physiology, School of Medicine, Mashhad University of Medical Sciences, Mashhad, Iran

ARTICLE INFO

Keywords:
Ferula asafoetida
Extract
Oleo-gum-resin
Smooth muscle
Relaxant effect

ABSTRACT

Asafoetida (*Ferula asafoetida*) an oleo-gum-resin belongs to the Apiaceae family which obtained from the living underground rhizome or tap roots of the plant. *F. assa-foetida* is used in traditional medicine for the treatment of variety of disorders. Asafoetida is used as a culinary spice and in folk medicine has been used to treat several diseases, including intestinal parasites, weak digestion, gastrointestinal disorders, asthma and influenza. A wide range of chemical compounds including sugars, sesquiterpene coumarins and polysulfides have been isolated from this plant. This oleo-gum-resin is known to possess antifungal, anti-diabetic, anti-inflammatory, anti-mutagenic and antiviral activities. Several studies investigated the effects of *F. asafoetida* gum extract on the contractile responses induced by acetylcholine, methacholin, histamine and KCl on different smooth muscles. The present review summarizes the information regarding the relaxant effect of asafetida and its extracts on different smooth muscles and the possible mechanisms of this effect.

Implication for health policy/practice/research/medical education:
foetida and its essential oil on different types of smooth muscle on contracted tissues induced by various contractile agents have been shown. The different mechanisms of relaxant effects of *F. assa-foetida* including inhibitory effects of muscarinic receptors and histamine (H_1) receptors as well as β-adrenoceptors stimulatory effects on calcium channels have also been reported. It might be beneficial spastic conditions.

Introduction

Asafoetida (*F. asafoetida* L.) belongs to the Apiaceae family which is obtained from the exudates of the living underground rhizome or tap roots of the plant. *F. asafoetida* or gum-resin is known as "Anghouzeh", "Khorakoma" and "Anguzakoma" in Iran (1). It has been used in traditional medicine and as a spice in different foods in India and Nepal (1).

Recently, emphases are focused on the novel therapeutic agents from medicinal plants and many people prefer medicinal plants to chemical drugs (2). *F. assa-foetida* is a wild native plant in Iran and *F. asafoetida* gum extract has been used in Iranian traditional medicine for abdominal pain, constipation and diarrhea treatment. It is also used for the treatment of asthma, influenza, stomachache, epilepsy, flatulence and intestinal parasites (3-5). Aphrodisiac, diuretic and sedative effects have been described for this plant (6). Several pharmacological effects including antiviral (7), antifungal (8), antioxidant (7), cancer chemoprevention (9), antispasmodic (10), hypotensive (10) and anti-diabetic (11) effects have been reported for *F. asafetida.*

Several fractions such as gum fraction (25%) and resin (40–64%, which contain ferulic acid esters (60%), free ferulic acid (1.3%), coumarin derivatives (e.g. umbelliferone), volatile oils (3%–17%) including sulphur-containing

***Corresponding author**: Mohammad Hossein Boskabady, M.D., Ph.D., Neurogenic Inflammation Research Centre and Dept. of Physiology, School of Medicine, Mashhad, Post Code 9177948564, Iran.
Email: boskabadymh@mums.ac.ir, mhboskabady@hotmail.com

compounds (3,12) were isolated from plant. E-1-propyl sec-butyl disulfide, as the major component, and 25 other compounds were identified in the hydrodistilled oil of Iranian Ferula assa-foetida oil (13). E-1-propenyl sec-butyl disulfide (40.0%) and germacrene B (7.8%) are the major components of Ferula assa-foetida. Therefore, only two components constituted more than 70% of the oil using supercritical carbon dioxide under optimum conditions with extraction yield, based on hydrodistillation (13).
Umbelliprenin is a member of prenylated coumarins that present in Ferula species, which its chemoprevention activity on the cancer was reported (14). In addition, a concentration-dependent response of 25, 50, 100, 200, and 400 μM umbelliprenin was decreased in DNA damage induced by H2O2 (15).
F. asafoetida is traditionally used for the treatment of asthma and angina pectoris (16), bronchitis, whooping cough and pneumonia in children (17-19). The observed relaxant effect of *F. asafoetida* on tracheal smooth muscle may indicate its bronchodilator effect (20).
Anticoagulant action of *Ferula asafoetida* gum extract has also been suggested (21). The beneficial effects of gum have been achieved from *Ferula asafoetida* in gastrointestinal and hemodynamic disorders (10). In addition, the relaxant effects of its gum extract on blood pressure were recorded from the anaesthetized rats (10). The present review summarizes the information regarding the relaxant effect of asafetida and its extracts on different smooth muscles and the possible mechanisms of this effect.

Methods

This review article was prepared by searching for the terms: *Ferula asafetida*, smooth muscles, umbelliprenin and relaxant effects. Information on *Ferula asafetida* was collected via search and studies in electronic databases including ISI Web of Knowledge, Medline/Pubmed, Sciencdirect, Embase, Scopus, Biological Abstracts, Chemical Abstracts and Google Scholar.

Results

The relaxant effect of various preparations of *Ferula asafetida* and its constituents on different types of smooth muscles were demonstrated which reviewed in the following sections:

Relaxant effects on tracheal smooth muscle

In previous studies, the relaxant effect of *F. assa-foetida* on smooth muscle of the tracheal chain (*in vitro*) was shown (20). Some constituents of the gum resin including carvacrol have inhibitory effect on muscarinic receptors of tracheal smooth muscle (22). In addition, we showed the relaxant effect of *F. asafoetida* extract by inhibitory effect for the plant on histamine (H_1) receptors of tracheal smooth muscles in the tracheal smooth muscle (23).
The *Ferula sinaica* (another species from *Ferula* genus) root extract also inhibited the contractions of rabbit tracheal and contractions of guinea pig tracheal smooth muscle induced by acetylcholine and histamine stimulation, respectively (24).
The relaxant effects of *F. asafoetida* and umbelliprenin on contracted smooth muscle by methacholine and KCL on the tracheal smooth muscle were also observed (25).
The relaxant effects of the extracts of *F. assa-foetida* and its constituents on tracheal smooth muscles are summarized in Table 1.

Relaxant effects on gastro-intestinal and urogenital smooth muscle

F. asafoetida gum extract reduces the spontaneous contraction of the isolated guinea-pig ileum (10). The inhibitory effects of *Ferula sinaica* (another species from *Ferula* genus) root extract on rabbit jejunum, guinea pig ileum, and guinea-pig uterine smooth muscle contractions by acetylcholine were also reported (24).
The spasmolytic and antispasmodic action of *F. assa-foetida* seed's essential oil against contractile induced by cumulative concentrations of acetylcholine were reported to be stronger than asafoetida which might be due to the higher concentration of the constituents in the oil (26).
The relaxant effect of the extracts of *F. assa-foetida* and its constituents on Gastro-intestinal and urogenital smooth muscle are summarized in Table 2.

Relaxant effects on vascular smooth muscle

The results of a study demonstrated that *F. asafoetida* gum extract (0.3-2.2 mg/100 g body weight) remarkably reduced the mean arterial blood pressure in anesthetized normotensive rats which at higher doses, the duration of the depressor response to extract was long-lasted (10). The

Table 1. Relaxant effect of the extracts and constituents of *F. assa-foetida* on tracheal smooth muscle

Extract, Constituent	Dose, Conce.	Method for Tissue smooth muscle contraction (TSM)	Response	Ref.
Aqueous extract	2, 5 and 10 mg/mL	KCl (60 mmol/L)	0.85, 5.13, 10.17	(25)
		Methacholine (10 μmol/L)	31.6, 65.72, 91.07	(25)
Umbelliprenin	0.04, 0.2 and 0.4 mg/mL	KCl (60 mmol/L)	-2.42, -0.53, 8.97	(25)
		methacholine (10 μmol/L)	8.59, 18.86, 26.28	(25)
Aqueous-ethanolic extract	2.5, 5, 10	Methacholine (range 0.1 - 1000 μM)	97, 83, 80	(32)
Aqueous extract	2, 5 and 10 mg/ml	10 μM methacholine → preincubated tissues by propranolol and chlorpheniramine	34, 59, 80	(20)
		10 μM methacholine → preincubated tissues by propranolol,	42, 75, 100	(20)

Table 2. Relaxant effect of the extracts of *F. assa-foetida* and its constituents on gastro-intestinal and urogenital smooth muscle

Extract, Constituent	Dose, Conce.	Method for Tissue smooth muscle contraction (TSM)	Response	Ref.
Aqueous extract	1, 2, 3, 5 and 7 mg/ml	Spontaneous contractions	-83, 68, 54 , 21, 9	(10)
		KCl (28 mM)	0, 3, 18, 23, 29	(10)
		Acetylcholine (25 μM)	3, 5, 20, 25, 29	(10)
		Histamine (25 μM)	4, 8, 32, 40, 53	(10)
Aqueous extract	0.1%, 0.2%, 0.3%	Acetylcholine (100 μM)	0, 50, 62	(26)
Essential oil	0.1%, 0.2%, 0.3%	Acetylcholine (100 μM)	20, 70, 85	(26)

inhibitory effects of *F. sinaica* root extract on contractions of rabbit aorta induced by norepinephrine stimulation were also observed (24).

The potent vasodilatation properties of *F. assa-foetida* extracts upon arterial rings were demonstrated (27). Kassis *et al.* demonstrated that the masculine property of this extract had mainly an endothelial-mediated effect and a secondary direct effect on arterial smooth muscle cells (27). In addition aphrodisiac effects of "masculine" extract at high doses were demonstrated by increase in penile erection episodes in the controlled rat studies. Similar effects of *Ferula hermonis* (related species) at a dose of 12 mg/kg in rats also were reported (28). The antioxidant and vasodilatation properties of masculine at concentrations of 0.05 and 0.2 mg/ml respectively were recorded (27).

Possible mechanisms of the relaxant effect of *Ferula asafoetida* on smooth muscles

The relaxant effect of the extract in smooth muscle might occurred by different mechanisms. For example, smooth muscle contractile tone can be relaxed by increased levels of adenosine 3,5-cyclic adenosine-monophosphate (cAMP) (29). In addition, one study showed that indomethacin (a cyclooxygenase inhibitor) remarkably inhibited the relaxant effect of *F. asafoetida* gum extract in isolated guinea-pig ileum which suggested that cyclooxygenase metabolites (e.g. prostaglandins such as PGE2, PGD2 and PGI2) might be involved in this relaxation (10). Different possible mechanisms responsible for the relaxant effect of *F. asafoetida* on smooth muscles are reviewed in this section.

Calcium channel blocking effect

The relaxant effects of the *F. asafoetida* gum extract on tracheal, vascular, gastro-intestinal and urogenital smooth muscles have been suggested that, this natural product reduces the cytosolic Ca^{2+} in a non-specific manner. Ca^{2+} ions gain access to the cytoplasm through voltage-activated or receptor-operated calcium channels (30). KCl induced contraction by an increase in K^+ and depolarization of smooth muscle fibers, leading to increased influx of calcium through L type voltage-operated channels (31).

The anti-cholinergic and anti-muscarinic effect of the plant

The inhibitory effect (antagonism effect) of extract on muscarinic receptors was previously suggested (32). Acetylcholine induced contraction via M3 subtype of muscarinic receptor in the muscle (33).

The inhibitory effect of acetylcholine on the existence and function of these muscarinic receptor subtypes was investigated in rabbit trachea in vitro on muscarinic system (34). The lower maximum response to methacholine has been revealed in experiments with high plant concentration indicating that non competitive antagonistic effect of the extract on muscarinic receptors (32).

Histaminic (H1 receptor) antagonistic activity

Contraction induced by histamine which happens via H_1 receptor activation has been suggested (33). The relaxant effects of extract on isolated guinea-pig ileum preparations precontracted by histamine were higher than contraction induced by acetylcholine (10). The inhibitory effect of acetylcholine by histamine (H_1) receptors was suggested (35). In a previous study, the contribution of H_1 receptors inhibitory in incubated tracheal smooth muscle with chlorpheniramine was observed (23).

Stimulatory effect on β2- adrenoceptors

The stimulatory effects of β agonists on β-adrenergic receptors in bronchi were suggested (36). In a previous study, the contribution of β-adrenergic receptors in incubated tracheal smooth muscle with propranolol (β-adrenergic receptors antagonist), the stimulatory effect of extract in β-adrenergic was observed (32).

Conclusion

F. asafoetida gum has been used in traditional medicine. The relaxant effects of *F. assa-foetida* and its essential oil on different types of smooth muscle on contracted tissues induced by various contractile agents have been shown. The different mechanisms of relaxant effects of *F. assa-foetida* including inhibitory effects of muscarinic receptors and histamine (H_1) receptors as well as β-adrenoceptors stimulatory effects on calcium channels have been reported.

Authors' contributions

Mohammad Reza Khazdair: Design of the study and preparation of the paper. Mohammad Hossein Boskabady: Help in design of the study and English editing of the paper.

Conflict of interests

There is no conflict of interest.

Founding/Support

None.

References

1. Iranshahy M, Iranshahi M. Traditional uses, phytochemistry and pharmacology of asafoetida (Ferula assa-foetida oleo-gum-resin)-A review. J Ethnopharmacol 2011; 134(1): 1-10.
2. Fernch D. Ethnobothany of the Umbelliferae. In: Heywood VH (Ed.), The Chemistry and Biology of the Umberifella. London: Academic press; 1971. p. 285-412.
3. Takeoka G. Volatile Constituents of Asafoetida, Aroma Active Compounds in Foods. ACS Publications; 2001. p. 33-44.
4. Lee CL, Chiang LC, Cheng LH, Liaw CC, Abd El-Razek MH, Chang FR, *et al.* Influenza A (H(1)N(1)) Antiviral and Cytotoxic Agents from Ferula assa-foetida. J Nat Prod 2009; 72(9): 1568-72.
5. Evans WC. Trease and Evans Pharmacognosy. London: WB Saunders; 2002. p. 286.
6. Zargari A. Medicinal Plants. 6th ed. Tehran: Tehran University Publications; 1996.
7. Dehpour AA, Ebrahimzadeh MA, Fazel NS, Mohammad NS. Antioxidant activity of the methanol extract of Ferula assafoetida and its essential oil composition. Grasasy Aceites 2009; 60(4): 405-12.
8. Angelini P, Pagiotti R, Venanzoni R, Granetti B. Antifungal and allelopathic effects of Asafoetida against Trichoderma harzianum and Pleurotus spp. Allelopat J 2009; 23(1): 357-68.
9. Saleem M, Alam A, Sultana S. Asafoetida inhibits early events of carcinogenesis: a chemopreventive study. Life Sci 2001; 68(16): 1913-21.
10. Fatehi M, Farifteh F, Fatehi-Hassanabad Z. Antispasmodic and hypotensive effects of Ferula asafoetida gum extract. J Ethnopharmacol 2004; 91(2-3): 321-4.
11. Abu-Zaiton AS. Anti-diabetic activity of Ferula assafoetida extract in normal and alloxan-induced diabetic rats. Pak J Biol Sci. 2010; 15(13): 97-100.
12. Kajimoto T. Sesquiterpenoid and disulphide derivatives from Ferula assa-foetida. Phytochemistry 1989; 28: 1761-3.
13. Khajeh M, Yamini Y, Bahramifar N, Sefidkon F, Pirmoradei MR. Comparison of essential oils compositions of Ferula assa-foetida obtained by supercritical carbon dioxide extraction and hydrodistillation methods. Food Chem 2005; 91: 639-44.
14. Iranshahi M, Shahverdi AR, Mirjani R, Amin G, Shafiee A. Umbelliprenin from Ferula persica roots inhibits the red pigment production in Serratia marcescens. Z Naturforsch 2004; 59: 506-8.
15. Soltani S, Mosaffa F, Iranshahi M, Karimi Gh, Malekaneh M, Haghighi F, Behravan J. Evaluation of antigenotoxicity effects of umbelliprenin on human peripheral lymphocytes exposed to oxidative stress. Cell Biol Toxicol 2009; 25(3): 291-6.
16. Srinivasan K. Spices as influencers of body metabolism: an overview of three decades of research. Food Res Int 2005; 38(1): 77-86.
17. Kapoor LD. Handbook of Ayurvedic Medicinal Plants. 1st ed. Washington, DC: CRC Press; 2001.
18. Ross IA. Medicinal plants of the world: chemical constituents, traditional, and modern medicinal uses. Totowa, NJ: Humana Press; 2005.
19. Appendino G, Maxia L, Bascope M, Houghton PJ, Sanchez-Duffhues G, Munoz E, *et al.* A meroterpenoid NF-kappaB inhibitor and drimanesesquiterpenoids from Asafetida. J Nat Prod 2006; 69(7): 1101-4.
20. Gholamnezhad Z, Byrami G, Boskabady MH, Iranshahi M. Possible mechanism(s) of the relaxant effect of asafoetida (*Ferula assa-foetida*) oleo-gum-resin extract on guinea-pig tracheal smooth muscle. Avicenna J Phytomed 2012; 2(1): 10-6.
21. Leung AY. Encyclopedia of Common Natural Ingredients used in Food, Drugs and Cosmetics. New York: Wiley; 1980.
22. Boskabady MH, Jafari Z, Pouraboli I. The effect of carvacrol on muscarinic receptors of guinea pig tracheal chains. Phytother Res 2011; 25(4): 530-5.
23. Kiyanmehr M, Boskabady MH, Khazdair MR, Hashemzehi M. The beta-adrenergic and histamine (h1) receptor blockade affects inhibitory effect of *ferula assafoetida* on muscarinic receptors of tracheal smooth muscle. In Press (J Med Sci).
24. Aqel MB, Al-khalil S, Afifi F. Effects of a Ferula sinaica root extract on the uterine smooth muscle of rat and guinea pig. J Ethnopharmacol 1991; 31: 291-7.
25. Bayrami G, Boskabady MH, Iranshahi M, Gholamnezhad Z. Relaxant effects of asafoetida extract and its constituent umbelliprenin on guinea-pig tracheal smooth muscle. Chin J Integr Med 2013 Dec 12.
26. Bagheri S, Hejazian Sh, Dashti-R M. The relaxant effect of seed's essential oil and oleo-gum-resin of ferula assa-foetida on isolated rat's ileum. Ann Med Health Sci Res 2014; 4(2): 238-41.
27. Kassis E, Fulder S, Khalid-Khalil, Hadieh B, Nahhas F, Saad B, *et al.* Efficacy and safety assessments of ferula assa-foetida l., traditionally used in greco-arab herbal medicine for enhancing male fertility, libido and erectile function. Open Complement Med J 2009; 1: 102-9.
28. Boskabady MH, Jandaghi P. Relaxant effects of carvacrol on guinea pig tracheal chains and its possible mechanisms. Pharmazie 2003; 58(9): 661-663.
29. Berridge MJ. The interaction of cyclic nucleotides and calcium in control of cellular activity. Adv Cyclic Nucl Res 1975; 6: 1-98.
30. Triggle DJ. Calcium ions and respiratory smooth

muscle function. Brit J Clin Pharmacol 1985; 20: 213s-9s.

31. Gilani AH, Janbaz KH, Zaman M, Lateff A, Tariq SR, Ahmad HR. Hypotensive and spasmolitic activites of crude extract of cyperus scariosus. Arch Pharmacol Res 1994; 17 (3): 145-9.
32. Khazdair MR, Boskabady MH, Kiyanmehr M, Hashemzehi M, Iranshahi M. The effects of *Ferula assafoetida* on muscarinic receptors of guinea-pig tracheal smooth muscle. In press (Jundishapur J Nat Pharm Prod).
33. Zavecz JH, Yellin TO. Histamine receptors in the myenteric plexus-longitudinal muscle of the response to electrical stimulation. J Pharmacol Exp Therap 1982; 223: 177-82.
34. Loenders B, Rampart M, Herman AG. Selective M3 muscarinic receptor inhibits smooth muscle contraction in rabbit trachea without increasing the release of acetylcholine. J Pharmacol Exp Ther 1992; 263(2): 773-7.
35. Popa VT, Somani P, Simon P, SimonV. The effect of inhaled verapamil on resting bronchial tone and airway constriction by histamine and acetylcholine in normal and asthmatic subjects. Am Rev Respir Dis 1984; 130(6): 106-13.
36. Linden A, Bergendal A, Ullman A, Skoogh BE, Lofdahl CG. Salmetrol, formetrol, and salbutamol in the isolated guinea-pig trachea: differences in maximum relaxant effect and potency but not in functional antagonism. Thorax 1993; 48(5): 547-53.

31

Effect of *Valeriana officinalis* hydroalcoholic extract on *Giardia lamblia* cysts

Mona Mohamadi[1], Bahman Khalili[2*], Simin Taghipur[1], Fatemeh Drees[3]

[1]Clinical Biochemistry Research Center, Shahrekord University of Medical Sciences, Shahrekord, Iran
[2]Cellular and Molecular Research Center, Shahrekord University of Medical Sciences, Shahrekord, Iran
[3]Medical Plants Research Center, Shahrekord University of Medical Sciences, Shahrekord, Iran

ARTICLE INFO

Keywords:
Giardia lamblia
Valeriana officinalis
Hydroalcoholic extract
In vitro

ABSTRACT

Introduction: *Giardia lamblia* is an important and prevalent parasitic cause of diarrhea and gastroenteritis. Regarding the significance of giardiasis treatment particularly by medicinal plants and *G. lamblia* resistance to chemical drugs, this study was conducted to study in vitro effect of *Valeriana officinalis* hydroalcoholic extract on *G. lamblia* cysts.
Methods: In this experimental, laboratory study the hydroalcoholic extract of *V. officinalis* at concentrations of 12.5, 25, 50, 100, and 200 mg/mL was applied on *G. lamblia* cysts. The findings were compared with controls.
Results: Mean results of the effect of *V. officinalis* hydroalcoholic extract at different concentrations on *G. lamblia* cysts after 1, 6 and 24 hours demonstrated that the extract at all concentrations caused a notable decrease in alive cysts, with more intensive effect at 100 and 200 mg/mL concentrations and 100% fatality after 1 hour. As the extract concentration decreased, the speed of *G. lamblia* cysts inhibition declined.
Conclusion: *V. officinalis* hydroalcoholic extract might be recommended as an effective compound for removing *G. lamblia* protozoan cysts, although further studies are needed to show this effect on human.

Implication for health policy/practice/research/medical education:
Valeriana officinalis might be used as an effective compound for removing *Giardia lamblia* protozoan cysts. Separation and recognition of the effective compound(s) is recommended.

Introduction

Giardia lamblia is an important and prevalent parasitic cause of diarrhea and gastroenteritis and giardiasis is a significant health problem worldwide. *G. lamblia* is known as the most common human intestinal protozoa especially in temperate regions, and exists in animals including birds, amphibians, rodents, some mammals, and human (1). In Iran, *G. lamblia* prevalence has been reported 10.9%, the highest contribution in intestinal parasitic infections nationwide (2).

This protozoan parasite is a main factor for epidemic diarrhea due to contaminated food and water. The prevalence of *G. lamblia* infection differs by age, geographic area, health conditions, and water situation. *G. lamblia* exists in 2 forms, trophozoite and cyst, and eating 100 or more cysts results in infection. Parasitic cyst is excreted through feces and causes infection. Cyst takes some days to some months to be excreted through feces. The children of under 10 years comprise the population at the highest risk of infection. However, the patients of any ages could present with mild diarrhea, flatulence, loss of appetite, crampy abdominal pain, epigastric tenderness, fatty stools, and malabsorption (3,4).

A variety of drugs is currently being taken for treatment of giardiasis, including metronidazole, albendazole, quinacrine, furazolidone, all of which lead to adverse effects particularly in children and women (5,6). Incidence of resistance to these drugs has been already demonstrated for *G. lamblia* and hence the research has been seeking to find compounds with fewer or no side effects (7,8).

In this regard, human beings have long used medicinal plants to treat diseases, which has been developed and

***Corresponding author**: Bahman Khalili, Medical Plants Research Center, Shahrekord University of Medical Sciences, Shahrekord, Iran. Email: bahman@skums.ac.ir evolved throughout centuries. By World Health Organization (WHO) report, over 80% of global population, particularly in developing countries and remote areas where health and safety facilities are lacking use medicinal plants to meet their basic healthcare needs (9). This wide welcome could be due to a number of reasons including fewer side effects, less cost of medicinal herbs, patients' and higher tendency thanks to traditional medicine recommendations, and use of these drugs by past generations as well as further agreement with normal physiological functions of the human body (10).

Of medicinal plants, cat grass (*Valeriana officinalis*) is a herbaceous perennial plant of the family Valerianaceae. *V. officinalis* root and rhizome contain valuable active essential substances and iridoid compounds called valepotriates. Valepotriates are a group of volatile compounds with sedative property. This plant has a variety of species containing other compounds such as alkaloids, flavonoids, tannins, gums, resins, and mucilage. In medicine this plant is taken as sedatives and analgesics as well as for the treatment of muscle cramps, irritable bowel syndrome, bloating, and headaches caused by stress and anxiety. Also it works for removing parasites and helminths, fixing constant hiccups, and treating stomachache of neural origin and liver diseases (11,12).

No study has been yet conducted to investigate *V. officinalis* effect on *G. lamblia* specifically. Therefore the present study was conducted to study the effect of *V. officinalis* on *G. lamblia* cysts in comparison to metronidazole and furazolidone.

Materials and Methods

The present experimental, laboratory study was conducted in 2014-2015 in laboratories of Department of Parasitology and Medical Plants Research Center of Shahrekord University of Medical Sciences.

Preparation of hydroalcoholic *V. officinalis* extract by maceration

Firstly, unusable parts of the plant were set aside, cleaned, shadow-dried in special trays at room temperature, pulverized by an electric mill and then passed through a sieve no. 10. The obtained powder was mixed with ethanol 70% at 1/3 ratio and extracted per maceration for 72 hours. Then vacuum distillation process was run to remove all alcohol in the solution using rotary vacuum evaporator and the obtained extract was left to be used for later tests (13). Notably, dimethyl sulfoxide was used for further dissolution of *V. officinalis* extract.

Preparation of G. lamblia cysts

G. lamblia cysts were isolated by sucrose density gradient. Firstly 10-15 mL of distilled water was added to fresh stool samples containing the appropriate number of cysts in a disposable glass for preparation of a suspension and then the suspension was refined by a layer of wet gauze fabric. The tubes were centrifuged for 5 minutes and then the upper layers were set aside. This procedure was run in triplicate. Then 3 mL 0.85 sucrose solution and afterwards 3 mL of the prepared stool suspension were introduced into the tubes. Next, the tubes were centrifuged in 4°C refrigerator for 10 minutes. As a result, four layers per tube were formed in a way that *G. lamblia* cysts were compressed as a ring-shaped cloud in the middle layer.

The contents of cloud layer were closely taken out by a Pasteur pipette and transferred to another tube. Then, 3-5 mL distilled water was added to the samples and the tubes were centrifuged at 600 g for 5 minutes to isolate sucrose solution. Afterwards, the upper liquid was set aside and the obtained sedimentation was centrifuged at 600 g for 5 minutes. This procedure was run in duplicate. At the end the upper layer was discarded, the sedimentation containing the cysts was mixed with 1 mL distilled water, and the suspension was transferred to the microtubes and frozen at -20°C for later tests after they were covered with a parafilm (14).

Testing

Firstly *G. lamblia* cysts were tested with *V. officinalis* hydroalcoholic extract at a wide range of concentrations in a pilot study for the best fatality effect and 12.5, 25, 500, 100, and 200 mg/mL concentrations were adopted.

For tests, eight microtubes were placed into a special rock and 100 μL of the extract under study was poured into the first tube and 50 μL normal saline was introduced into the second to fifth tubes by a 100 μL sampler. Hence the extract concentration in the first tube was 200 mg/mL. Then 50 μL of the extract in the first tube was introduced into the second tube and mixed well with normal saline. The procedure was similarly run till the fifth tube and therefore the extract concentration in the first to fifth tube was 200, 100, 50, 25, and 12.5 mg/mL, respectively

In the next step, 50 μL of *G. lamblia* cysts suspension containing 5×10^4 cysts, counted by Theobar lam, was introduced into all the eight microtubes and then 100 μL dimethyl sulfoxide, instead of the extract, was poured into the sixth microtube as negative control and 100 μL metronidazole and furazolidone poured into the seventh and eighth mcrotube, respectively, as positive controls. Subsequently, the microtubes were incubated at 37°C for 1, 6, and 24 hours for provision of better temperature and time conditions for the extract's effect on *G. lamblia* cysts. Afterwards, eosin (0.1%) staining was used to investigate the fatality effect of the extract at different concentrations on *G. lamblia* cysts (15). To enhance the precision of the findings, any tests of the extract effect on the cysts were done in triplicate.

To select the appropriate concentration of metronidazole and furazolidone as positive control, these two drugs at different solution concentrations were exposed to *G. lamblia* cysts in different microtubes in a pilot study and then incubated under the conditions already described and the effectiveness of this solution on *G. lamblia* was tested in triplicate. Metronidazole at a concentration of 5 mg/mL with 40% fatality effect and furazolidone at a concentration of 25.6 mg/mL with 30% fatality effect had the greatest effect on cysts after 24 hours and hence they were selected as the desired concentrations for comparison with *V. officinalis* extract at different concentrations in each test.

For data analysis, descriptive statistics such as frequency, percentage, mean and standard deviation, and analytical statistics such as Repeated Measures analysis of variance (ANOVA) and Probit analysis in SPSS 20 were used. Level of significance was considered 0.05.

Results

Mean results of three tests of the effect of *V. officinalis* hydroalcoholic extract at different concentrations on *G. lamblia* cysts after 1, 6 and 24 hours demonstrated that the extract at all concentrations caused a remarkable decrease in alive cysts, with further effect at 100 and 200 mg/mL concentrations and a rapid, 100% fatality effect. As the extract concentration decreased, the speed of *G. lamblia* cysts inhibition declined so that the fatality effect was derived 84.00% and 69.3% at 25 and 12.5 mg/mL concentrations, respectively. Furthermore, with increasing time of exposure for each concentration, the fatality percentage in *G. lamblia* cysts increased at concentrations of 50, 25 and 12.5 mg/mL, so that mean fatality effect after 1 hour was derived 87.3%, 69.3%, and 54.7%, respectively, while it increased to 96.7%, 84.0%, and 69.3%, respectively, after 24 hours.

On the other hand, comparison of the effect of *V. officinalis* hydroalcoholic extract at 5 concentrations on *G. lamblia* cysts at different intervals with that of metronidazole and furazolidone as positive controls indicated that mean fatality effect of metronidazole and furazolidone after 24 hours was 47.33% and 30.00%, respectively. Therefore, *V. officinalis* hydroalcoholic extract, even at the smallest concentration, exerted a significantly higher fatality effect than these two drugs with pharmacologic concentration of 5 and 6.25 mg/mL respectively ($P<0.001$). This represents the high effect of *V. officinalis* extract on *G. lamblia* cysts (Table 1).

Figure 1 illustrates the effect trend of *V. officinalis* hydroalcoholic extract at different concentrations on *G. lamblia* cysts in comparison to metronidazole and furazolidone in triplicate.

Table 1. Mean fatality percentage of *Valeriana officinalis* hydroalcoholic extract at different concentrations on *Giardia lamblia* cysts in triplicate

Extract concentration (mg/mL)	Mean fatality effect at different intervals		
	1 h	6 h	24 h
200	100.0%	100.0%	100.0%
100	100.0%	100.0%	100.0%
50	87.3%	93.3%	96.7%
25	69.3%	75.3%	84.0%
12.5	54.7%	61.3%	69.3%
Positive control (metronidazole)	23.3%	33.3%	47.3%
Positive control (furazolidne)	22.0%	22.0%	30.0%
Negative control	0.0%	0.0%	0.0%

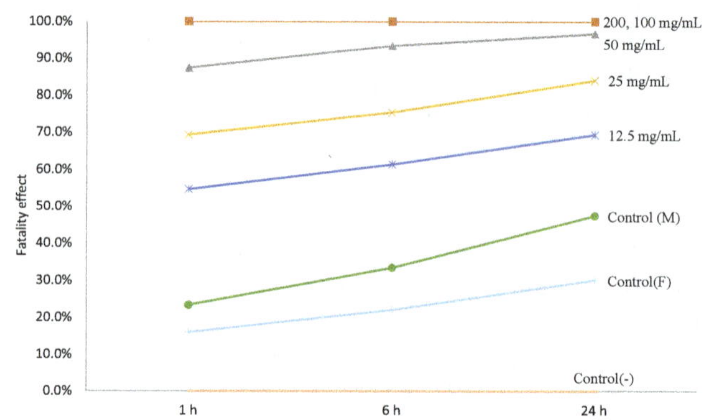

Figure 1. Effect trend of *Valeriana officinalis* hydroalcoholic extract at different concentrations on *Giardia lamblia* cysts at intervals under study (in triplicate).

Discussion

This study was conducted to study in vitro effect of *V. officinalis* hydroalcoholic extract on *G. lamblia* cysts. The anti parasitic effects of *V. officinalis* have not been yet investigated satisfactorily; however, its antifungal and antioxidant properties have been examined in some studies such as Saatchi et al study. Saatchi et al study demonstrated that alcoholic extract of *V. officinalis* and *Melissa officinalis* exhibited high antimicrobial and antioxidant activites and inhibited the growth of 10 fungi (16). In the present study *V. officinalis* hydroalcoholic extract had pronounced anti parasitic properties on *G. lamblia* protozoa.

Many studies have investigated medicinal plants effects on *G. lamblia* cysts. Rahimi-Esboei et al (17) studied in vitro effect of hydroalcoholic leek extract on *G. lamblia* cysts and found that the extract at 100 and 50 mg/mL concentrations after 24 hours had the highest (99% and 96%) fatality effect (respectively) on *G. lamblia* cysts. Similarly, *V. officinalis* hydroalcoholic extract at 100 and 50 mg/mL concentrations, in the present study, had the highest (100% and 96.67%) fatality effect (after 1 hour and 24 hours, respectively) on *G. lamblia* cysts.

In Shahabi et al study (18), copticum extract at 200 mg/mL concentration caused the death of all *G. lamblia* cysts after 1 hour, consistent with our findings of *V. officinalis* extract at 100 mg/mL in the present study.

In Safarnejad et al study (19), savory methanol extract at 200 mg/mL concentration exerted an 84.3% fatality effect on *G. lamblia* cysts after 1 hour, smaller than the fatality effect of *V. officinalis* in the present study.

Conclusion

Overall the findings of the present study indicated that *V. officinalis* hydroalcoholic extract had a high fatality effect on *G. lamblia* cysts and therefore could be recommended as an effective compound for removing *G. lamblia* protozoan cysts. However further research is needed for clinical application of *V. officinalis* extract, including study of effective chemicals in *V. officinalis* extract and controlled trial of laboratory animals and, if the property of interest was demonstrated, humans.

Acknowledgments
Hereby we gratefully thank the respectful officials at Department of Parasitology, Medical Plants Research Center, and Research and Technology Deputy of Shahrekord University of Medical Sciences for assistance in this study.

Authors' contributions
All contributed to the conception of the work, approval of the final version of the manuscript, and agreed for all aspects of the work. BKh conducted the study, contributed in preparation of the first draft and revising the final draft. FD contributed to statistical analysis.

Conflict of interests
The authors declared no competing interests.

Ethical considerations
Ethical issues (including plagiarism, misconduct, data fabrication, falsification, double publication or submission, redundancy) have been completely observed by the authors.

Funding/Support
This paper was derived from MSc thesis of Medical Parasitoly and financially supported by Shahrekord University of Medical Sciences, Shahrekord, Iran (grant No. 1618, date: 22/06/2014).

References

1. Markell EK, John DT. Medical parasitology. 14th ed. Philadelphia: WB Saunders; 2006:63-70.
2. Sayyari A, Imanzadeh F, Bagheri Yazdi S, Karami H, Yaghoobi M. Prevalence of intestinal parasitic infections in the Islamic Republic of Iran. East Mediterr Health J. 2005;11(3):377-383.
3. Gharavi MJ. Text Book of Clinical Parasitology (in Persian). 4th ed. Tehran: Mirmah; 2011.
4. Saebi E. Protozoal Disease in Iran (In Persian). 4th ed. Tehran: Ayiizh; 2009: 79-92.
5. Hellgren U, Ericsson O, Aden Abdi Y, Gustafsson LL. Handbook of Drugs for Tropical Parasitic Infections. CRC Press; 1995.
6. Harris J, Plummer S, Lloyd D. Antigiardial drugs. Appl Microbiol Biotechnol. 2001;57(5-6):614-619.
7. Edwards DI. Nitroimidazole drugs-action and resistance mechanisms I. Mechanism of action. J Antimicrob Chemother. 1993;31(1):9-20.
8. Edwards DI. Nitroimidazole drugs-action and resistance mechanisms II. Mechanisms of resistance. J Antimicrob Chemother. 1993;31(2):201-210.
9. Zargari A. Herbal Plants (in Persian). 8th ed. Tehran: University of Tehran Press; 2011.
10. Corns CM. Herbal remedies and clinical biochemistry. Ann Clin Chem. 2003;40(5):489-507.
11. Davazdah Emami S, Majnoon Hoseini N. Agriculture and manufacturing of herbs and spices (in Persian). Tehran: University of Tehran Press; 2011: 148-53.
12. Zahedi MJ, Heidari M, Mohajeri M. Study the effect of *Valeriana Officinalis* and *Echium Amoenum* on the liver and renal function tests in rats (in Persian). J Kerman Univ Med Sci. 2004;11(1):22-27.
13. Hausen MA, Menna-Barreto RF, Lira DC, de Carvalho L, Barbosa HS. Synergic effect of metronidazole and pyrantel pamoate on *Giardia lamblia*. Parasitol Int. 2011;60(1):54-58.
14. Babaei Z, Oormazdi H, Rezaie S, Rezaeian M, Razmjou E. Giardia intestinalis: DNA extraction approaches to improve PCR results. Exp Parasitol. 2011;128128(2):159-162.
15. Farsangi MH, Sahebani N, Movahed A, Tahmasebi R, Raiani M. Lethal effect of *Thymus vulgaris* on *Giardia* cyst; in vitro (in Persian). Iran South Med J. 2002;4(2):88-95.
16. Saatchi A, Kadivar M, Soleimaninejad S. Antioxidant and antifungal effects of ethanol extracts of *Melissa officinalis* and *Valeriana officinalis* (In Persian).18th National Congress on Food Technologhy; 2008 Oct 15-16; Mashhad, Iran.
17. Rahimi-Esboei B, Gholami S, Azadbakht M, Ziaei H. Effect of Hydroalcholic extract of *Artemisia annua* on cysts of *Giardia lamblia* in in vitro (in Persian). J Mazandaran Univ Med Sci. 2012;22(90):72-80.
18. Shahabi S, Ayazi Roozbehani F, Kamalinejad M, Abadi A. Anti-giardia activity of *Carum copticum* on *Giardia lamblia* cysts in vitro (In Persian). Pejouhesh Dar Pezeshki. 2008;32(4):303-307.
19. Safarnejad Tameshkel F, Khatami Nejad M, Nasrollahi A, Rahdari P, Gholam Hossein Poor F, Rahnavard A. The antimicrobial effect of methanol extracts of *Eucalyptus*, *Satureia hortensis* and *Heracleum glabrescens* on *Giardia cysts* (in Persian). Med Lab J. 2012;6(2):21-27.

32

The effects of celery leave extract on male hormones in rats

Wesam Kooti[1], Maryam Ghasemi-boroon[2], Mehri Ghafourian[3], Majid Asadi-Samani[4*], Mahmoud Harizi[2], Naim Sharafi-Ahvazi[1], Reza Afrisham[2]

[1]Member of Student Research Committee, Kurdistan University of Medical Sciences, Sanandaj, Iran
[2]Member of Student Research Committee, Ahvaz Jundishapur University of Medical Sciences, Ahvaz, Iran
[3]Health Research Institute, Research Center of Thalassemia & Hemoglobinopathy, Department of Immunology, Ahvaz Jundishapur University of Medical Sciences, Ahvaz, Iran
[4]Medical Plants Research Center, Shahrekord University of Medical Sciences, Shahrekord, Iran

ARTICLE INFO

Keywords:
Apium graveolens
Side effects
Luteinizing hormone
Rat

ABSTRACT

Introduction: Celery (*Apium graveolens*) belongs to the Umbelliferae family, and has a plenty of nutritional and pharmaceutical applications. The presence of phytoestrogenic compounds has been reported in this plant. These compounds may affect the pituitary-gonad axis. The aim of the present study was to evaluate the efficacy of hydro-alcoholic extracts of celery leaves on serum levels of testosterone, LH and FSH in male rats.
Methods: In this experimental study, 32 male Wistar rats were divided into four groups, eight rats included in each. The control group did not receive any treatment. The placebo group received distilled water and the case groups received 200 and 300 mg/kg/B.W of hydro-alcoholic celery leaf extract for 20 consecutive days by oral administration. After completion of the treatment, the rats were anesthetized and blood sampling from their heart was carried out. Then, serum levels of testosterone, LH and FSH were measured using immunoassay methods. The obtained data were analyzed by the SPSS using the statistical ANOVA test.
Results: The level of LH in the case group receiving 200 mg/kg B.W of celery extract showed a significant decrease compared with the control and placebo groups ($P<0.05$). The level of FSH and testosterone in case groups did not show any significant difference in comparison with the control group ($P>0.05$).
Conclusion: The result of the present study shows that in the administered dose, celery extract does not have any considerable side effect on the secretion of hormones in male rats.

Implication for health policy/practice/research/medical education:
Celery (*Apium graveolens*) does not cause any hormonal impairment in male rats; so, as celery improves fertility, its consumption might be useful in the treatment of infertility.

Introduction

The importance of fertility and procreation as a factor for survival of the human race is not hidden from anyone (1). According to documents the use of the herbs has a long history in order to fertility regulation (2). Nowadays the effect of plant-derived chemicals on the endocrine system and the activity of sexual organs have induced a great interest (3).
Among the medicinal herbs in indigenous systems of medicine it can be pointed to the numerous health benefits of celery. Celery (*Apium graveolens* L.) is a plant, belonging to the parsley descent (Umbelliferae), an herbaceous, biennial, and branched stem plant, with a height of 20 to 60 cm (4). This plant is native to the Mediterranean region that is also cultivated in other parts of the world (5). In laboratory studies celery has been referred for antifungal effects (6), anti-hyperlipidemic activities (7,8) and anti-inflammatory effects (9). This herb is rich in antioxidant compounds such as flavonoids (e.g. apiin and apigenin), as well as vitamins E and C (10,11). The sperm plasma membrane is susceptible to oxidative damage due to large amounts of polyunsaturated fatty acids leading to decreased sperm motility and viability (12). Antioxidant compounds may enhance the sperm function and also

***Corresponding author**: Majid Asadi-Samani, Medical Plants Research Center, Shahrekord University of Medical Sciences, Shharekord, Iran. Email: biology_2011@yahoo.com improve fertility. In this regard, celery extract, due to its antioxidant contents has been pointed for inhibiting the liposomal peroxidation (13) and protection of testes against sodium valproate (14). Also some reports suggest the efficacy of the extracts on the male reproductive system (15,16). In this study we aimed to evaluate hormonal impairment in male rats after oral administration of hydro-alcoholic extracts of celery leaves.

Materials and Methods

In this experimental study, 32 male Wistar rats, with a weight range of 170–200 g, purchased from the Animal Reproduction and Breeding Center of Ahvaz University of Medical Sciences were used. The animals were kept in plastic cages in a room with optimal temperature and appropriate environmental situations and with the environmental temperature of 22 to 24°C, and a period of 12 hours darkness and 12 hours light. The animals were provided food and water indefinitely. All other conditions of rat maintenance were remained identical during the investigation.

Preparation of hydro-alcoholic extraction of celery

Celery pant was purchased from a well-known store in Ahvaz, and then evaluated and confirmed as *A. graveolens*. The leaves were then dried in the shade and milled; soon after. Powders were stored in a refrigerator until extraction.

In order to prepare 50 g of hydro-alcoholic extract, the orally administrable celery were dissolved in 200 ml of 70% ethanol and the solution was kept at room temperature for three days. During these three days the solution was stirred several times to separate the extract, and after 72 hours, the mixture filtered with a filter paper. The extract solution was spread on a glass surface at room temperature to evaporate the solvent. The dried extract powder was obtained by scraping them from the glass surface, and then stored at 4°C until the use (17). The 200 and 300 mg/kg/B.W. concentrations were prepared from the powder of celery leaf extract, using distilled water as a solvent.

Grouping of animal and extract administration

Rats were divided into four groups including eight rats in each: control, placebo, case 1 and case 2 groups. The control group did not receive any treatment. The placebo group received 1 ml distilled water (as the solvent of the extract); and the case groups 1 and 2 received 200 and 300 mg/kg/B.W of hydro-alcoholic extract of celery, for 20 consecutive days, by gavage, respectively (18). One day after the last administration, rats were anesthetized with xylazine and ketamine, thereafter, blood sampling from the heart was done. Then each sample centrifuged at 3000 RPM for 15 minutes to separate the serum from the clot. After separation the serum from the clot, using a sampler, the samples were frozen and maintained in -20°C. Serum levels of LH, FSH and testosterone were measured by immunohistochemistry methods.

Statistical analysis

The data obtained from the hormone measurement were analyzed by variance one-way ANOVA using SPSS 15 software and the comparative LSD test, considering the significance level of $P \leq 0.05$.

Results

The effect of hydro-alcoholic extract of celery leaf on serum level of FSH

The comparison of the mean FSH serum level (mIU/ml) in case groups receiving different doses of hydro-alcoholic extract of celery leaf with the placebo and control groups did not show any significant difference ($P>0.05$; Figure 1).

The Effect of hydro-alcoholic extract of celery leaf on serum level of LH

The investigation of mean serum level of LH (mIU/ml) in different groups involved in this research demonstrated that the administration of the celery leaf extract at the dose of 200 mg/kg causes a significant reduction of LH in comparison with the placebo and control groups ($P<0.05$). However, any significant difference was not seen between the 300 mg/kg extract receiving group with the control and placebo groups ($P>0.05$; Figure 2).

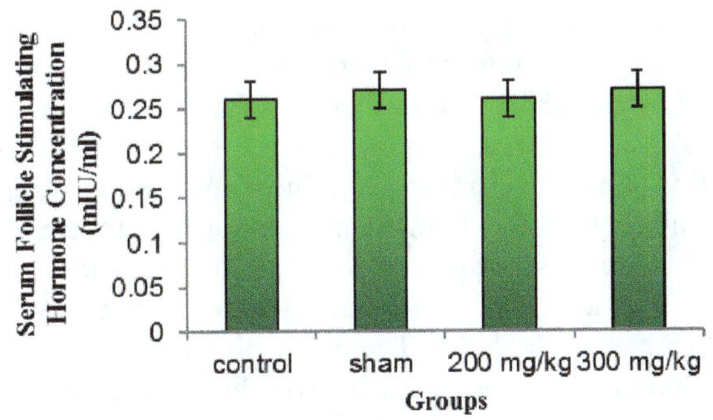

Figure 1. The comparison of the effect of celery leaf hydro-alcoholic extract on the average serum level of FSH in case and control groups

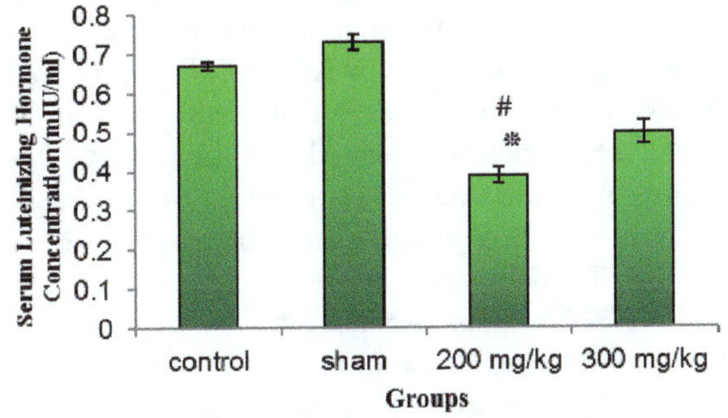

Figure 2. The comparison of celery hydro-alcoholic extract effect on serum level of LH in case and control groups; *Significant difference with respect to the control group ($P<0.05$); #Significant difference with respect to the sham group ($P<0.05$)

The Effect of hydro-alcoholic extract of celery leaf on serum level of testosterone

Based on the presented results in Figure 3, the investigation of the effect of different doses of celery leaf hydro-alcoholic extract on serum level of testosterone (ng/ml) in the 200 and 300 mg/kg extract receiving groups did not show any significant difference with the control and placebo groups (P>0.05).

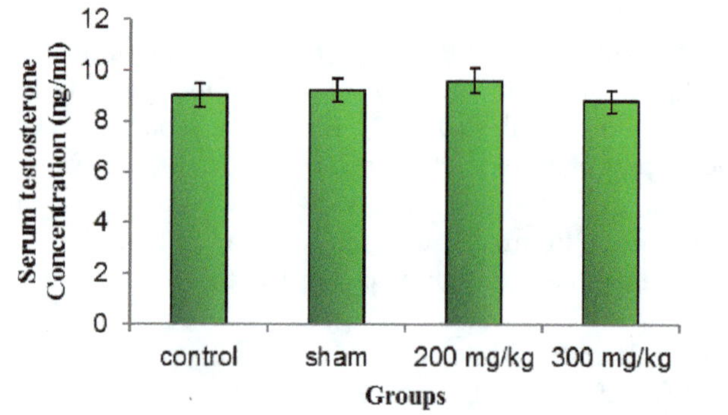

Figure 3. The comparison of celery leaf hydro-alcoholic extract effect on the average serum level of testosterone in the case and control groups

Discussion

The present study was carried out with the purpose of investigation of celery hydro-alcoholic extract effect on pituitary-gonad hormonal axis. The results of this study demonstrated a significant reduction in serum level of LH in case group compared with the control group. These findings were in accordance with the results of the study performed by Modaresi *et al.* (19). In a research carried out by Mokhtari *et al.*, on *Coriandrum sativum* L plant belonging to Apiaceae family, it was shown that the hydro-alcoholic extract of *Coriandrum sativum* L seed has led to a reduction in serum gonadotropins in the treatment group compared with the control group (20). Moreover, in the research done by Hemayatkhah Jahromi *et al.* the reduction of serum LH was observed after treatment with the hydro-alcoholic extract of *Citrus aurantifolia* peel. Among the important compounds of these two plants are flavonoids and coumarins (21).

The existence of phytoestrogenic compounds such as flavonoids and coumarins was demonstrated in celery extract by phytochemical studies (22). Phytoestrogens are natural plant-derived compounds with the structure and function similar to estrogen (23). These compounds result in inhibition of the human and animal gonadotropin secretion and the hypothalamus-pituitary-gonad axis arrest, by affecting the hypothalamic gonadotropin producing cells (24,25). Therefore, the decreased LH secretion can be attributed to extract of the phytoestrogenic compounds (11).

According to the findings of the present study, FSH serum level in the case groups did not show any significant difference in comparison with the control and placebo groups that is in agreement with the findings of Kerishchi *et al.* (26). It could be due to the modulatory effects of some factors such as inhibin, activin and follistatin, which play a role in regulation and modulation of FSH via a central effect on gonadotropin releasing hormone (27). On the other hand, the results of the researches carried out by the other scientists showed that the probability of occurrence of a mutation in LH receptors in Leydig cells is high, however, these mutations occur merely in Sertoli cells (28,29). Therefore, another reason for the lack of the changes in FSH, may be probably due to the changes in receptor activity after the administration of the extract.

In this study, serum level of testosterone was measured, as well. The findings demonstrated that serum level of testosterone did not have any significant difference in case group compared with the placebo and control groups. Kerishchi *et al.* showed that the administration of 100 and 300 mg/kg of the extract does not have any effect on serum levels of testosterone and gonadotropins through the investigation of the effect of celery seed extract on the pituitary-gonad axis in Syrian mouse (26). This result is in agreement with the results of the present study. However, the increase in serum level of testosterone in the group receiving 200 mg/kg celery seed extract has been also another result of this research.

Moreover, the results of the various studies might be due to the differences in the methods of experiments, such as the used extract, the routes of administration the extract, the extraction techniques, the duration of treatment and the animal species of the experiment.

The secondary phenol metabolites of plants affect the hormonal networks such as pituitary-gonad axis. Lack of the changes in higher doses may be the result of the feedback regulation of this network on LH and FSH hormones, followed by the modulation of testosterone, as well (30). Furthermore, the antioxidants lead to the modulation of the hormone concentrations via changing the levels of O2 in the body and ATP metabolism (31). FSH and LH hormones act synergistically. These two hormones affect Sertoli cells, and lack of each hormone leads to impaired spermatogenesis (32). Considering the role of testosterone in spermatogenesis and the important secondary effects on sexual organs, it may be concluded that it is the most important reproduction factor in testis (20).

Conclusion

Since in the present study serum levels of FSH and testosterone did not show any considerable changes, it seems that consumption of this plant does not cause any hormonal impairment in males; and probably does not have any side effect on the fertility. However, more investigations are required in this field. In order to improve the validity of the obtained results, it is recommended that the effects of other celery extracts on sexual hormone levels be evaluated using other solvents. On the other hand, the clinical effects could be investigated through preparation of the appropriate formulation of the effective extracts.

Acknowledgments
We hereby thank Mr. Esrafil Mansuri and Dr. Abdolkazem Neysi (the specialists of statistics of Shahid Chamran University) due to their unsparing collaboration. The results are obtained by the proposed research project approved by the Research Committee No. 91s45 implemented in Ahvaz Jundishapur University of Medical Sciences and funded by the deputy of research.

Authors' contributions
All the authors wrote the manuscript equally.

Conflict of interests
The authors declared no competing interests.

Ethical considerations
Ethical issues (including plagiarism, misconduct, data fabrication, falsification, and double submission) have been completely observed by the authors.

Funding/Support
The presented results were obtained by the implemented research project No. 91s45 that was approved by the Student Research Committee of Ahvaz University of Medical Sciences and Health Services; and has been with the expenses of this deputy.

References

1. Yakubu M, Akanji M, Oladiji A. Male sexual dysfunction and methods used in assessing medicinal plants with aphrodisiac potentials. Phcog Rev 2007; 1(1): 49.
2. Talukder S, Hossain M, Sarker S, Khan M. Investigation into effect of crude mixture of abrus precatorius seed on hypothalamopituitary gonadal axis and development of antifertility in male rats. Bangladesh J Agr Res 2011; 36(1): 103-9.
3. Yakubu MT. Effect of Cnidoscolous aconitifolius (Miller) IM Johnston leaf extract on reproductive hormones of female rats. Iran J Reprod Med 2008; 6(3): 149-55.
4. Sivashanmugam MUA, Jagannath P. Induction of Apoptosis and Cytotoxic Activities of Apium graveolens Linn. Using in vitro Models. Middle-East J Sci Res 2011; 9(1): 90-4.
5. Fu N, Wang Q, Shen H-L. De Novo Assembly, Gene Annotation and Marker Development Using Illumina Paired-End Transcriptome Sequences in Celery (Apium graveolens L.). PloS One 2013; 8(2): e57686.
6. Momin RA, Nair MG. Mosquitocidal, nematicidal, and antifungal compounds from Apium graveolens L. seeds. J Agric Food Chem 2001; 49(1): 142-5.
7. Mansi K, Abushoffa AM, Disi A, Aburjai T. Hypolipidemic effects of seed extract of celery (Apium graveolens) in rats. Pharmacogn Mag 2009; 5(20): 301.
8. Kooti W, Ghasemiboroon M, Asadi-Samani M, Ahangarpoor A, Noori Ahmad Abadi M, Afrisham R, *et al.* The effects of hydro-alcoholic extract of celery on lipid profile of rats fed a high fat diet. Adv Environ Biol 2014; 8(9): 325-30.
9. Mencherini T, Cau A, Bianco G, Della Loggia R, Aquino RP, Autore G. An extract of Apium graveolens var. dulce leaves: structure of the major constituent, apiin, and its anti-inflammatory properties. J Pharm Pharmacol 2007; 59(6): 891-7.
10. Fazal SS, Singla RK. Review on the Pharmacognostical & Pharmacological Characterization of Apium Graveolens Linn. Indo Global J Pharm Sci 2012; 2(1): 36-42.
11. Kooti W, Ali-Akbari S, Asadi-Samani M, Ghadery H, Ashtary-Larki D. A review on medicinal plant of Apium graveolens. Adv Herb Med 2014; 1(1): 48-59.
12. Sikka SC. Oxidative stress and role of antioxidants in normal and abnormal sperm function. Front Biosci 1996; 1: 78-86.
13. Popovic M, Kaurinovic B, Trivic S, Mimica-Dukic N, Bursac M. Effect of celery (Apium graveolens) extracts on some biochemical parameters of oxidative stress in mice treated with carbon tetrachloride. Phytother Res 2006; 20(7): 531-7.
14. Hamza AA, Amin A. Apium graveolens modulates sodium valproate-induced reproductive toxicity in rats. J Exp Zool Part A 2007; 307(4): 199-206.
15. Kooti W, Ghasemiboroon M, Ahangarpoor A, Hardani A, Amirzargar A, Asadi Samani M, *et al.* The effect of hydro-alcoholic extract of celery on male rats in fertility control and sex ratio of rat offspring. J Babol Univ Med Sci 2014; 16(4): 43-9.
16. Kooti W, Ghasemiboroon M, Asadi-Samani M, Ahangarpoor M, Zamani M, Amirzargar A, *et al.* The effect of hydro-alcoholic extract of Celery leaves on the delivery rate (fertilization and stillbirths), the number, weight and sex ratio of rat off spring. Adv Environ Biol 2014; 8(10): 824-30.
17. Gharib Naseri MK, Zareei M, Amiri O. Spamolitic effect of Vitis vinifera leaf hydroalcoholic extract on rat colon. Iran J Basic Med Sci 2006; 9(1): 41-9.
18. Khaki A, Fathiazad F, Nouri M, Khaki AA, Ozanci CC, Ghafari-Novin M, *et al.* The effects of Ginger on spermatogenesis and sperm parameters of rat. Iran J Reprod Med 2009; 7(1): 7-12.
19. Modaresi M, Ghalamkari G. The Effect of Celery (Apium graveolens) Extract on the Reproductive Hormones in Male Mice. APCBEE Procedia 2012; 4, 99-104.
20. Mokhtari M, Jowhari H, Yazdanpour F. Effects of hydro-alcoholic seed extract of Coriandrum sativum L. on pituitary-ovary hormones in rat. Med Sci J Islamic Azad Univ Tehran Med Branch 2013; 22(4): 243-73.
21. Hemayatkhah Jahromi V, Farajmand M , Azhdari S, Ghaedi Sh, Farzam M, Kargar jahromi H. Effect of hydroalcoholic extract of Citrus aurantifolia peel on serum level of testosterone, FSH, LH and testis tissue in adult male rats. Int J Biol Pharm Allied Sci 2013;

2(6): 1307-15.

22. Fazala SS, Ansarib MM, Singlac RK, Khand S. Isolation of 3-n-Butyl Phthalide & Sedanenolide from Apium graveolens Linn. Indo Global J Pharma Sci 2012; 2(3): 258-61.
23. Panjehshahin M, Panahi Z, Dehghani F, Talaei Khozani T. The effects of hydroalcoholic extract of Actinidia chinensis on sperm count and motility, and on the blood levels of estradiol and testosterone in male rats. Arch Iran Med 2005; 8(3): 211-6.
24. McGarvey C, Cates PS, Brooks AN, Swanson IA, Milligan SR, Coen CW, *et al.* Phytoestrogens and gonadotropin-releasing hormone pulse generator activity and pituitary luteinizing hormone release in the rat. Endocrinology 2001; 142(3): 1202-8.
25. Karimi Jashni H, Najmadini N, Hooshmand F. Effect of alcoholic extract of Aloe vera plant on serum testosterone and gonadotropin levels in rats. J Jahrom Univ Med Sci 2012; 10(2): 2.
26. Kerishchi P, Nasri S, Amin Gh, Tabibian M. The effects of Apium graveolens extract on sperm parameters and H-G hormonal axis in mice. Proceedings of the 20th Congress of Physiology and Pharmacology 2011; Hamadan, Iran.
27. Azarnioushan F, Khatamsaz S, Sadeghi H. The effects of hydroalcoholic extract of Dorema Aucheri on blood concentration of gonadotropin and androgen hormones in adult male rats. Armaghan Danesh 2009; 14: 63-70.
28. Mokhtari M, Shariati M, Ghahramani R. Effect of Trigonella foenum-graecum L. seed extract on concentration of testosterone and spermatogenesis in rats. J Med Plants Res 2008; 7(25): 12-20.
29. Mokhtari M. Effect of selegiline on concentration of testosterone and spermatogenesis in rats. Asian J Anim Vet Adv 2007; 2(4): 229-33.
30. Azarniushan F., Karami M, Gholizdeh L, Davare K, the effect of ethanol extracts of Dorema aucheri on thyroid hormones in rats. J Shahrekord Univ Med Sci 2010; 12(2): 84-6.
31. Panda S, Kar A. Amelioration of l-thyroxin-induced hyperthyroidism by coumarin (1, 2-benzopyron) in female rats. Clin Exp Pharmacol Physio 2007; 34(11): 1217-9.
32. Mclachlan RI, O'Donnell L, Meachem SJ, Stanton PG, De Krester DM, Pratis K, *et al.* Identification of specific sites of hormonal regulation in spermatogenesis in rats, monkeys and man. Recent Prog Horm Res 2002; 57: 149-79.

Hypoglycemic effect of *Satureja montanum* L. hydroethanolic extract on diabetic rats

Naser Mirazi[1]*, Maryam Rezaei[2], Mahmoud Mirhoseini[2]

[1]Department of Biology, Faculty of Basic Sciences, Bu-Ali Sina University, Hamedan, Iran
[2]Medical Plants Research Center, Shahrekord University of Medical Sciences, Shahrekord, Iran

ARTICLE INFO

Keywords:
Satureja montanum L.
Diabetes
Streptozocin
Rat

ABSTRACT

Introduction: Diabetes is one of the most prevalent metabolic disorders which is associated with several complications in different organs. Nowadays, medicinal herbs are being widely used to treat diseases. This study was conducted to study the hypoglycemic effect of *Satureja montanum* in diabetic male rats.
Methods: In this study 42 male Wistar rats were randomly assigned to 7 equal groups including control, diabetic control, treatments 1, 2, and 3, metformin-treated diabetic, and healthy treated with *Satureja montanum*. To induce diabetes streptozotocin (STZ) at 60 mg/kg was intraperitoneally (ip) administered. The animals were treated daily with *Satureja montanum* extract (ip) for one week and their blood glucose was measured daily.
Results: *Satureja montanum* extract could significantly decrease blood glucose. The greatest effect of the extract was seen on day 8 at 800 mg/kg ($P<0.001$). *Satureja montanum* extract caused a significant increase in serum insulin compared to the control group ($P<0.001$).
Conclusion: The findings of this study indicate that *Satureja montanum* hydroethanolic extract is able to significantly decrease blood glucose of diabetic rats possibly with a stimulatory effect on beta cells.

Implication for health policy/practice/research/medical education:
Satureja montanum hydroethanolic extract can significantly enhance blood insulin of diabetic rats, decreasing blood glucose, hence, it might be beneficial in diabetic patients.

Introduction

Diabetes is one of the most prevalent metabolic disorders which is associated with several complications in different organs (1). This disease is characterized by hyperglycemia and disorder of metabolism of carbohydrates, lipids, and proteins. Diabetes is one of the most prevalent and costly chronic diseases worldwide and is increasing in prevalence because of variations in lifestyle and also improved healthcare in communities, leading to enhanced survival (2).
Insulin is one of the hormones contributing differently to metabolism and other body processes. Insulin controls the storage and metabolism of carbohydrates, proteins, and lipids. It also enhances active transfer of glucose from tissue cell membrane of lipid and muscle, is involved in converting glucose and intracellular free fatty acids into reserves of glycogen and triglycerides, increases conversion of hepatic glucose into glycogen, and inhibits glucose output from liver. Intravenous administration of insulin causes stimulation of growth hormone through decreasing glycemia (3).
Inadequate monitoring of blood sugar, genetic predisposition including family history, smoking, obesity, physical inactivity, hypertension, and hyperlipidemia are some of the risk factors for diabetes (4).
Free radicals are chemically active molecules. The production of free radicals in cells is a natural process of body metabolic reactions. Normally, these radicals are removed by the enzymes and antioxidant compounds in the body. Lack of balance between contribution of antioxidant defense and increased production of free radicals leads to conditions called oxidative stress. The diabetes-derived hyperglycemia causes intensified indices of oxidative stress such as membrane lipids peroxidation (5).
Medicinal herbs are considered as a very suitable alterna-

***Corresponding author:** Naser Mirazi; Department of Biology, Faculty of Basic Sciences, Bu-Ali Sina University, Hamedan, Iran. Email: mirazi205@gmail.com tive to synthetic drugs because of easy access, fewer side effects, and less cost. Plant-derived biological substances are a subdiscipline of modern pharmacotherapy of diseases (6). Summer savory, scientifically called *Satureja montanum*, is a medicinal herb from Lamiaceae.

This genus consists of approximately 30 species, of which 12 occur in and 8 are exclusively unique to Iran (7). In traditional medicine, analgesic and disinfectant properties have been mentioned for *Satureja montanum* (8). *Satureja montanum* is used to treat thoracic diseases, cough, thinness, and rheumatologic and neurological pains (9). Use of *Satureja montanum* leaf extract causes decrease in hypercholesterolemia (10). Some studies have demonstrated its anti-inflammatory and antimicrobial properties, as well (11,12).

Aerial parts of *Satureja montanum* have many applications in food and pharmacologic industries and could be used as a strong and natural alternative to synthetic antioxidants (13).

Studies have demonstrated that *Satureja montanum* extract protects reproductive system against cyclophosphamide toxicity through antioxidant and androgenic activities and is used as a supplement in patients with hepatitis (14). Zeidán-Chuliá et al study demonstrated antioxidant, antimicrobial, and anti-inflammatory properties of *Satureja montanum* (15).

In light of the significance of study of diabetes and no investigation of *Satureja montanum* hydroalcoholic extract on diabetes as a significant and prevalent disease, this study was conducted to study the hypoglycemic effect of *Satureja montanum* extract in diabetic male Wistar rats.

Materials and methods

Plant preparation and extraction

Satureja montanum was obtained from the Herbarium unit of Agriculture of Jihad Organization of Hamadan province and was transferred to laboratory after identification by a botanist in Agricultural Research Center of Hamadan province. After the plants were cleaned, they were shadow-dried in air. The leaves were separated and pulverized by a meal. Two hundred grams of the obtained powder was stored in ethylic alcohol 80% in refrigerator for a week. Then the contents were filtered by a filter paper and the obtained solution was concentrated by rotary at 55 rpm at 60°C. After concentration, the resulting extract was placed under the hood for two days to completely dry. The prepared extract was kept in freezer at -20°C for later uses.

Laboratory animals

In this study, 42 animals were kept in Animal House of Research Laboratory of Faculty of Sciences, Bu-Ali Sina University, Hamadan at 22±2°C under 12 hours dark/light cycles with free access to water and food. For adaptation to laboratory conditions, the animals were kept in the laboratory for one week before the study. The protocol was confirmed in Ethical Committee of Bu-Ali Sina University and all ethical standards of animal experimentation (National Institutes of Health, 1985) were followed in the present study.

The rats were randomly assigned to eight equal groups consisting of healthy control, diabetic control intraperitoneally (i.p) administered with streptozotocin (STZ) at 60 mg/kg once, healthy group administered with the extract at 400 mg/kg, diabetic groups i.p administered with various doses of the extract (at 200, 400, and 800 mg/kg) daily for 8 days, and diabetic group treated with gavage metformin at 500 mg/kg daily.

To induce diabetes, STZ (Sigma Co.) at 60 mg/kg was administered i.p. Three days after administration, the rats' glycemia was measured and those with blood glucose over 250 mg/dL were considered as diabetic. The diabetic rats had diabetes symptoms such as polydipsia, diuresis, and weight loss.

After the diabetes was confirmed in the groups of interest, the animals were treated with the extract for one week. The animals were i.p administered with the extract at specified doses according to the grouping on a daily basis. Glycemia was measured and recorded at 3 steps, prior to STZ administration, after diabetes induction on a daily basis for one week, and at the completion of tests. All the animals were sacrificed with no suffering according to ethical principles of animal experimentation and their blood samples were collected. The level of serum insulin was measured by radioimmunoassay kit (Diasorin, Italy). The used kit was compatible with rats' insulin.

The data of studied groups were analyzed by SPSS and expressed as mean ± SEM. For comparison, one-way analysis of variance (ANOVA) was used and for inter-group comparisons Tukey test was used. The level of significance was considered $P < 0.05$.

Results

Seventy-two hours after STZ administration, glycemia increased significantly in the groups administered with STZ compared to the control group not receiving STZ ($P < 0.001$). Treatment with *Satureja montanum* leaf hydroethanolic extract could significantly decrease glycemia in diabetic rats in a dose-dependent manner.

These findings indicated that glycemia decreased significantly in the diabetic rats treated with *Satureja montanum* leaf hydroethanolic extract at 200 mg/kg on day 5 compared to the diabetized control group ($P < 0.01$). Moreover glycemia decreased significantly in the diabetic rats treated with *Satureja montanum* leaf hydroethanolic extract at 400 and 800 mg/kg compared to the diabetic control group ($P < 0.001$). The difference in glycemia between the diabetic group treated with the extract at high dose and the control group was not significant, between metformin-treated diabetic group and control group was significant ($P < 0.001$), and between metformin-treated diabetic group and the groups treated with *Satureja montanum* leaf hydroethanolic extract at low and moderate doses was not significant. On the other hand, the difference between metformin-treated group and control group was derived significant ($P<0.001$; Figure 1).

These findings indicated that glycemia decreased significantly in the diabetic rats treated with *Satureja montanum* leaf hydroethanolic extract at 200 mg/kg on day 6 compared to the diabetic control group ($P<0.01$). The difference remained significant compared to the control group ($P<0.001$). Moreover, glycemia decreased significantly in the diabetic rats treated with *Satureja montanum* leaf hydroethanolic extract at 400 or 800 mg/kg compared to the diabetic control group and the group treated with the extract at 200 mg/kg ($P<0.001$), but the difference in glycemia between the group treated with the extract at 400 mg/kg and the control group with increased glycemia remained significant ($P<0.001$). The difference in glycemia between the diabetic group treated with the extract at high dose and the control group was not significant, between metformin-treated diabetic group and control group was significant ($P<0.001$), and between metformin-treated diabetic group and the groups treated with *Satureja montanum* leaf hydroethanolic extract at low and moderate doses was not significant. On the other hand, the difference between metformin-treated group and control group was derived significant ($P<0.001$; Figure 2).

These findings indicated that glycemia decreased significantly in the diabetic rats treated with *Satureja montanum* leaf hydroethanolic extract at different doses on day 8 were similar to day 6 (Figure 3).

The variations in glycemia in any studied groups at different days indicated that *Satureja montanum* leaf hydroethanolic extract caused a significant, dose-dependent decrease in glycemia in the rats. This decrease was obtained highest for metformin at day 6, and a significant increase in the rats' glycemia was seen from day 7 afterwards com-

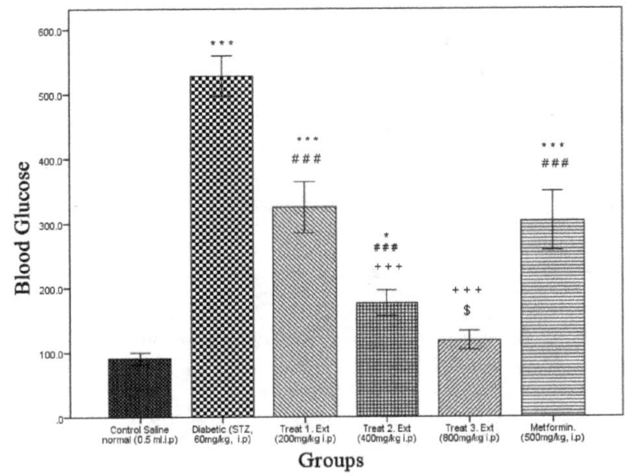

Figure 2. Comparison of glycemia in different groups at day 6 of the study; mean ± standard error of measurement express the data of male Wistar rats (n = 6); * represents the significance of variation in glycemia of the animals in different groups after treatment in comparison to the control group ($^{***}P<0.0001$, $^{*}P<0.05$); # represents the significance of variation in glycemia of the animals in different groups in comparison to the untreated diabetized group ($^{###}P<0.001$); + represents the significance of variation in glycemia of the animals in different groups in comparison to the group administered with the extract at low dose (200 mg/kg) ($^{+++}P<0.001$); $ represents the significance of variation in glycemia of the animals in the group administered with the extract at high dose (800 mg/kg) in comparison to those in the group administered with the extract at moderate dose (400 mg/kg) ($P<0.05$).

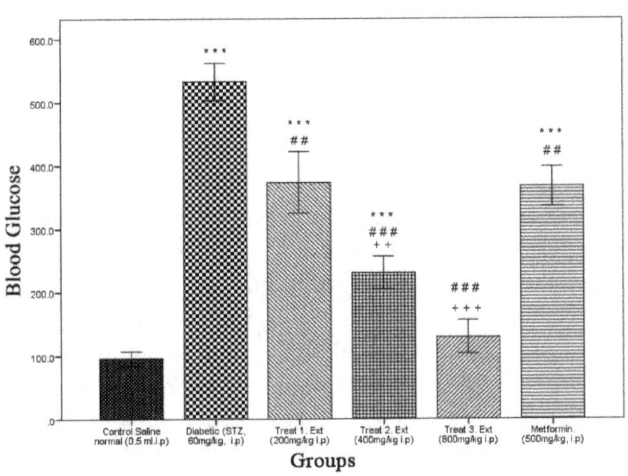

Figure 1. Comparison of glycemia in different groups at day 5 of the study; mean ± standard error of measurement express the data of male Wistar rats (n = 6); * represents the significance of variation in glycemia of the animals in different groups after treatment in comparison to the control group ($^{***}P<0.001$); # represents the significance of variation in glycemia of the animals in different groups in comparison to the untreated diabetized group ($^{##}P<0.01$, $^{###}P<0.001$); + represents the significance of variation in glycemia of the animals in different groups in comparison to the group administered with the extract at low dose (200 mg/kg) ($^{++}P<0.01$, $^{+++}P<0.001$).

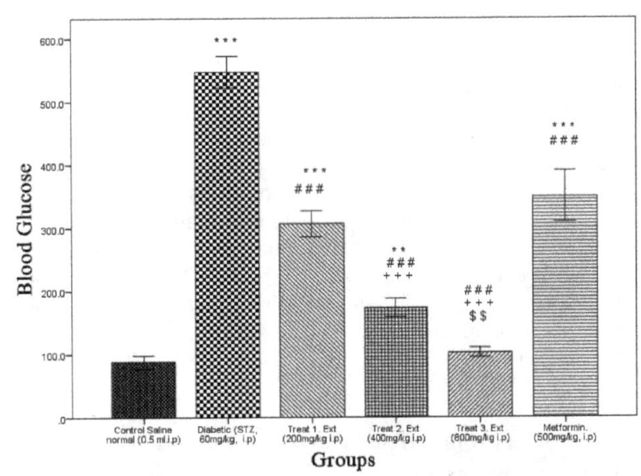

Figure 3. Comparison of glycemia in different groups at day 8 of the study; mean ± standard error of measurement express the data of male Wistar rats (n = 6); * represents the significance of variation in glycemia of the animals in different groups after treatment in comparison to the control group ($^{***}P<0.001$); # represents the significance of variation in glycemia of the animals in different groups in comparison to the untreated diabetized group ($^{###}P<0.001$); + represents the significance of variation in glycemia of the animals in different groups in comparison to the group administered with the extract at low dose (200 mg/kg) ($^{+++}P<0.001$).

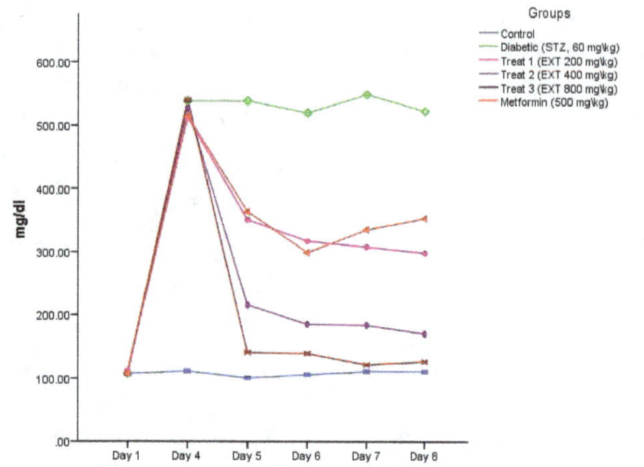

Figure 4. Comparison of glycemia in different groups at different days of the study.

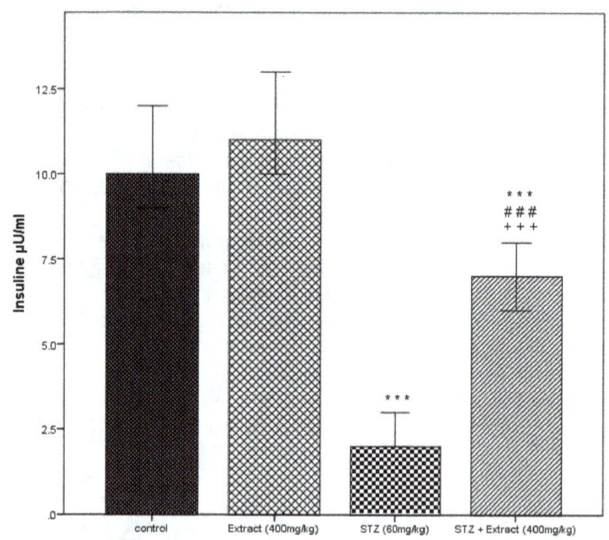

Figure 5. Comparison of serum insulin among control group, the group treated with extract at moderate dose, untreated diabetic group, and diabetic group treated with extract at moderate dose; mean ± standard error of measurement express the data of male Wistar rats (n = 6); * represents the significance of variation in serum insulin of the animals in groups in comparison to the control group (*** $P < 0.001$); # represents the significance of variation in serum insulin of the animals in different groups in comparison to the healthy, extract-treated group (### $P < 0.001$); + represents the significance of variation in serum insulin of the animals in different groups in comparison to diabetic, untreated group (200 mg/kg) (+++ $P < 0.001$).

pared to the groups treated with *Satureja montanum* leaf hydroethanolic extract at low, moderate, and high doses ($P < 0.001$; Figure 4). The variations in serum insulin in the groups treated with *Satureja montanum* leaf hydroethanolic extract indicated that *Satureja montanum* leaf hydroethanolic extract at 400 mg/kg caused no significant difference in the treated healthy group. However, *Satureja montanum* leaf hydroethanolic extract at 400 mg/kg caused a significant increase in serum insulin in diabetic group compared to the diabetic control group ($P < 0.001$). However the increase in insulin in this group decreased significantly compared to the control group and the control group treated with the extract at 400 mg/kg ($P < 0.001$; Figure 5).

Discussion

The findings of this study indicated that i.p administration of *Satureja montanum* hydroalcoholic extract in short-term significantly affected the glycemia in the studied animals in a positive manner. *Satureja montanum* hydroethanolic extract at low, moderate, and high doses caused a significant decrease blood glucose of the rats with STZ-induced diabetes in a dose-dependent manner.

The studies have indicated oxidative stress and inflammatory damages are caused by hyperglycemic conditions in diabetes (16). The incidence of oxidative stress is higher in the patients with diabetes than the individuals in control group. The production rate of free radicals increases in the patients with diabetes while antioxidant resistance declines in them. As a result, oxidative stress increases in these patients (12). The induction of diabetes in rats caused decline in activity of antioxidant enzymes, superoxide dismutase and glutathione peroxidase, in the studied groups. Prolonged diabetes caused decline in catalase, glutathione reductase, GSH-Px and SOD (17).

In traditional medicine, *Satureja montanum* is used as a supplement for patients with diabetes. Studies have indicated that *Satureja montanum* essence could decline free radicals (17,18). In addition, antioxidant, antimicrobial, and anti-inflammatory properties have been confirmed for *Satureja montanum* (12,13,19). Containing several phenolic compounds with strong antioxidant and anti-inflammatory effects, *Satureja montanum* can reduce diabetes-derived oxidative stress. A study found that *Satureja montanum* exerted stronger antioxidant properties than *Mentha piperita* extract. Many studies have pointed to anti-inflammatory and antimicrobial properties of *Satureja montanum* (20).

A study has demonstrated that *Satureja montanum* contains mucilage compounds, resin, and tannin. Moreover limonene 1 and 8 and cineole are other single ring monoterpenes in *Satureja montanum*. Borneol and camphor have been reported as other monoterpenes in this plant (21). Antioxidant property of *Satureja montanum* ethanol extract, which is enhanced as the extract's concentration increases, has been also demonstrated (22). Furthermore some studies have found that *Satureja montanum* essence's antioxidant property is enhanced as its concentration increases (23).

Studies have indicated that there are phenolic monoterpenes such as thymol, and gamma-terpinene in *Satureja montanum*. In addition, *Satureja montanum* extract has been reported to contain carvacrol (24,25). A study has demonstrated that *Satureja montanum* essence' ability to prevent linoleic acid oxidation was very high and approximately equal to BTH's (26).

In light of the present study's and other studies' findings,

Satureja montanum could exert anti diabetic properties because of strong antioxidant and anti-inflammatory properties and suppressing oxidative stress following diabetes. As mentioned previously, as the *Satureja montanum* extract concentration increases, its antioxidant property is enhanced. This finding is consistent with the present study as the *Satureja montanum* extract anti diabetic property was enhanced with increase in its concentration. Hence *Satureja montanum* could prevent increase in glycemia in the studied rats through high antioxidant and anti-inflammatory activity.

As mentioned above, *Satureja montanum* antioxidant effects and hence high anti-inflammatory activity demonstrated in several studies could contribute to diabetogenetic process of STZ and prevent its further effects, facilitating the process of recovery and rearrangement of insulin-producing cells. These findings demonstrated that the rate of insulin secretion in the diabetic animals treated with *Satureja montanum* leaf extract increased significantly compared to the diabetic group. Since the destruction of pancreatic islets beta cells and cell DNA is caused after STZ administration, the *Satureja montanum* extract is thought to contribute to protecting or repair damaged pancreas tissue against inflammation and necrosis due to STZ by increasing the activity of dismutase superoxide and glutation peroxidase, and therefore cell stimulation was furthered and pancreatic islets tissue was restored.

The findings of the present study indicated that *Satureja montanum* could significantly affect the diabetes course and prevent increase in glycemia and insulin in STZ-diabetic adult male rats. However further and more advanced equipment lacking in the present study is needed to explain the cell and enzyme mechanisms, and further studies are strongly recommended to remove the limitations of the present study. Altogether, if the potentially involved mechanisms in this process are explained, *Satureja montanum* could be used as a strong anti-diabetic medication and/or natural anti diabetic drugs with fewer side effects could be supplemented by extraction of *Satureja montanum* effective compounds.

Acknowledgements

This paper was derived from MSc thesis of Maryam Rezaei. The authors of this manuscript gratefully thank Dr. Ramazan Kalvandi, botanist at Agricultural Research Center of Hamadan province, for making generous efforts to scientifically identify the plant and respectful authorities of Faculty of Basic Sciences of Bu-Ali Sina University for providing the necessary arrangements for implementing this thesis.

Authors' contributions

All the authors wrote the manuscript equally.

Conflict of interests

The authors declared no competing interests.

Ethical considerations

Ethical issues (including plagiarism, misconduct, data fabrication, falsification, double publication or submission, redundancy) have been completely observed by the authors.

Funding/Support

This paper was financially supported by Department of Biology, Faculty of Basic Sciences, Bu-Ali Sina University, Hamedan, Iran, with registered code number: 2125476, 20/sept/2014.

References

1. Artola A, Kamal A, Ramakers GM, Biessels GJ, Gispen WH. Diabetes mellitus concomitantly facilitates the induction of long term depression and inhibits that of long-term potentiation in hippocampus. Eur J Neurosci. 2005;22(1):169-178.
2. Taheri E, Saedisomeolia A, Djalali M, Qorbani M. The relationship between serum 25-hydroxy vitamin D concentration and lipid profile in type 2 diabetic patients and healthy subjects. J Diabetes Metab Disord. 2012;11(1):16-20.
3. Daneman D. Type 1 diabetes. Lancet. 2006; 367(9513): 847-858.
4. Kucukatay V, Ağar A, Gumuslu S, Yargiçoğlu P. Effect of sulfur dioxide on active and passive avoidance in experimental diabetes mellitus: relation to oxidant stress and antioxidant enzymes. Int J Neurosci. 2007; 117(8):1091-1107.
5. Rains JL, Jain SK. Oxidative stress, insulin signaling, and diabetes. Free Radic Biol Med. 2011;50(5):567-575.
6. Mohajeri D, Doustar Y, Rezaei A, Mesgari-Abbasi M. Hepatoprotective effect of ethanolic extract of Crocus sativus L. (Saffron) stigma in comparison with silymarin against rifampin induced hepatotoxicity in rats. Zahedan J Res Med Sci. 2011;12(5):53-59.
7. Fathi A, Sahari MA, Zangiabadi M, Barzegar M. Application of Satureja hortensis L. and Zataria multiflora Boiss. Essentiol oils as two natural antioxidants in soybean oil during microwave heating. Journal of Medicinal Plants. 2011;10(39):13-20.
8. Omidbaigi R. Approaches to Production and Processing of Medicinal Plants. Vol 2. Tehran, Iran: Tarrahan-e-Nashr; 1997.
9. Teimouri M, Bahar Z, Mirza MA. Antimicrobial activity of essential oil of Satereja laxiflora L. Koch before and after flowering. Iranian Journal of Medicinal and Aromatic Plants. 2003;13:49-68.
10. Hajhashemi V, Ghannadi A, Pezeshkian SK. Antinocicieptive and anti-inflammutory effect of Satureja hortensis L., extracts and essential oil. Ethnopharmacol. 2002;82(2-3):83-87.
11. Tabatabaei Rasti AR, Khalighi A, Kashi A, Asnaashari S, Bamdad Moghadam S, Delazar A. Antioxidant

activity and chemical composition of essential oil of Satureja sahendica Born. Pharm Sci. 2007;3:1-6.
12. Najafian, S, Zahedifar M. Antioxidant activity and essential oil composition of Satureja hortensis L. as influenced by sulfur fertilizer. J Sci Food Agric. 2015;95(12):2404-8.
13. Djenane D, Yangüela J, Amrouche T, Boubrit S, Boussad N, Roncalés P. Chemical composition and antimicrobial effects of essential oils of Eucalyptus globulus, Myrtus communis and Satureja hortensis against Escherichia coli O157:H7 and Staphylococcus aureus in minced beef. Food Sci Technol Int. 2011;17(6):505-515.
14. Shojaee-Aliabadi S, Hosseini H, Mohammadifar MA, et al. Characterization of antioxidant-antimicrobial κ-carrageenan films containing Satureja hortensis essential oil. Int J Biol Macromol. 2013;52:116-24.
15. Zeidán-Chuliá F, Keskin M, Könönen E, et al. Antibacterial and antigelatinolytic effects of Satureja hortensis L. essential oil on epithelial cells exposed to Fusobacterium nucleatum. J Med Food. 2015;18(4): 503-506.
16. Saadat M, Pournourmohammadi S, Donyavi M, Khorasani R, Amin G, Nazar Salehnia A. Alteration of rat hepatic glycogen phosphorylase and phosphoenolpyruvate carboxykinase activities by Satureja khuzestanica Jamzad essential oil. J Pharm Pharm Sci. 2004;7:310-314.
17. Vosough-Ghanbari S, Mohammadirad A, Yasa N, Basiri S, Esmaily H, Abdollahi M. Improvement by Satureja khuzestanica essential oil of malathion-induced red blood cells acetylcholinesterase inhibition and altered hepatic mitochondrial glycogen phosphorylase and phosphoenolpyruvate carboxykinase activities. Pestic Biochem Physiol. 2007;89:124-129.
18. Mahboubi M, Kazempour N. Chemical composition and antimicrobial activity of Satureja hortensis and Trachyspermum copticum essential oil. Iran J Microbiol. 2011;3(4):194-200.
19. Ghazanfari G, Minaie B, Yasa N, Ashtaral NL, Mohammadirad A, Nikfar S. Biochemical and histopathological evidences for beneficial effects of Satureja khuzestanica Jamzad essential oil on the mouse model of inflammatory bowel disease. Toxicol Mech Methods. 2006;16:365-372.
20. Boyer F, Vidot JB, Dubourg AG, Rondeau P, Essop MF, Bourdon E. Oxidative stress and adipocyte biology: focus on the role of AGEs. Oxid Med Cell Longev. 2015;2015:534873.
21. Calcutt NA, Freshwater JD, Mizisin AP. Prevention of sensory disorders in diabetic Sprague-Dawley rats by aldose reductase inhibition or treatment with ciliary neurotrophic factor. Diabetologia. 2004;47(4):718-724.
22. Yagihashi S. Pathology and pathogenetic mechanisms of diabetic neuropathy. Diabetes/Metabolism Reviews. 1995;11(3):193-225.
23. Pasaoglu H, Sancak B, Bukan N. Lipid peroxidation and resistance to oxidation in patients with type 2 diabetes mellitus. Tohoku J Exp Med. 2004;203(3): 211-218.
24. Vlassara H. Recent progress in advanced glycation end products and diabetic complications. Diabetes. 1997;46:19-25.
25. Mata AT, Proenca C, Ferreira AR, Serralheiro ML, Nogueira JM, Araujo ME. Antioxidant and antiacetylcholinesterase activities of five plants used as Portuguese food spices. Food Chem. 2007;103(3): 778-786.
26. Kulisic T, Radonic A, Milos M. Inhibition of lard oxidation by fractions of different essential oils. Grass y Aceites. 2005;56(4):284-291.

Clastogenic effect of *Picrorhiza kurroa* rhizome extract on cultured human peripheral blood lymphocytes

Acharya Balkrishna[1,2], Hemanth Kumar Manikyam[2], Vinay K Sharma[2], Niti Sharma[2*]

[1]University of Patanjali, Haridwar, Uttarakhand 249402, India
[2]Patanjali Natural Coloroma Pvt Ltd, Haridwar, Uttarakhand 249404, India

ARTICLE INFO

Keywords:
Picrorhiza kurroa
Rhizome
Chromosome aberration
Human peripheral blood lymphocytes

ABSTRACT

Introduction: The *Picrorhiza kurroa* rhizome has a long history of use in Indian Ayurvedic and Chinese system of medicine for the treatment of a wide spectrum of diseases. Today it is viewed as an important therapeutic target in both Western and Eastern medicinal systems. This work was aimed to study the clastogenic effect of *Picrorhiza kurroa* rhizome extract on cultured human peripheral blood lymphocytes.
Methods: Hydroalcoholic extract of rhizome was prepared and mammalian chromosomal aberration test was conducted using cultured human peripheral blood lymphocytes. The study was performed in two independent phases where the human peripheral blood lymphocytes were exposed to various of the extract in absence and presence of metabolic activation system for a continuous and short duration.
Results: *Picrorhiza kurroa* rhizome extract did not induce chromosome aberration up to 2500 μg/mL in final culture concentration in the presence (1% v/v) and absence of metabolic activation.
Conclusion: *Picrorhiza kurroa* rhizome extract is completely safe to be used as a medicine since it manifest its healing effects without causing genotoxicity.

Implication for health policy/practice/research/medical education:
The genotoxicity of *Picrorhiza kurroa* rhizome extract was studied in the human peripheral blood lymphocytes. The results suggest that it is a safe plant to be used as a medicine since it manifest its healing effects without causing genotoxicity.

Introduction

Picrorhiza kurroa Royle ex. Benth belongs to Scrophularaceae family and is commonly called Kutki or Kutka. It is a well-recognized herb in the Ayurvedic and Chinese traditional medicine. It is a wonder herb with hepatoprotective (1-4), anticholestatic (5), antioxidant (6), antidiabetic (7) and immune-modulating properties (8-10). The leaves, root and rhizome of *Picrorhiza* are effective in numerous ailments namely liver and upper respiratory tract illnesses, chronic diarrhea, malaria, jaundice, epilepsy, paralysis, rheumatoid arthritis and skin diseases (11-14). In rats with malaria, *Picrorhiza* reestablished depleted glutathione levels helping to conserve a normal oxidation-reduction balance (15).
Additionally, *Picrorhiza* extract has been found to be useful in dealing with viral hepatitis symptoms as it has favorable anti-hepatitis B surface antigen potential (16).
Nowadays plants or plant extracts have important therapeutic applications in both Western and Eastern medicinal systems. However, some of them are potentially toxic, mutagenic or carcinogenic. Thus, to evaluate potential genotoxicity of the standardized hydro-alcoholic extract of *Picrorhiza kurroa* rhizome, mammalian chromosomal aberration test was conducted on cultured human peripheral blood lymphocytes.

Material and Methods

Material

Picrorhiza kurroa rhizomes were procured from Patanjali Natural Coloroma Pvt Ltd and stored in ambient conditions for further study. The other solvents and chemicals were purchased from Sigma-Aldrich, India.

Extraction

The rhizomes of the plant were dried in shade for about 3 weeks and ground using a mixer to a coarse powder. Using a soxhlet extraction method, the powder of dried rhizome was processed with petroleum ether (40-50°C) for 18 h in

***Corresponding author:** Niti Sharma,
Email: nitivinay@yahoo.co.in

order to remove fat and unwanted components. The treated powder was further processed with hydro-alcoholic solution (60:40) by using the same extraction procedure for 18h. The extract was evaporated to dryness in a rotary flash evaporator at a temperature not exceeding 60°C, then stored in an air tight container.

Test system

Human venous blood from healthy adult donors lacking current viral infections was collected and used for the study. The study was conducted in accordance to the procedures and recommendations of OECD Guideline 473, updated and adopted July 1997.

The study was conducted in two independent phases:

Initial Chromosome Aberration Assay (Phase I)

Confirmatory Chromosome Aberration Assay (Phase II)

Based on the results of solubility, it was tested up to the highest concentration 2500 μg/mL (both phases of the experiment). Dose range finding study was conducted as an integral part of the chromosomal aberration assay. A range of soluble dose concentrations ranging viz., 2500, 1250, 625, 312.5, 156.3, 78.1, 39.1, 19.5, 9.8 and 4.9 μg/mL was applied in the initial chromosome aberration assay.

In the first phase of the experiment, the proliferating human lymphocytes (72 ± 2 hours after the initiation of whole blood culture) were exposed at various doses of the Test Sample (4.9, 9.8, 19.5, 39.1, 78.1, 156.3, 312.5, 625, 1250 and 2500 μg/mL) in the absence and presence of metabolic activation system (1% v/v) for a short duration (about 4-hour exposure).

In the second phase of the experiment, the proliferating human lymphocytes (72 ± 2 hours after the initiation of whole blood culture) were exposed at diverse dose levels of the Test Sample (2500, 1500, 1000, 750 and 500 μg/mL) in the absence of metabolic activation system for a continuous treatment (up to 1.5 normal cell cycle length). One set of the proliferating human lymphocytes were exposed at various dose levels of Test Sample (2500, 1500, 1000, 750 and 500 μg/mL) in presence of metabolic activation system (1% v/v) for a short duration (about 4-hour exposure).

In both the phases (Experimental Phase 1 & 2) the treated cells were harvested at about 1.5 cell cycle length after treatment (22 hours). Mitomycin C and Cyclophosphamide were used as positive control substances for experiments without and with S9, respectively.

During harvesting of cell cultures, the cells were treated with metaphase arresting agent (Colchicine) 2 hours prior to harvesting. Later the cells were hypotonically treated, fixed in acetomethonol fixative and metaphase spreads were prepared by hanging drop method. The slides were stained with 5% Giemsa solution.

The metaphase cells were analyzed microscopically for the presence of chromosome aberrations if any, and a minimum number of 1000 cells per sample were screened randomly and number of metaphases was recorded in different fields to determine the mitotic index. The number of aberrant cells with one or more aberrations excluding gaps and the number of aberrant cells with one or more aberrations including gaps was recorded separately to calculate percent aberrant cells.

Results

Initial chromosome aberration assay

The initial chromosomal aberration was conducted with about 4-hour exposures to standardized *Picrorhiza kurroa* rhizome extract (Test Sample), in the presence and absence of S9 metabolic activation system. The assay was carried out with ten dose levels of the Test Sample viz., 2500, 1250, 625, 312.5, 156.3, 78.1, 39.1, 19.5, 9.8 and 4.9 μg/mL in the final culture. The result of mitotic indices at all the ten concentrations of the Test Sample was found to be comparable to the vehicle control group. The results of chromosome aberrations including gap and chromosome aberration excluding gap at various dose concentrations (2500, 1250, 625 μg/mL) did not reveal any induction of chromosome aberrations when compared to the vehicle control groups (Tables 1 and 2).

The results of the positive control, Mitomycin C (2.0 μg/mL; in the absence of metabolic activation) and Cyclophosphamide (60 μg/mL; in the presence of metabolic activation 1% v/v) significantly increased the number of structural chromosome aberrations when compared to vehicle control groups.

Therefore, it is clear from the results of the initial chromosomal aberration assay that *Picrorhiza kurroa* rhizome extract, in the presence and absence of S9 metabolic activation system does not induce chromosome aberrations at concentrations tested. However, the positive control groups showed an increase in the frequency of aberrant cells and thus demonstrated sensitivity of the test system.

Confirmatory chromosome aberration assay

The confirmatory assay was performed after the results of the initial trial were known. The clear negative result of the initial chromosome aberration assay was further confirmed for the evidence of clastogenicity, if any.

Assay without S9 activation-continuous exposure

Three days after culture initiation, the cultures were treated with the Test Sample, in the absence of metabolic activation at various dose concentrations (2500, 1500, 1000, 750 and 500 μg/mL) along with concurrent vehicle and positive controls. Incubation at 37 ± 2°C was continued until the time of harvest. The results of mitotic indices at all the five concentrations of the Test Sample were found to be comparable to the vehicle control group. No cytotoxicity was observed at any of the dose levels of the Test Sample, in the absence of metabolic activation. The results of chromosome aberrations including gap and chromosome aberration excluding gap at various concentrations (2500, 1500, 1000 μg/mL) did not reveal any induction of chromosome aberrations when compared to the vehicle control groups.

The results of the positive control, Mitomycin C (2.0 μg/mL) in the absence of metabolic activation showed a

Table 1. Mitotic Index observed in experimental phase 1 both in absence and presence of metabolic activation (10% v/v)

In presence of metabolic activation (10% v/v)			In absence of metabolic activation		
Dose levels (µg/mL)	Mitotic index[a]	% Mitotic Index	Dose levels (µg/mL)	Mitotic index	% Mitotic index
0.0 (VC)	13.052 ± 1.01	NA	0.0 (VC)	14.706 ± 0.73	NA
60 (CPA)	10.325 ± 0.73	79	2 (MMC)	8.345 ± 0.30	57
2500 (TS)	12.864 ± 0.43	99	2500 (TS)	13.339 ± 1.22	91
1250 (TS)	11.596 ± 0.45	89	1250 (TS)	14.782 ± 1.30	101
625 (TS)	11.97 ± 0.77	92	625 (TS)	14.222 ± 0.07	97
312.5 (TS)	11.511 ± 0.15	88	312.5 (TS)	14.179 ± 0.81	96
153.25 (TS)	11.692 ± 0.06	90	153.25 (TS)	13.951 ± 0.12	95
78.13 (TS)	11.785 ± 0.01	90	78.13 (TS)	13.493 ± 0.13	92
39.06 (TS)	12.448 ± 0.64	95	39.06 (TS)	14.025 ± 0.67	95
19.53 (TS)	11.420 ± 0.75	87	19.53 (TS)	13.458 ± 0.00	92
9.77 (TS)	12.345 ± 0.34	95	9.77 (TS)	13.290 ± 0.15	90
4.88 (TS)	11.882 ± 0.22	91	4.88 (TS)	14.180 ± 0.03	107

Abbreviations: CPA, Cyclophosphamide (Positive control); MMC, Mitomycin C (Positive control), TS, Test Sample, VC, vehicle control (Dimethyl sulfoxide)

[a] Mitotic index = Number of metaphase cells/total number of cells screened × 100.

Table 2. Mitotic index observed in experimental phase II with exposure of whole blood culture to short term treatment (4 ± 1 hour) in presence of metabolic activation system (10% v/v)

Dose Levels (µg/mL)	Mitotic index	% Mitotic index
0.0 (VC)	13.052 ± 1.01	NA
60 (CPA)	10.325 ± 0.73	79
2500 (TS)	12.864 ± 0.43	99
1500 (TS)	11.596 ± 0.45	89
1000 (TS)	11.97 ± 0.77	92
750 (TS)	11.511 ± 0.15	88
500 (TS)	11.692 ± 0.06	90

Abbreviations: CPA, Cyclophosphamide (Positive control); TS, Test Sample, VC, vehicle control (Dimethyl sulfoxide).

considerable increase in the number of structural chromosome aberrations when compared to vehicle control groups (Tables 3-5).

Therefore, confirmatory chromosome aberration assay clearly indicate that the Test Sample, in the absence of S9 metabolic activation system does not induce chromosome aberrations at the concentrations tested. However, the positive control group showed an increase in the frequency of aberrant cells and thus demonstrated sensitivity of the test system.

Assay with S9 activation–short exposure

The confirmatory chromosome aberration assay was conducted with about 4-hour exposures to the Test Sample, in the presence of activation system. The assay was carried out at five concentrations of the Test Sample (2500, 1500, 1000, 750 and 500 µg/mL).

The results of mitotic indices at all the five concentrations of the Test Sample, were found to be comparable to the vehicle control group. No cytotoxicity was observed at any of the dose levels of the Test Sample in the presence of metabolic activation. The results of chromosome aberrations including gap and chromosome aberration excluding gap at various dose concentrations (2500, 1500, 1000 µg/mL) in the presence of metabolic activation did not reveal any induction of chromosome aberrations when compared to

Table 3. Mitotic index observed in experimental phase II with exposure of whole blood culture to continuous treatment (22 hours) in absence of metabolic activation system.

Dose Levels (µg/mL)	Mitotic index[a]	% Mitotic index
0.0 (VC)	13.052 ± 1.01	NA
2 (MMC)	10.325 ± 0.73	79
2500 (TS)	12.864 ± 0.43	99
1500 (TS)	11.596 ± 0.45	89
1000 (TS)	11.97 ± 0.77	92
750 (TS)	11.511 ± 0.15	88
500 (TS)	11.692 ± 0.06	90

Abbreviations: MMC, Mitomycin C (Positive control), TS, Test Sample, VC, vehicle control (Dimethyl sulfoxide).

[a] Mitotic index = Number of metaphase cells/total number of cells screened × 100.

Table 4. Chromosome aberration analysis in experimental phase I with exposure of whole blood culture to short term treatment (4 ± 1 hour) in absence of metabolic activation system

Dose Levels (µg/mL)	% Aberrated cells (structural)		% Numerical aberration
	Including Gap	Excluding gap	
0.0 (VC)	2.00 ± 0.71	0.50 ± 0.71	0.20 ± 0.71
2 (MMC)	12.00 ± 0.41	12.00 ± 0.41	0.00 ± 0.00
2500 (TS)	1.50 ± 0.71	0.50 ± 0.71	0.00 ± 0.00
1250 (TS)	0.50 ± 0.41	0.50 ± 0.71	0.00 ± 0.00
625 (TS)	0.50 ± 0.71	0.00 ± 0.00	0.00 ± 0.00

Abbreviations: MMC, Mitomycin C (Positive control), TS, Test Sample, VC, vehicle control (Dimethyl sulfoxide).

Table 5. Chromosome aberration analysis in experimental phase II with exposure of whole blood culture to continuous treatment (22 hours) in absence of metabolic activation system

Dose Levels (µg/mL)	% Aberrated cells (structural)		% Numerical aberration
	Including Gap	Excluding gap	
0.0 (VC)	1.50 ± 0.71	1.50 ± 0.71	0.00 ± 0.00
2 (MMC)	13.00 ± 1.41	12.00 ± 0.00	0.00 ± 0.00
2500 (TS)	1.00 ± 0.00	0.50 ± 0.71	0.00 ± 0.00
1250 (TS)	0.50 ± 0.71	0.50 ± 0.71	0.00 ± 0.00
625 (TS)	0.50 ± 0.71	0.50 ± 0.71	0.00 ± 0.00

Abbreviations: MMC, Mitomycin C (Positive control), TS, Test Sample, VC, vehicle control (Dimethyl sulfoxide).

Table 6. Chromosome aberration analysis in experimental phase I with exposure of whole blood culture to short term treatment (4±1 hour) in presence of metabolic activation system (10% v/v)

Dose Levels (μg/mL)	% Aberrated cells (structural)		% Numerical aberration
	Including Gap	Excluding gap	
0.0 (VC)	1.50 ± 0.71	0.50 ± 0.71	0.20 ± 0.71
2 (MMC)	12.5 ± 0.71	12.00 ± 1.41	0.00 ± 0.00
2500 (TS)	1.50 ± 0.71	0.50 ± 0.71	0.00 ± 0.00
1250 (TS)	1.00 ± 0.00	0.50 ± 0.71	0.00 ± 0.00
625 (TS)	0.50 ± 0.71	0.50 ± 0.71	0.00 ±0.00

Abbreviations: MMC, Mitomycin C (Positive control), TS, Test Sample, VC, vehicle control (Dimethyl sulfoxide).

Table 7. Chromosome aberration analysis in experimental phase II with exposure of whole blood culture to short term treatment (4±1 hour) in presence of metabolic activation system

Dose Levels (μg/mL)	% Aberrated cells (structural)		% Numerical aberration
	Including Gap	Excluding gap	
0.0 (VC)	1.00 ± 0.41	0.50 ± 0.71	0.20 ± 0.71
2 (MMC)	11.50 ± 0.71	9.50 ± 0.71	0.00 ± 0.00
2500 (TS)	1.50 ± 0.71	0.50 ± 0.71	0.00 ± 0.00
1250 (TS)	0.50 ± 0.71	0.00 ± 0.00	0.00 ± 0.00
625 (TS)	1.00 ± 0.00	0.50 ± 0.71	0.00 ± 0.00

Abbreviations: MMC, Mitomycin C (Positive control), TS, Test Sample, VC, vehicle control (Dimethyl sulfoxide).

the vehicle control groups.

In the presence of metabolic activation (1%v/v), the positive control (60 μg/mL Cyclophosphamide) showed a significant increase in the number of structural chromosome aberrations when compared to vehicle control groups (Tables 1, 2, 6, and 7).

Therefore, it is clear from the results of the confirmatory chromosome aberration assay that Test Sample, in the presence of S9 metabolic activation system does not induce chromosome aberrations at the concentrations tested. However, the positive control group (Cyclophosphamide) showed an increase in frequency of aberrant cells and thus demonstrated sensitivity of the test system (Figures 1-8).

Discussion

For chromosomal aberration studies, mammalian cells were cultured in vitro, exposed to a test substance, harvested, and the occurrence of chromosome aberrations was measured. Human peripheral blood lymphocytes do not normally divide but they are stimulated to divide in culture by exposure to Phytohemagglutinin (PHA) (17). At predetermined intervals after exposure to the Test Sample, the lymphocytes were treated with metaphase arresting substance, Colcemid. Later the cells were collected, stained, and investigated for the presence of chromosomal aberrations.

Several mutagenic agents did not directly interact with the DNA but did so after being converted to active intermediates by liver enzymes (18). Due to limited capacity of human lymphocytes to metabolize the test sample an external metabolic activation system (rat liver S9 homogenate)

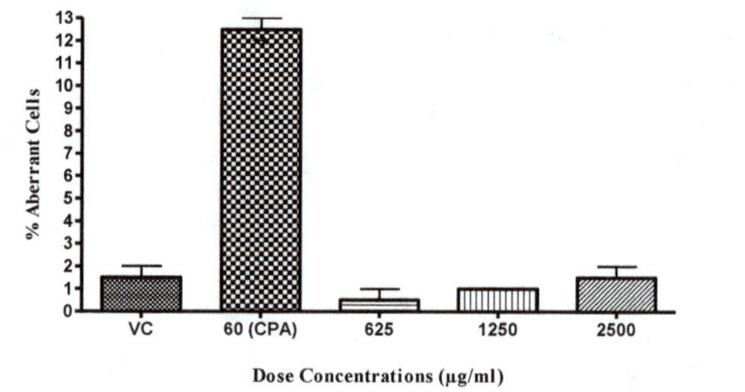

Figure 1. Experimental phase 1 percent aberrant cells observed with metabolic activation (including gap) at various concentrations of Test Sample.

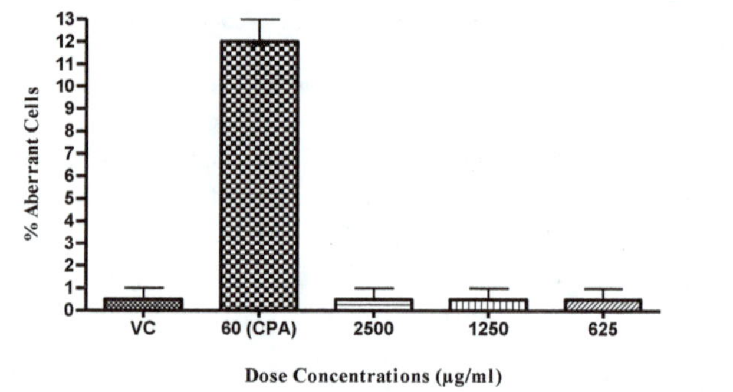

Figure 2. Experimental phase 1 percent aberrant cells observed with metabolic activation (excluding gap) at various concentrations of Test Sample.

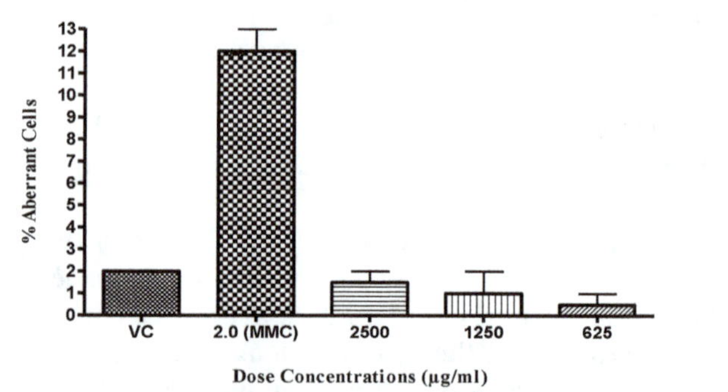

Figure 3. Experimental phase 1 percent aberrant cells observed without metabolic activation (including gap) at various concentrations of Test Sample

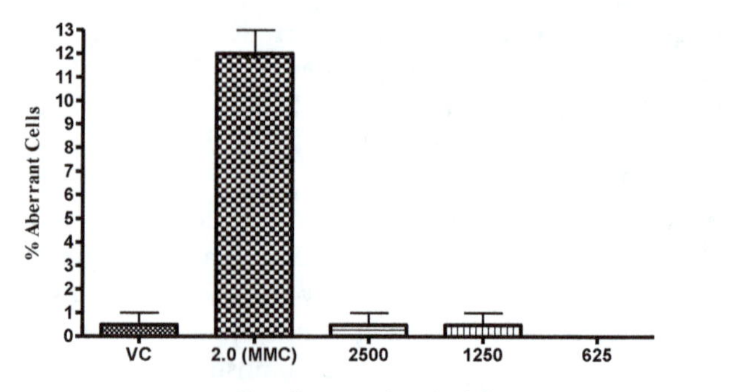

Figure 4. Experimental phase 1 percent aberrant cells observed without metabolic activation (excluding gap) at various concentrations of Test Sample

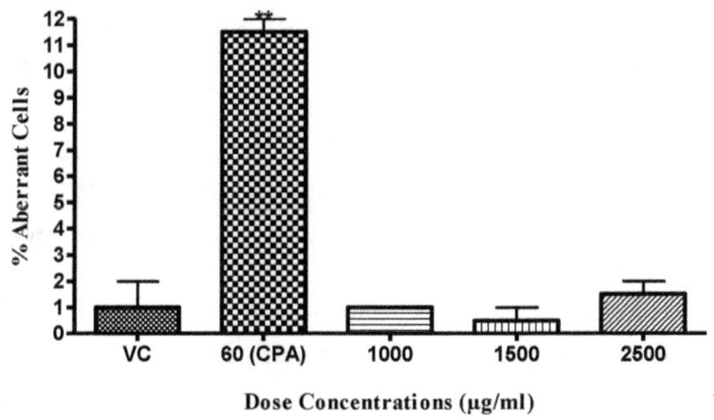

Figure 5. Experimental phase II percent aberrant cells observed with metabolic activation (including gap) at various concentrations of Test Sample

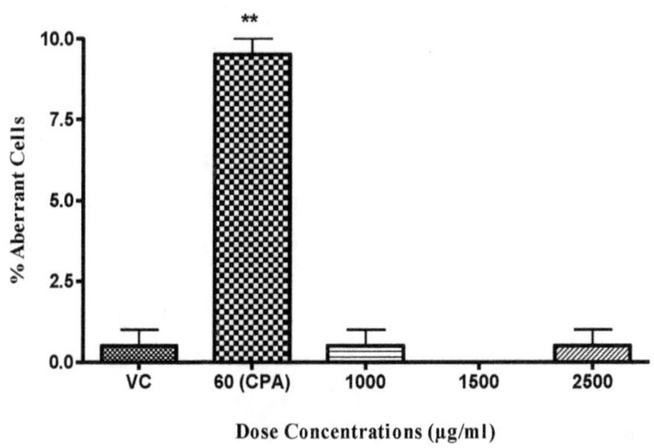

Figure 6. Experimental phase II percent aberrant cells observed with metabolic activation (excluding gap) at various concentrations of Test Sample

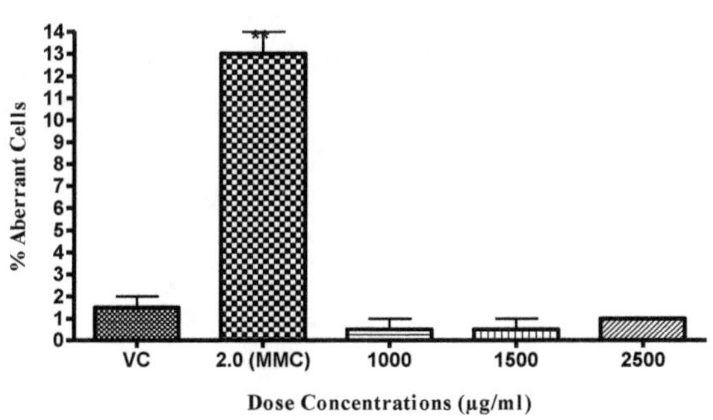

Figure 7. Experimental phase II percent aberrant cells observed without metabolic activation (including gap) at various concentrations of Test Sample.

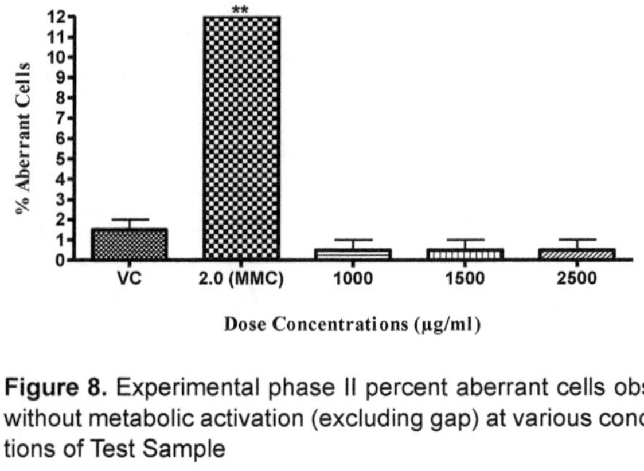

Figure 8. Experimental phase II percent aberrant cells observed without metabolic activation (excluding gap) at various concentrations of Test Sample

was incorporated to further improve the conversion as well as the ability of the assay to identify the clastogenic metabolic intermediates (19,20).

Numerical aberrations (a change in the number of chromosomes from the normal number of 46 for human lymphocytes) are not determined by this study plan.

Conclusion

From the results of this study, it is concluded that the hydro-alcoholic extract of *Picrorhiza kurroa* rhizome does not induce chromosome aberration up to 2500 µg/mL in final culture concentration both in presence (1% v/v) and absence of metabolic activation. Therefore, *Picrorhiza kurroa* rhizome extract can be used as a safe Ayurvedic medicine since it manifest its healing effects without causing genotoxicity. Nevertheless, more scientific data on in vivo activities in human is required to clarify the use of *Picrorhiza kurroa* as a therapeutic medicine.

Acknowledgements

The authors are thankful to Patanjali Natural Coloroma Pvt Ltd. and Patanjali Ayurveda Ltd., Haridwar, India for providing lab facility and support for the research work.

Authors' contributions

ABK conceived of the study, participated in its design and coordination and helped to draft the manuscript. HKM participated in the designing experimental protocol and performed the statistical analysis. VKS and NS participated in its design and coordination and helped to draft the manuscript. All authors read and approved the final manuscript.

Conflict of interests

The authors declared no competing interests.

Ethical considerations

The authors have been entirely regarded ethical issues such as plagiarisms, data assembly, double publication or submission.

Funding/Support

This research was financially supported by Patanjali Natural Coloroma Pvt Ltd, Haridwar.

References

1. Verma PC, Basu V, Gupta V, Saxena G, Rahman LU. Pharmacology and chemistry of a potent hepatoprotective compound Picroliv isolated from the roots and rhizomes of Picrorhiza kurroa Royle ex benth. (kutki). Curr Pharma Biotechnol. 2009;10(6):641-9.
2. Shetty SN, Mengi S, Vaidya R, Vaidya ADB. A study of standardized extracts of Picrorhiza kurroa Royle ex Benth in experimental nonalcoholic fatty liver disease. J Ayur Integr Med. 2010;1(3):203-10.
3. Arsul VA, Wagh SR, Mayee RV. Hepatoprotective activity of livergen, a polyherbal formulation against

carbon tetrachloride induced hepatotoxicity in rats. Int J Pharm Pharmaceut Sci. 2011;3(3):228-31.

4. Singh H, Sharma YK. Clinical evaluation of the hepatoprotective effect of Katuki (Picrorhiza kurroa Royle ex Benth.) processed in Guduchi (Tinospora cordifolia Wild.) Miers in patients receiving lipid lowering drugs (Statins). Indian J Trad Know. 2011; 10(4):657-60.
5. Shukla B, Visen PK, Patnaik GK. Choleretic effect of Picroliv, the hepatoprotective principle of Picrorhiza kurroa. Planta Medica. 1991;57(1):29-33.
6. Kant K, Walia M, Agnihotri VK, Pathania V, Singh B. Evaluation of antioxidant activity of Picrorhiza kurroa (Leaves) extracts. Indian J Pharm Sci. 2013; 75(3):324-29.
7. Husain GM, Rai R, Rai G, Singh HB, Thakur AK, Kumar V. Potential mechanism of anti-diabetic activity of Picrorhiza kurroa. TANG. 2014;4(4):e27.
8. Siddiqui NA, Singh S, Siddiquei MM, Khan TH. Immunomodulatory effect of Withania somnifera, Asparagus racemosus and Picrorhiza kurroa roots. Int J Pharmacol. 2012;8(2):108-14.
9. Hussain A, Shadma W, Maksood A, Ansari SH. Protective effects of Picrorhiza kurroa on cyclophosphamide-induced immunosuppression in mice. Pharmacog Res. 2013;5(1):30-5.
10. Nagarathna PK, Reena K, Reddy S, Wesley J. Review on immunomodulation and immunomodulatory activity of some herbal plants. Int J Pharmaceut Sci Rev Res. 2013;22(1):223-30.
11. Khare CP. Indian Herbal Remedies: Rational Western Therapy, Ayurvedic and Other Traditional Usage. Springer Science & Business Media; 2011.
12. Irshad S, Mannan A, Mirza B. Antimalarial activity of three Pakistani medicinal plants. Pak J Pharmaceut Sci. 2011;24(4):589-91.
13. Banyal HS, Devi R, Devi N. Picrorhiza kurrooa Royal Ex Benth exhibits antimalarial activity against Plasmodium berghei Vincke and Lips. Asian J Biol Sci. 2014;7:72-5.
14. Pathan D, Ambavade S. Anticonvulsant activity of ethanolic extract of Picrorhiza kurroa. Pharmacophore. 2014;5(1):141-6.
15. Wang H, Zhao W, Choomuenwai V, Andrews KT, Quinn RJ, Feng Y. Chemical investigation of an antimalarial Chinese medicinal herb Picrorhiza scrophulariiflora. Bioorg Med Chem Lett. 2013;23(21):5915-8.
16. Jeyakumar R, Rajesh R, Meena B, et al. Antihepatotoxic effect of Picrorhiza kurroa on mitochondrial defense system in antitubercular drugs (isoniazid and rifampicin)-induced hepatitis in rats. J Med Plants Res. 2008;2(1):17-19.
17. Poole A, Leslie GB. A Practical Approach to Toxicological Investigations. Cambridge University Press; 2009.
18. Kim D, Guengerich FP. Cytochrome P450 activation of arylamines and heterocyclic amines. Annu Rev Pharmacol Toxicol. 2005;45:27-49.
19. Madle S, Obe G. In vitro testing of an indirect mutagen (cyclophosphamide) with human leukocyte cultures: activation with liver microsomes and use of a dialysis bag. Mut Res. 1977;56:101-4.
20. Madle S, Obe G. Methods for analysis of the mutagenicity of indirect mutagens/carcinogens in eukaryotic cells. Hum Genet. 1980;56:7-20.

Polyphenolic burden and *in vitro* antioxidant properties of *Moringa oleifera* root extracts

Ioanna Karagiorgou[1,2], Spyros Grigorakis[3], Stavros Lalas[2], Dimitris P. Makris[1*]

[1]School of Environment, University of the Aegean, Mitr. Ioakim Street, Myrina – 81400, Lemnos, Greece
[2]Department of Food Technology, Technological Educational Institute (T.E.I.) of Thessaly, N. Temponera Street, Karditsa – 43100, Greece
[3]Food Quality & Chemistry of Natural Products, Mediterranean Agronomic Institute of Chania (M.A.I.Ch.), International Centre for Advanced Mediterranean Agronomic Studies (CIHEAM), P.O. Box 85, Chania-73100, Greece

ARTICLE INFO

Keywords:
Antioxidants
Moringa oleifera roots
Polyphenols

ABSTRACT

Introduction: *Moringa oleifera* is a small tree with very significant nutritional but also pharmacological properties and various preparations from almost all parts of the plant (leaves, fruit, stems, bark, roots) are used in folk medicine for treating several ailments. This study aimed to investigating the polyphenolic burden and *in vitro* antioxidant properties of *M. oleifera* root extracts, obtained with solvents covering a range of polarities.
Methods: Lyophilised *Moringa oleifera* roots were extracted with solvents of increasing polarity, including ethyl acetate, butanol, methanol and water. The generated extracts were screened for polyphenolic load and antioxidant activities, by determining the total polyphenol, total flavonoid, total flavanol, antiradical activity and reducing power. Liquid chromatography-mass spectrometry was also employed to obtain some evidence regarding the nature of the main constituents.
Results: The results indicated that both aqueous and methanolic extracts were the richest in total polyphenols, but the aqueous extract also exhibited high reducing power. The liquid chromatography-diode array-mass spectrometry analysis also revealed that the major substances occurring in the aqueous extract were relatively polar molecules, but the mass spectral data were ambiguous to assign tentative structures.
Conclusion: Polar solvents, such as water, may be effectively used to recover high amounts of *M. oleifera* root phenolics, which possess important antioxidant properties.

Implication for health policy/practice/research/medical education:
In spite the concrete evidence regarding the pharmacological potential of *Moringa oleifera* root extracts, the data available to-date on the polyphenolic composition of this tissue are particularly limited. It is anticipated that this study will further expand the knowledge pertaining to the major polyphenol classes occurring in fractions of *M. oleifera* root extracts, with respect to composition, polarity and *in vitro* antioxidant properties.

Introduction

Moringa oleifera Lam (syn. *M. ptreygosperma* Gaertn.), referred to as the 'drumstick tree' or the 'horse radish tree', is one of the most widely distributed species of a monogeneric family Moringaceae (1). *M. oleifera* is an important food commodity and the leaves, fruits, flowers and immature pods of this tree are used as a nutritive vegetable in many countries, being rich in β-carotene, phenolics, protein, vitamin C, calcium and potassium etc.
In addition to its high nutritional value, *M. oleifera* is also important for its medicinal properties. Various parts of this plant such as the leaves, roots, seeds, bark, fruits, flowers and immature pods act as cardiac and circulatory stimulants, possess anitumor, antipyretic, antiepileptic, anti-inflammatory, antiulcer, antispasmodic, diuretic, antihypertensive, cholesterol lowering, antioxidant, antidiabetic, hepatoprotective, antibacterial and antifungal activities, and are routinely used in folk medicine for the treatment of different ailments in several countries (2,3). Regarding the roots, they have been found to possess several distinct pharmacological properties and root preparations are used for the cure of bronchitis, stomatitis,

***Corresponding author:** Dimitris P. Makris, Assistant Professor; Email: dmakris@aegean.gr urinary discharges and asthma (4). However, despite the aforementioned activities, *M. oleifera* roots extracts have been scarcely investigated with regard to their polyphenolic content and composition, hence the data available in the literature are particularly limited. Therefore, this study had a scope to illustrate some aspects of the polyphenolic composition and antioxidant potency of *M. oleifera* root extracts. To the best of our knowledge, the present study is the first investigation reporting on the polyphenolic burden and *in vitro* antioxidant properties of *M. oleifera* root extracts, obtained with solvents covering a range of polarities.

Materials and methods

Chemicals

Ferric chloride hexahydrate ($FeCl_3$ $6H_2O$) was from Acros Organics (New Jersey, USA). Gallic acid, Folin-Ciocalteu reagent, rutin (quercetin 3-*O*-rutinoside), ascorbic acid, 2,2-diphenyl-*β*-picrylhydrazyl (DPPH•) radical, *p*-(dimethylamino)-cinnamaldehyde (DMAC), (+)-catechin and 2,4,6-tripyridyl-s-triazine (TPTZ) were from Sigma Chemical Co. (St. Louis, MO). Aluminium chloride ($AlCl_3$) was from Fisher Scientific (New Jersey, USA).

Plant material

M. oleifera roots were obtained from an experimental plantation (Karditsa prefecture, Central Greece). Roots were washed well to remove soil debris, cut into small pieces with a sharp cutter and lyophilised (mean moisture content 81.4%). The lyophilised material was pulverised in a laboratory blender and kept in sealed plastic tubes, at – 40°C, until used.

Batch extraction procedure

An amount of 1 g of lyophilised material was mixed with 20 mL of solvent (water, methanol, butanol, ethyl acetate) in a stoppered plastic tube. The material was subjected to extraction under stirring at 600 rpm, with a teflon-coated magnetic stirrer, for 180 minutes, at room temperature (23 ± 1°C). Following extraction, samples were centrifuged in a table centrifugator (Hermle, Wehingen, Germany) at 10 000 rpm for 10 minutes. The clear supernatant was used for further analysis.

Determination of total polyphenol yield (Y_{TP})

A previously reported protocol was used (5). Briefly, 0.78 mL of distilled water, 0.02 mL of sample and 0.05 mL of Folin-Ciocalteu reagent were mixed. After exactly 1 minute, 0.15 mL of aqueous sodium carbonate 20% was added, and the mixture was vortexed and allowed to stand at room temperature in the dark, for 60 minutes. The absorbance was read at 750 nm (A_{750}) and the total polyphenol concentration (C_{TP}) was calculated from a calibration curve, using gallic acid as a standard (25-500 mg L^{-1}). Yield in total polyphenols (Y_{TP}) was determined as mg gallic acid equivalents (GAE) per g of dry weight (dw), using the following equation:

$$Y_{TP}(mg\ GAE\ g^{-1}\ dw) = \frac{C_{TP} \times V}{m} \quad (1)$$

Where *V* is the volume of the extraction medium (L) and *m* the dry weight of the lyophilized material (g).

Determination of total flavonoid yield (Y_{TFn})

A previously published methodology was employed (6). An aliquot of 0.25 mL sample was mixed with 0.75 mL $AlCl_3$ reagent [0.16% (w/v) $AlCl_3$ and 5% (v/v) acetic acid in methanol] and allowed to stand for 30 minutes, at room temperature. The absorbance was obtained at 415 nm (A_{415}) and the total flavonoid concentration (C_{TFn}) was calculated from a calibration curve, constructed with rutin (quercetin 3-*O*-rutinoside) as the calibration standard (10-160 mg L^{-1}). Yield in total flavonoids (Y_{TFn}), expressed as mg rutin equivalents (RtE) per g of dry weight was determined using Eq. (1).

Determination of total flavanol yield (Y_{TF})

Total flavanols were determined following derivatization with DMAC, based on a previously established protocol (7), with modifications. Briefly, an aliquot of 0.02 mL sample was mixed with 0.88 mL HCl (2M in MeOH) and 0.1 mL DMAC (0.1% in MeOH). The mixture was left to react for 15 minutes and then the absorbance was read at 640 nm. The total flavanol concentration (C_{TF}) was calculated from a calibration curve, constructed with (+)-catechin as the calibration standard (1-80 mg L^{-1}). Yield in total flavanols (Y_{TF}), expressed as mg catechin equivalents (CtE) per g of dry weight was determined using Eq. (1).

Determination of the reducing power (P_R)

A methodology reported previously was used (5). Sample (0.05 mL) appropriately diluted with methanol was mixed thoroughly with 0.05 mL $FeCl_3$ solution (4 mM in 0.05M HCl), and incubated for 30 minutes in a water bath at 37°C. Following this, 0.9 mL TPTZ solution (1 mM in 0.05M HCl) were added, and the absorbance was recorded at 620 nm after exactly 10 minutes. P_R was determined as μmol ascorbic acid equivalents (μmol AAE) per g of dw.

Determination of the antiradical activity (A_{AR})

The assay was performed on the basis of a well-established protocol (8). A volume of 0.025 mL sample was mixed with 0.975 mL DPPH solution (100 μM in methanol) and the absorbance at 515 nm was read immediately after mixing ($A_{515(i)}$) and after exactly 30 minutes ($A_{515(f)}$). The A_{AR} was determined using the following equation:

$$A_{AR}(\mu mol\ DPPH\ g^{-1}\ dw) = \frac{C_{DPPH}}{C_{TP}} \times (1 - \frac{A_{515(f)}}{A_{515(i)}}) \times Y_{TP} \quad (2)$$

Where C_{DPPH} is the initial molar concentration of DPPH (μmol L^{-1}) and C_{TP} is the total polyphenol concentration of the extract, expressed as mg GAE L^{-1}. Results were expressed as μmol DPPH per g of dry weight.

Qualitative liquid chromatography-diode array-mass spectrometry (LC-DAD-MS)
A previously described method was used (8). A Finnigan MAT Spectra System P4000 pump was used coupled with a UV6000LP diode array detector and a Finnigan AQA mass spectrometer. Analyses were carried out on an end-capped Superspher RP-18, 125×2 mm, 4 μm, column (Merck, Germany), protected by a guard column packed with the same material, and maintained at 40°C. Analyses were carried out employing electrospray ionization (ESI) at the positive ion mode, with acquisition set at 5 and 50 eV, capillary voltage 4 kV, source voltage 25 V, detector voltage 650 V and probe temperature 400°C. Eluent (A) and eluent (B) were 2% acetic acid and methanol, respectively. The flow rate was 0.33 mL min^{-1}, and the elution programme used was as follows: 0-2 minutes, 0% B; 2-52 minutes, 100% B; 60 minutes, 100% B.

Statistics

All extractions were carried out in duplicate. All determinations were carried out at least in triplicate and values were averaged. Statistical differences among values were ascertained by performing Student's *t* test, at least at a 95% significance level. Statistics was performed with Microsoft™ Excel 2010 and SigmaPlot™ 12.0.

Results

In this study, the assessment of the polyphenolic content of the extracts obtained was based on the determination of three representative indices, the Y_{TP}, Y_{TFn} and Y_{TF}. As can be seen in Table 1, the highest Y_{TP} was achieved with methanol, but water extraction provided Y_{TP} of comparable magnitude. Extracts of butanol and ethyl acetate were much poorer and the corresponding Y_{TP} values were by 88.6 and 96.2% lower compared with that of methanolic extract. Unlike Y_{TP}, the Y_{TFn} determined for the water extract was 92.7% higher compared with that of methanol, suggesting that the flavonoid fraction occurring in *M. oleifera* roots might consist of compounds with relatively high polarity. This claim was corroborated by the fact that extracts obtained with both butanol and ethyl acetate, which are even less polar solvents, were also poor in flavonoids. Regarding Y_{TF}, a level of 3.24 mg CtE g^{-1} dw was determined in the methanolic extract (Table 1) and it was statistically higher that the levels found in all other extracts ($P < 0.05$). Nevertheless, it is to be noted that the water extract also had Y_{TF} of 2.87 mg CtE g^{-1} dw, as opposed to butanol and ethyl acetate extracts, which had Y_{TF} lower than 0.28 mg CtE g^{-1} dw. This outcome suggested that the flavanol fraction is rather represented by relatively polar constituents.

P_R determination showed that the water extract was by far the most effective, yielding levels that were by 80.9%, 81.44% and 85% higher than the corresponding of methanol, butanol and ethyl acetate extracts (Figure 1), which did not exhibit large differences and their P_R varied from 1.06 to 1.35 μmol AAE g^{-1} dw. The order of efficacy was also very similar with regard to A_{AR}, and the water extract was by 78.9% and 88.2% more effective than the butanol and ethyl acetate extracts. However, a major difference was observed with the methanol extract, which displayed 11.5% higher A_{AR} compared with the water extract (Figure 2).

The LC-MS analysis confirmed that the major phenolics occurring in the extracts obtained were quite polar, since the principal peaks detected were eluted very early. However, three minor peaks were also detected at longer retention times (Table 2), indicating the presence of less polar substances too. The peak eluted at 1.75 minutes yielded a molecular ion with $m/z = 649$, but no derivative ions could be identified. The peak with retention time 2.13 minutes gave a distinct mass spectrum with a molecular ion at $m/z = 543$ and several fragment ions (Table 2). Finally, the peak at 3.50 minutes showed a molecular ion at $m/z = 553$ with no derivative ions.

Discussion

The highest Y_{TP} level found in this study (7.19 mg GAE g^{-1} dw) was close to 10.10 mg GAE g^{-1} dw (9), but significantly higher than 2.20 mg GAE g^{-1} dw (10), reported for methanolic extracts of *M. oleifera* roots. Furthermore, based on Y_{TFn} obtained with the solvents used, it was concluded that this class of polyphenols might consist of polar compounds. This assumption is also supported by other investigations, which demonstrated that *M. oleifera* root extracts obtained with 80% aqueous methanol contained higher amounts of total flavonoids, compared with extracts obtained with either pure methanol or ethanol (10).

Table 1. Y_{TP}, Y_{TFn}, and Y_{TF} achieved by extracting lyophilised *M. oleifera* roots with solvents of variable polarity[a]

Extract	Y_{TP} (mg GAE g^{-1} dw)	Y_{TFn} (mg RtE g^{-1} dw)	Y_{TF} (mg CtE g^{-1} dw)
Water	7.02 ± 0.10	2.73 ± 0.05[b]	2.87 ± 0.06
Methanol	7.19 ± 0.15[b]	0.20 ± 0.01	3.24 ± 0.06[b]
Butanol	0.82 ± 0.02	0.09 ± 0.00	0.28 ± 0.02
Ethyl acetate	0.27 ± 0.01	0.17 ± 0.01	0.03 ± 0.00

[a] All extractions were carried out under stirring (600 rpm) for 180 min, at ambient temperature ($T = 23 \pm 2$°C) and solvent-to-solid ratio of 20 mL g^{-1}. Results are given as average values of triplicate determination (±SD).
[b] Indicates statistically different values ($P < 0.05$).

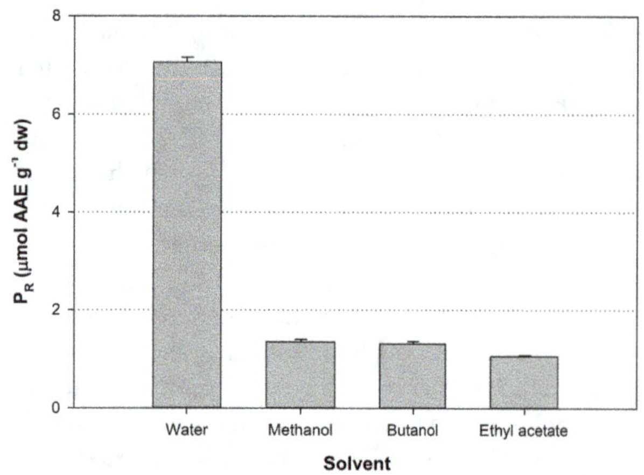

Figure 1. Reducing power (P_R) of *M. oleifera* root extracts obtained with solvents of variable polarity. All extractions were carried out under stirring (600 rpm) for 180 minutes, at ambient temperature (T = 23 ± 2°C) and solvent-to-solid ratio of 20 mL g^{-1}. Results are given as average values of triplicate determination (±SD).

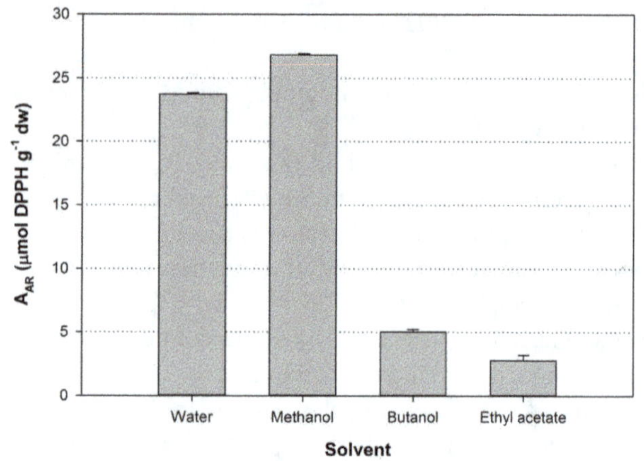

Figure 2. Antiradical activity (A_{AR}) of *M. oleifera* root extracts obtained with solvents of variable polarity. All extractions were carried out under stirring (600 rpm) for 180 minutes, at ambient temperature (T = 23 ± 2°C) and solvent-to-solid ratio of 20 mL g^{-1}. Results are given as average values of triplicate determination (±SD).

Table 2. UV-vis and mass spectral characteristics of the main polyphenolic phytochemicals tentatively identified in *M. oleifera* root aqueous extracts

Peak	Rt (min)	λ_{max} (nm)	$[M+H]^+$ (*m/z*)	Other ions (*m/z*)
1	1.75	292	649	-
2	2.13	258	543	485, 381, 365, 323
3	3.50	292	553	-
4	17.00	256, 362	479	303
5	41.00	240, 278	579	301
6	41.50	240, 278	579	301

The Y_{TFn} determined in the extract obtained with 80% methanol was 2.94 mg catechin equivalents g^{-1} dw, which is very close to 2.73 mg RtE g^{-1} dw determined in this study (Table 1). However, other studies failed to detect flavonoids in water extracts of *M. oleifera* roots, but reported levels of 0.18 mg g^{-1} dw in extracts obtained with methanol (9). This value is similar to Y_{TFn} found in this study for the methanolic extract (0.20 mg RtE g^{-1} dw), but also the extract with ethyl acetate (0.17 mg RtE g^{-1} dw). Contradictory results were also reported by earlier examinations, where methanolic extracts (11) but also ethanolic extracts (12) of *M. oleifera* roots were shown to be free from flavonoids. In addition, all the extracts obtained were found to give positive response to reaction with DMAC, indicating the presence of flavanols, since this reagent is very specific and does not react with any other class of flavonoids (13,14). Although there are no similar reports in the literature, there have been claims for the presence of proanthocyanidins in methanolic extracts of *M. oleifera* roots (15).

The evaluation of the antioxidant potency of the extracts was carried out on the basis of two complementary tests, namely the reducing power (P_R) and the antiradical activity (A_{AR}). It has been pointed out that extracts deriving from different plant tissues, thus possessing significantly different polyphenolic composition, may have almost identical response to these two tests and yield highly correlated values (16). However, the first tests examines the ability of the compounds in question (polyphenols) to exchange electrons in a purely redox reaction, but hydrogen transfer mechanisms cannot be detected. To the contrary, the use of DPPH in the measurement of A_{AR} may also assess the ability of antioxidants to donate hydrogen atoms, depending on the conditions (17).

Apparently, the differences in the antioxidant potency of the extracts could reflect to some extent the differences found in the polyphenolic composition. In particular, the high A_{AR} of the methanolic extract could be justified by the higher flavanol concentration, because flavanols have been proven very powerful antioxidants in several systems (18) and their content has been significantly correlated with A_{AR} in grape seed extracts, but correlation with P_R was not consistent (19). Other studies demonstrated that the various forms of flavanols (monomers, type of dimers) affected in an important manner the scavenging ability of DPPH•, indicating flavanol dimers to be more efficient than monomers (20). Further to that, mixture effects resulting in synergism or antagonism amongst the various polyphenols occurring in the extracts could not be ruled out. Evidence emerged from studies on the A_{AR} of mixtures with pure compounds (21) but also with plant extracts (22) demonstrated the manifestation of antagonistic effects, as a result of regeneration of a compound with higher oxidation potential, at the expense of another with lower oxidation potential, by donating H atoms. Mixture effects, based on the estimation P_R, of pure antioxidants (23) or antioxidants in combination with extracts (24) were in the same line.

Regarding the polyphenolic composition, it could be speculated that substances eluted early are rather simple phenolics, as judged by the UV characteristics given in Table 2. On the other hand, the compound eluted at 17 minutes showed a typical flavonol spectrum and on the basis of the mass spectral data it could be tentatively assigned to quercetin 3-*O*-glucuronide. Likewise, the peaks eluted at 41-41.5 minutes were tentatively identified as flavanol derivatives (25).

Conclusion

The polyphenolic composition of *M. oleifera* roots remains largely unexamined, despite the considerable volume of literature highlighting its important pharmacological properties. The present study represents a first approach to this issue, by screening some widely used solvents of increasing polarity with regard to their potential in extracting polyphenols from lyophilised *M. oleifera* roots. The results indicated that water extracts were the richest in total polyphenols, displaying strong antioxidant activity. The liquid chromatography-mass spectrometry study confirmed that the major in *M. oleifera* roots are quite polar, but minor substances corresponding to flavonoids were also detected.

Authors' contributions

IK: Laboratory experimentation and antioxidant tests; SG: Sample handling, LC-MS analysis, and data handling; SL: Raw material handling and laboratory experimentation; DPM: Paper writing, data handling, data interpretation, and statistics.

Conflict of interests

The authors declared no competing interests.

Ethical considerations

Ethical issues (including plagiarism, misconduct, data fabrication, falsification, double publication or submission, redundancy) have been completely observed by the authors.

Funding/Support

This research was financially supported jointly by the University of the Aegean and the T.E.I. of Thessaly.

References

1. Anwar F, Latif S, Ashraf M, Gilani AH. Moringa oleifera: a food plant with multiple medicinal uses. Phytother Res. 2007;21(1):17-25.
2. Farooq F, Rai M, Tiwari A, Khan AA, Farooq S. Medicinal properties of Moringa oleifera: An overview of promising healer. J Med Plants Res. 2012; 6(27):4368-4374.
3. Kumar PS, Mishra D, Ghosh G, Panda CS. Medicinal uses and pharmacological properties of Moringa oleifera. Int J Phytomed. 2010;2(3):210-216.
4. Goyal BR, Agrawal BB, Goyal RK, Mehta AA. Phytopharmacology of Moringa oleifera Lam.: an overview. Nat Prod Rad. 2007; 6(4):347-353.
5. Karakashov B, Grigorakis S, Loupassaki S, Mourtzinos I, Makris DP. Optimisation of organic solvent-free polyphenol extraction from Hypericum triquetrifolium Turra using Box–Behnken experimental design and kinetics. Int J Ind Chem. 2015;6(2):85-92.
6. Makris DP, Passalidi V, Kallithraka S, Mourtzinos I. Optimisation of polyphenol extraction from red grape pomace using aqueous glycerol/tartaric acid mixtures and response surface methodology. Prep Biochem Biotechnol. 2015. doi: 10.1080/10826068.2015.1015562.
7. Makris DP, Boskou G, Chiou A, Andrikopoulos NK. An investigation on factors affecting recovery of antioxidant phenolics and anthocyanins from red grape (Vitis vinifera L.) pomace employing water/ethanol-based solutions. Am J Food Technol. 2008; 3(3):164-173.
8. Shehata E, Grigorakis S, Loupassaki S, Makris DP. Extraction optimisation using water/glycerol for the efficient recovery of polyphenolic antioxidants from two Artemisia species. Separ Purif Technol. 2015; 149:462-469.
9. Satish A, Reddy PV, Sairam S, Ahmed F, Urooj A. Antioxidative Effect and DNA protecting property of Moringa oleifera root extracts. J Herbs Spices Med Plants. 2014;20(3):209-220.
10. Sultana B, Anwar F, Ashraf M. Antioxidant activity and total phenolic content of Moringa oleifera leaves. Molecules. 2009;14(6):2167-2180.
11. Gupta M, Kanti Mazumder U, Chakrabarti S. CNS activities of methanolic extract of Moringa oleifera root in mice. Fitoterapia. 1999;70(3):244-250.
12. Raj AJ, Gopalakrishnan VK, Yadav SA, Dorairaj S. Antimicrobial activity of Moringa oleifera (Lam.) root extract. J Pharm Res. 2011;4(5):1426-1430.
13. McMurrough I, McDowell J. Chromatographic separation and automated analysis of flavanols. Anal Biochem. 1978;91(1):92-100.
14. Treutter D. Chemical reaction detection of catechins and proanthocyanidins with 4-dimethylaminocinnamaldehyde. J Chrom A. 1989; 467:185-93.
15. Atawodi SE, Atawodi JC, Idakwo GA, et al. Evaluation of the polyphenol content and antioxidant properties of methanol extracts of the leaves, stem, and root barks of Moringa oleifera Lam. J Med Food. 2010; 13(3):710-716.
16. Makris DP, Boskou G, Andrikopoulos NK. Polyphenolic content and in vitro antioxidant characteristics of wine industry and other agri-food solid waste extracts. J Food Compos Anal. 2007;20(2):125-32.
17. Magalhães LM, Segundo MA, Reis S, Lima JL. Methodological aspects about in vitro evaluation of antioxidant properties. Anal Chim Acta. 2008;613(1): 1-19.
18. Hagerman AE, Riedl KM, Jones GA, et al. High molecular weight plant polyphenolics (tannins) as

biological antioxidants. J Agric Food Chem. 1998; 46(5):1887-1892.

19. Karvela E, Makris DP, Kalogeropoulos N, Karathanos VT, Kefalas P. Factorial design optimisation of grape (Vitis vinifera) seed polyphenol extraction. Eur Food Res Technol. 2009;229(5):731-742.
20. Villaño D, Fernández-Pachón M, Moyá M, Troncoso A, García-Parrilla M. Radical scavenging ability of polyphenolic compounds towards DPPH free radical. Talanta. 2007;1(1):230-235.
21. Aoun M, Makris D. Binary mixtures of natural polyphenolic antioxidants with ascorbic acid: impact of interactions on the antiradical activity. Int Food Res J. 2012;19(2):603-606.
22. Karvela E, Makris DP, Karathanos VT. Implementation of response surface methodology to assess the antiradical behaviour in mixtures of ascorbic acid and α-tocopherol with grape (Vitis vinifera) stem extracts. Food Chem. 2012;132(1):351-359.
23. Aoun M, Makris DP. Use of response surface methodology to evaluate the reducing power in binary solutions of ascorbic acid with natural polyphenolic antioxidants. Int J Food Studies. 2013;2(2):238-251.
24. Karvela E, Makris DP. Assessment of the reducing effects in mixtures of grape (Vitis vinifera) seed extracts with α-tocopherol using response surface methodology. J Microbiol Biotechnol Food Sci. 2012;2(2):771-87.
25. Tzima K, Kallithraka S, Kotseridis Y, Makris DP. Kinetic modelling for flavonoid recovery from red grape (Vitis vinifera) pomace with aqueous lactic acid. Processes. 2014;2(4):901-11.

Collection and assessment of traditional medicinal plants used by the indigenous people of Dastena in Iran

Habib-allah Mohammadi[1*], Seyed-Ebrahim Sajjadi[1], Mostafa Noroozi[2], Mahmoud Mirhosseini[3]

[1]Department of Pharmacognosy, School of Pharmacy, Isfahan University of Medical Sciences, Isfahan, Iran
[2]Isfahan Center for Research of Agricultural Science and Natural Resources, Isfahan, Iran
[3]Medical Plants Research Center, Shahrekord University of Medical Sciences, Shahrekord, Iran

ARTICLE INFO

Keywords:
Herbs
Traditional uses
Ethnobotany
Iran

ABSTRACT

Introduction: Nowadays, traditional and herbal medicines have attracted the attention of researchers all around the world and despite the development of synthetic drugs, demand for plant-based medicines is growing. The main reason for this growing trend is increasing public concerns about the adverse effects of synthetic medicines. Traditional medicine and ethnobotany are two important issues that should be noted to achieve effective herbal medicines with considerable therapeutic effects. Traditional medicine is based on experience of people over centuries and ethno-botany is based on recognition of the native plants. Iran has very high plant diversity because of its different climate, ecosystems and soil conditions. Regarding increasing demand for medicinal plants, this study aimed to collect some native plant varieties growing in Dastena and to review some of local and folk application of these plants.
Methods: In the present study, the plant species were collected during two consecutive years (2013-2014) and systematically identified. The traditional and local uses of collected plants were questioned through interviews with local people.
Results: In this study, 90 plant species belonging to 30 families were collected and identified. They had various therapeutic effects. Lamiaceae and Asteraceae families had the highest use among the collected plants.
Conclusion: Results of this study showed that herbal medicines in this area are mostly used to treat digestive and respiratory system disorders. They have economical values and should be studied and explored more detailed.

Implication for health policy/practice/research/medical education:
Dastena medicinal plants are mostly used to treat digestive and respiratory system disorders. They have economical values and should be studied and explored more detailed.

Introduction

Iran has an excellent history of traditional medicine, dating back to the Old Babylonian and Assyrian periods. Throughout the centuries, Iranian traditional medicine has played a prominent role in the health of Iranian people and also entire population of the world (1). The origin of Iranian traditional medicine dates back to the age of Avicenna and his book of Canon. Latin translation of the canon has been taught at European colleges for centuries and played an invaluable contribution to world medicine (2). Traditional medicine is taking inspiration from nature to solve human problems. Ancient Iranian medicine uses temperament diagnosis in order to indicate the health status of people. Physiologically, it attributes the number of human diseases to the person to dystemperament (3). Iranian traditional medicine has a direct link with traditional nutrition. It designed a nutritional scheme for Iranian people based on climate, agricultural resources and experiences gained during the long period (4).

Ethno-botanical study is documentation of non-written traditional information in order to ensure a more rational use of resources and effective protection of biodiversity and cultural information (5). During the first half of the 20th century, ethno-botany was merely descriptive and most of researches in this field have only provided long lists of plants and their uses. However, during the past 50 years, ethno-botany has become less purely descriptive and more analytical. Therefore, researchers are con-

***Corresponding author:** Habib-allah Mohammadi; Department of Pharmacognosy, School of Pharmacy, Isfahan University of Medical Sciences, Isfahan, Iran. Email: Habibmohamadi2000@gmail.com fronted with other theoretical questions. For example, the study of ways in which different cultures classify plant can be useful in cognitive processes such as categorization and classification (2).

Before past two decades, all drugs had natural and mainly plant origin but rapid advances in scientific medicine and technology reduced their use in comparison to the past. Therefore medicinal plants were replaced by synthetic drugs. Today, due to increased concerns about synthetic drugs and their unwanted side effect, researcher's attention has been shifted toward medicinal plant (2).

Adverse side effects associated with consumption of synthetic drug such as "thalidomide incident" in Europe was one of the most important reason for public approach to the medicinal plant (6).

Iran has a wide range of medical experiences because of long historical precedent and diversity of race, ethnicity, language, and climate. The herbal medicines are considered to be of great importance especially, for tribes and residents settled in the impassable part of the Iran. Gaining experiences and transferring them from one generation to the next is the important issue (7). On the other hand, climatic and environmental variability between regions leads to growth of different types of plant species. Iran is one of the few countries in the world that has such a rather large diversity. Regarding large diversity and distribution of medicinal plants in Iran, botanical research and collection of data obtained from other researches can provides a good recognition of this great treasure for us and future generation (8).

Dastena is one of cities of the province of Chahar-Mahal-va-Bakhtiyari in Iran, located 47 kilometers (29 miles) west of the center of the Chahar-Mahal-va-Bakhtiyari. The city's altitude is approximately 2000 meters above sea level. This city supports great diversity because of its mountainous weather and soil type. This study aimed to collect some native plant varieties growing in this city and to review some of local and folk application of these plants. At first, medicinal plants species were collected and identified, then their local names and traditional and local application in medicine were studied (9).

Materials and methods

Plant specimens were collected from plains and mountains from May 2013 to September 2014. In some cases, local people experiences were used to find the right place of plants. We tried to use standard methods in order to collect medicinal plants. Plants with traditional application in medicine were harvested through consulting with local people and experts (10,11). After collection, plant specimens were identified and approved by Mr. Mustafa Noroozi based on morphological and anatomical characters listed in textbook of plant taxonomy (12-18). The herbarium specimens of plant were recorded at the Herbarium of the Faculty of Pharmacy and Pharmaceutical Sciences, Isfahan University of Medical Sciences, Isfahan, Iran. It should be noted that information about local and traditional applications of plants were collected during and after the sampling through an interviews. 37 individuals including 15 farmers, 2 medicinal plants sellers and 20 native who had knowledge about medicinal plants were interviewed. They were asked for local names and traditional applications of plants.

Results

A total of 90 species were collected from Dastena city, which belonged to 30 families. Lamiaceae (20 species), Asteraceae (12 species) and Fabaceae (7 species) were dominant families. The aerial parts of the plants are most commonly used by the indigenous people of Dastena region. In Dastena city, traditional medicines are mostly used to treat digestive and respiratory system disorders, although they are also used to treat variety of diseases. Since Chaharmahal-va-Bakhtiari and Kohghiluyeh-va-Boyer Ahmad are placed in close aproximity and on the other hand two of them are located along the central Zagross mountains, there are some similarities in respect with traditional application of plants. So, according to what is said, we used of one ethnobotanical study in Kohghiluyeh va Boyer Ahmad to complete some cells of result table. Scientific and Persian names (19) of collected plants as well as used parts of plants, native name and their applications are shown in Table 1.

The most parts of the plants that were frequently used by native people include aerial parts (38%), leaf (14.2%), flowers (13.3%), seeds (8.8%) and roots (7%) (Figure 1). Medicinal plants in Dastena are mostly used to treat digestive system disorders (23%), respiratory system infections (13.5%), nervous system disorders (11%) and infections (1%) (Figure 2).

Discussion and Conclusion

This study led to the introduction of 90 plant species used by local people. It should be noted that a few of these applications are now common among local people but most of them were already common. Traditional medicine has become forgotten over time and today's generation pays little attention to it. Therefore there is a need to protect this precious treasure and transfer it to the next generation. In Dastena, Asteraceae and Lamiaceae were the most frequently used families. These families also had the highest frequency of use in Kohgiluyeh and Boyer-Ahmad (20). Medicinal plants have been used by local people of Dastena for various purposes. The parts of plant that were most frequently used by native peoples were aerial parts. Aerial parts especially leaves are photo synthetically active and produce large amounts of secondary metabolites. Moreover access to these parts is much easier than other parts. Previous study also showed that aerial parts of plants are more active than other parts. These can explain same results observed by different researchers in different parts of the world (20-22).

Use of medicinal herbs to overcome digestive system problems are also reported in several studies conducted in different parts of Iran (20-22). They are commonly used to treat digestive system disorders because they are edible

Table 1. Scientific, native and Persian names of collected plants as well as used parts of plants and their applications

Row	Scientific name	Family	Persian name	Local name	Parts used for medicinal purposes	Some local use
1	*Achillea wilhelmsii* C.Koch	Asteraceae	Bumadaran	Golberenjas	Flowering branches	Carminative, anti-nausea
2	*Adonis aestivalis* L.	Ranunculaceae	Cheshm khrus tabestani	Cheshm khrus	Aerial parts	Laxative, treatment of kidney stones
3	*Ajuga chamaecistus* Ging. *Subsp.*	Lamiaceae	Labdisi butei	Samsak	Aerial parts	Antipyretic
4	*Ajuga chamaecistus* Ging. *Subsp.*	Lamiaceae	Labdisi butei	Samsak	Aerial parts	Antipyretic
5	*Alcea koelzi* I. Riedl.	Malvaceae	Khatmiye lorestani	Gol khatmi	Flowers, roots	Soothing a sore throat, laxative
6	*Allium ampeloprasum* L.	Amaryllidaceae	Tare kuhi	Tara koei	Leaves and bulbs	Intestinal and urinary antiseptic, anti-rheumatism, Spice
7	*Allium austroiranicum* R.M.Fritsch.	Amaryllidaceae	Lepu	Lopu	Stem	Cooling tempers, seasoning of dairy products
8	*Allium hirtifolium* Boiss.	Amaryllidaceae	Musir	Musir	Leaves and bulbs	Seasoning of dairy products, reducing blood fat and sugar
9	*Allium schoenoprasum* L.	Amaryllidaceae	Piyaz kuhi	Sirdeng	Leaves and bulbs	Seasoning of food and salad, disinfectants digestive helper,
10	*Allyssum dasycarpum Steph.ex Willd.*	Brassicaceae	Ghodume mive korki	Ghoduma	Seed	Anti-cough
11	*Allyssum inflatum* Nyarady.	Brassicaceae	Ghodume bad karde	Ghoduma	Seed	Anti-cough
12	*Anchusa italica* Retz.	Boraginaceae	Gavzaban	Gol gov zoun	Aerial parts	Sedation, treatment of respiratory tract inflammation, laxative
13	*Anthemis odountostephana* Boiss.	Asteraceae	Babune taj dandani	Babuna	Flower	Anti-hair loss
14	*Artemisia aucheri* Boiss.	Asteraceae	Dermane kuhi	Derma	Flower	Stomach ache reliever
15	*Arum conophalloides* Ky.ex schott.	Araceae	Sheypuri	Kardim	Leaves	Elimination of seasonal allergies, used in a soup
16	*Asperugo procumbens* L.	Boraginaceae	Alaf chasbak	Chasbaki	Aerial parts	Sedation
17	*Astragalus adscendens* Boiss. & Hausskn.	Fabaceae	Gaz khansar	Gina Gazi	Resin	Treatment of diarrhea, treatment of burns
18	*Astragalus gossypinus* Fisch.	Fabaceae	katira	Gina katira	Resin	Laxative, anti-cough and treatment of hoarseness
19	*Avena sativa* L.	Poaceae	Jo do sar	Jo do sar	Seed	Nourishing the body, relieving fatigue
20	*Biebersteinia multifida* DC.	Graniaceae	Adamak	Bahman pich	Bulb	Superficial wounds, stomach disorders (20)
21	*Bromus tectorum* L.	Poaceae	Alaf bam	Alaf bum	Aerial parts	Healing of painful wound
22	*Capsella bursa-pastoris* (L.)Medicus.	Brassicaceae	Kise Keshish	Chalchalak	Leaves	Carminative, stomachache (20)
23	*Cardaria draba* (L.) Desv.	Brassicaceae	Ozmak	Moche	Seed, leaves	Seasoning of food, diuretic
24	*Centaurea depressa* M.B.	Astraceae	Gole gandom	Gole gandom	Flower	Diuretic, treatment of kidney stones
25	*Centaurea persica* Boiss.	Astraceae	Gole gandome farsi	Gole gandom	Flower	Diuretic, treatment of kidney stones
26	*Cerasus brachypetala* Boiss.	Rosaceae	Albaloye kuhestani	Albalo koei	Fruit	Controlling of blood pressure
27	*Cichorium intybus* L.	Astraceae	Kasni	Kashni	Root and flower	Stomach tonic, appetizer
28	*Cnicus benedictus* L.	Astraceae	Kharmoghadas	Kharshotor	Leaves	Treatment of kidney stones and bladder
29	*Crataegus azarolus* L.	Rosaceae	Zalzalake zard	Sista	Aerial parts	Cardiovascular tonic
30	*Descurainia sophia* (L.)Schur.	Brassicaceae	Khakshir irani	Khakiji	Seed	Appetizer, anti-heat stroke, anti-cough
31	*Dracocephalum kotschyi* Boiss.	Lamiaceae	Zarin giyah	Zarovi	Aerial parts	Anti-arthritic and rheumatic
32	*Echinophora platyloba* DC.	Apiaceae	Khosharize	Khoshoruza	Leaves	Seasoning of dairy product
33	*Equisetum arvensis* L.	Equisetaceae	Dom asbe sahraei	Dom asbi	Aerial parts	treatment of kidney stones

Table 1. Continued

34	*Eremostachys laevigata* Bunge.	Lamiaceae	Sonbol biyabaniye rafie	Gandal	Aerial parts	Insect repellent, lowering livestock fever
35	*Eremostachys macrophylla* Montbr & Auch.	Lamiaceae	Sonbole biyabani	Mer giyah	Seed, aerial parts	Wounds healing, creation love and affection between husband and wife
36	*Eryngium billardieri* F. Delaroche.	Apiaceae	Zool	KharZool	Root, stem	Treatment of constipation (20)
37	*Fibigia macrocarpa* Medicus.	Brassicaceae		Pulak	Aerial parts	Treatment of migraine headaches and sinus infections
38	*Ficus carica* L.	Moraceae	Anjir kuhi	Anchichak	Fruit	Laxative, abdominal strengthening
39	*Fritillaria imperialis* L.	Liliaceae	Lale vajegun	Ashke maryam	Bulbs	Treatment of abscess
40	*Glycyrrhiza glabra* L.	Fabaceae	Shirin bayan	Mejoo	Root	Treatment of digestive disorders and stomach ulcers
41	*Grammosciadium scabridum* Boiss.	Apiaceae	Shevid kuhi	Koru	Aerial parts	Sedation, treatment of stomach disorders and
42	*Gundelia tournefortii* L.	Astraceae	Kangar khoraki	Kangar	Flower, stem	Treatment of mouth ulcers and rheumatism, seasoning of dairy
43	*Hypericum scabrum* L.	Hypericaceae	Gole raei dayhami	Davasimi	Aerial parts	Woman infection, analgesic
44	*Leontica leontopetalum* L.	Podophyllaceae	Trob shir	Alaf shakhi	Aerial parts	Treatment of epilepsy
45	*Linum album* K.ex Boiss.	Linaceae	Katan sefid	Chakamdari	Aerial parts	Salves for bone fracture
46	*Lotus corniculatus* L.	Fabaceae	Yonje zard	Yonja	Aerial parts	Laxative, increasing blood
47	*Lycopus europaeus* L.	Lamiaceae	Paye gorg	Pa gorg	Aerial parts	Treatment of nervous disorders and anxiety
48	*Malva sylvestris* L.	Malvaceae	Panirak	Noon bengeshti	Flower	Anti-cough, soothing sore throat
49	*Marrubium astracanicum* Jacq.	Lamiaceae	Ferasione banafsh	Orishom mori	Aerial parts	Relieving stomach pain, joint pain (20)
50	*Marrubium cuneatum* Russell.	Lamiaceae	Ferasion tebi	Orishom mori	Aerial parts	Relieving stomach pain, joint pain (20)
51	*Mentha longifolia* (L.) Hudson.	Lamiaceae	Poone	Pina	Aerial parts	Carminative, treatment of menstrual disorders, flavoring of dairy
52	*Morina persica* L.	Morinacea	Khar aroos	Berenjak	Seed	General tonic
53	*Morus alba* L.	Moraceae	Tute sefid	Tit	Fruit	Laxative, dry instead of sugar for diabetics
54	*Nasturtium officinale* (L.) R. Br.	Brassicaceae	Bolagh oti	Ghegi, Mama cham. cham	Aerial parts	Antiparasitic, warm and wet nature
55	*Ononis spinosa* L.	Fabaceae	Khar khar	Khar khar	Root	Diuretic
56	*Papaver dubium* L.	Papaveraceae	Khashkashe harz	Khashkhashe harz	Flower	Anti-inflammation and abscess
57	*Parietaria judaica* L.	Urticaceae	Gush mush afshan	Marzanjush	Aerial parts	Menstruation disorder (20)
58	*Peganum harmala* L.	Zygophyllaceae	Esfand	Dinisht	Seed	Disinfecting the environment, removing the evil eye
59	*Phlomis olivieri* Benth.	Lamiaceae	Gush bare	Bale gush	Aerial parts	Seasoning of food and dairy
60	*Plantago lanceolata* L.	Plantaginaceae	Barhange sar nayzei	Bartang	Seed	Treatment of sinusitis and bronchitis
61	*Plantago major* L.	Plantaginaceae	Barhang	Bartang	Aerial parts, seed	Anti-inflammation, treatment of sinusitis and bronchitis
62	*Prangos acaulis (DC.) Bornm.*	Apiaceae	Jashire kutule	Feala	Aerial parts	Seasoning of yogurt and buttermilk
63	*Prangos ferulacea* (L.) Lindl.	Apiaceae	Jashir	Kharkul	Aerial parts	Analgesic, antiseptic
64	*Prangos uloptera* DC.	Apiaceae	Jashire sakhrei	Kharkul	Aerial parts	Carminative, invigorating
65	*Quercus brantii* Lindl.	Fagaceae	Balut	Balit	Fruit, bark	Plant skin for strengthening the stomach, plant fruit for treatment of diarrhea
66	*Rhamnus cornifolia* Boiss.&Hohen.	Ramnaceae	Gerduye kuhi	Gerdu koei	Bark	Skin problems
67	*Rheum ribes* L.	Polygonaceae	Rivas	Rivas	Stem	Strong laxative, anti-parasitic, appetizer
68	*Rosa damascena* Mill.	Rosaceae	Gol mohammadi	Gol sor	Flower	Constipation, seasoning of yogurt

Table 1. Continued

69	*Rumex crispus* L.	Polygonaceae	Torshak mavaj	Torshak	Aerial parts	As vegetable broth
70	*Salix alba* L.	Salicaceae	Bid	Bi	Bark, leaves	Jaundice treatment with leaves
71	*Salvia hydrangea* DC.	Lamiaceae	Maryam goliye tamashaei	Gol ovrune	Aerial parts	Treatment of colds, anti-stress
72	*Salvia reuterana* Boiss.	Lamiaceae	Maryam goliye esfahani	Shayna	Aerial parts	Treatment of colds
73	*Salvia virgata* Jacq.	Lamiaceae	Maryam goliye tarkei	Maryam goliye harz	Aerial parts	Sedative, carminative
74	*Sanguisobra minor* Scop.	Rosaceae	Toot rubahi	Gheytarun	Root, leaves	Oral infections and wounds, aiarrhea (20)
75	*Satureja bachtiarica* Bunge.	Lamiaceae	Marze bakhtiyari	Marza koei	Aerial parts	Seasoning of food and salad
76	*Scorzonera mucida* Rech. f. Aell. & Esfand.	Astraceae	Shange nal asbi	Shang	Aerial parts	Useful for sensitive skin, seasoning of dairy products
77	*Scrophularia striata* Boiss.	Scrophulariaceae	Gole maymuniye shiyar dar	Narmouk	Leaves	Joint pains, bone pains (20)
78	*Silene conoidea* L.	Caryophyllaceae	Silene mazrae ruy	Kashkul	Flower	Treatment of infections and sore eyes
79	*Stachys inflata* Benth.	Lamiaceae	Sonboleye arghavani	Gol murashk	Aerial parts	General tonic in weakness, fever reducing
80	*Stachys lavandulifolia* Vahl.	Lamiaceae	Chai kuhi	Ovlile pashmi	Aerial parts	Sedatives, anti-cough
81	*Stachys pilifera* Benth.	Lamiaceae	Sonboleye mu dar	Marze kuhi	Aerial parts	Treatment of colds and constipation (20)
82	*Tanacetum parthenium* (L.) Schultz-Bip.	Asteraceae	Babune gavi	Mokhalesa	Aerial parts	Anti-inflammatory, anti-flatulence, hot nature
83	*Tanacetum polycephalum* Schult-Bip.	Asteraceae	Minaye sakhrezi	Daramey-e pus	Aerial parts	Gastroenteritis (20)
84	*Teucrium polium* L.	Lamiaceae	Maryam nokhodi	Chez	Aerial parts	Hypoglycemic, wound antiseptic
85	*Thymus daenensis* Celak.	Lamiaceae	Avishane denaei	Ovshum	Aerial parts	Treatment of cold and sinusitis, treatment of women infections
86	*Trifolium pratens* L.	Fabaceae	Shabdare chamanzari	Shovare sor	Flower branch	Anti sputum, anti-cough
87	*Trifolium repens* L.	Fabaceae	Shabdare sefid	Shovar	Flower branch	Treatment of dermatitis, itching
88	*Tripleurospermum disciforme* (C.A.Mey.) Schults-Bip.	Astraceae	Babune kazeb	Mamasur suri	Aerial parts	Strengthen of stomach, antiseptic, seasoning of yogurt
89	*Valeriana sisymbryfola* Vahl.	Valerianaceae	Sonbolotibe kuhestani	Sonbolotib	Aerial parts	Sedative
90	*Ziziphora capitata* L.	Lamiaceae	Kakuti sarsan	Pina koei	Aerial parts	Tonic for the digestive system

and pass through the gastrointestinal tract and have most contact with it (20).

Among 90 collected species, In addition to medical and culinary purposes, 11 species have also used to flavor dishes. These species include *Allium ampeloprasum* L, *Allium austroiranicum* R.M. Fritsch, *Allium hirtifolium* Boiss, *Allium schoenoprasum* L, *Arum conophalloides* Ky.ex schott, *Cardaria draba* (L.) Des, *Gundelia tournefortii* L, *Mentha longifolia* (L.) Hudson, *Rosa damascene* Mill, *Scorzonera mucida* Rech.f.Aell. & Esfand, *Tripleurospermum disciforme* (C.A.Mey.) Schults-Bip. 5 species include *Echinophora platyloba* DC, *Phlomis olivieri* Benth, *Prangos acaulis (*DC.) Bornm, *Rumex crispus* L, *Satureja bachtiarica* Bunge were only edible and no therapeutic properties was mentioned for them.

A number of interviewees expressed incredibly weird facts about *Eremostachys macrophylla* Montbr & Auch with native name of Mehrgiyah. Local people said that, in the past, Mehrgiyah was used to create and develop love and affection between husband and wife. Plant powder or seed was poured into food and given to one of them. They said that Mehrgiyah consumer should avoid dairy products. In order to prevent consumer from dairy and fluids consumption, someone was asked to take care of them. Interviewees said that Mehrgiyah consumption make person thirsty and he starts to drink a lot of water and sore liquid and if he drink too much he will die after a month.

A story about its abuse which had been lead to someone death was also mentioned by one interviewee. Another non therapeutic application of this plant was insect repellent use.

Some of native plants in this region are become endan-

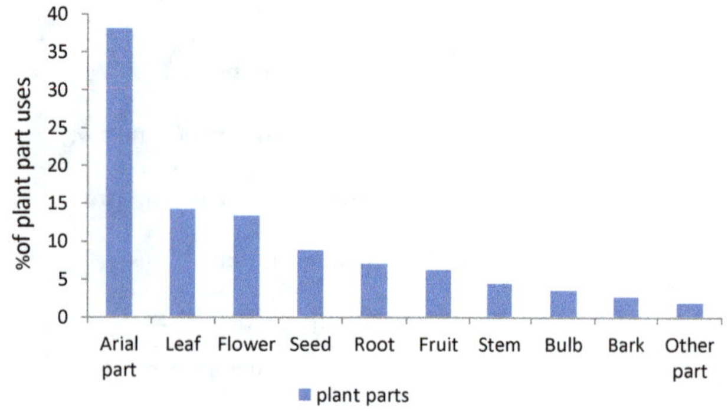

Figure 1. Different parts of plants used by local people of Dastena

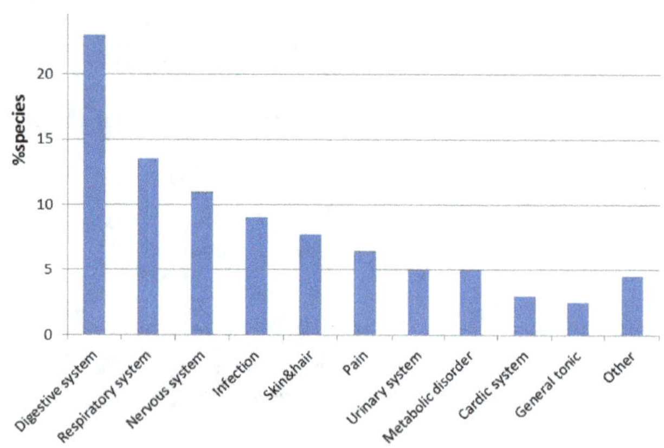

Figure 2. Percentage of species used for various diseases.

gered due to various factors like overgrazing and overharvesting. A few samples of *Crataegus azarolus* L, *Ficus carica* L. and *Quercus brantii* Lindl were reminded today and they are mainly found in private gardens with proper care. *Allium austroiranicum* Fritsch, *Allium hirtifolium* Boiss, *Allium schoenoprasum* L, *Dracocephalum kotschyi* Boiss, *Fritillaria imperialis L, Prangos acaulis Bornm*, and *Tanacetum parthenium* (L.) Schultz-Bip, were also declined considerably and samples are found in specific areas with no access for humans and livestock.

In conclusion, it can be seen that older people interviewed preferred to use herbal therapy and had considerable information but younger people preferred chemical ones and had less information. Dastena plants species have wide range of therapeutic applications in indigenous societies. Thus it is hoped and expected that this study brings valuable recognition and introduction about their therapeutic effects and applications and provides an appropriate management for their protection.

Authors' contributions

HM contributed to the conception and design of the work, drafting and revising the draft, approval of the final version of the manuscript, and agreed for all aspects of the work. SES contributed in the conception and design of the work, revising the draft, approval of the final version of the manuscript. MN contributed in the conception and design of the work. HM contributed in the translation and edition of article.

Conflict of interests

The authors declared no competing interests.

Ethical considerations

Ethical issues (including plagiarism, misconduct, data fabrication, falsification, double publication or submission, redundancy) have been completely observed by the authors.

Funding/Support

This research was financially supported by Isfahan University of Medical Sciences, Isfahan, Iran.

References

1. Amiri M, Joharchi M. Ethnobotanical investigation of traditional medicinal plants commercialized in the markets of Mashhad, Iran. Avicenna J Phytomed. 2013;3(3):254-271.
2. Sewell RD, Rafieian-Kopaei M. The history and ups and downs of herbal medicine usage. J HerbMed Pharmacol. 2014;3(1):1-3.
3. Mojahedi M, Naseri M, Majdzadeh R, et al. Reliability and validity assessment of Mizaj questionnaire: A novel self-report scale in Iranian traditional medicine. Iranian Red Crescent Med J. 2014;16(3):e15924.
4. Moradi H, Minaii B, Nikbakht Nasrabadi A, Siahpoosh M. Avicenna viewpoint about health preservation through healthy nutrition principles. Iranian J Publ Health. 2013;42(2):220-221.
5. Sharififar F, Moharam-Khani M, Moattar F, Babakhanloo P, Khodami M. Ethnobotanical study of medicinal plants of Joopar mountains of Kerman province, Iran. J Kerman Univ Med Sci. 2014;21(1): 37-51.
6. Nasri H, Shirzad H. Toxicity and safety of medicinal plants. J HerbMed Pharmacol. 2013;2(2):21-22.
7. Bahmani M, Zargaran A, Rafieian-Kopaei M, Saki M. Ethnobotanical study of medicinal plants used in the management of diabetes mellitus in the Urmia, northwest Iran. Asian Pac J Trop Med 2014;7(Suppl 1):348-354.
8. Asadbeigi M, Mohammadi T, Rafieian-Kopaei M, Saki K, Bahmani M, Delfan B. Traditional effects of medicinal plants in the treatment of respiratory diseases and disorders: an ethnobotanical study in the Urmia. Asian Pac J Trop Med. 2014;7(Suppl 1): S364-S368.
9. Ahanjide E. Tamadon-e dirine-ye Chaharmahal va Bakhtiari. Tehran, Iran: Amir; 1999:435-453.
10. Mardaninejad SH, Janghorban M, Vazirpour M. Collection and identification of medicinal plants used by the indigenous people of Mobarakeh (Isfahan), southwestern Iran. J Herb Drugs. 2013;4(1):23-32.
11. Jafari A. Iranian mountains and mountainletter. 1st ed. Tehran, Iran: Ecological and Gitalogical Administration; 1989.
12. Ghahreman A. Flora of Iran. Tehran: Research Institute of Forests and Pastures Press; 1975-2002. [In

Persian].
13. Mobin S. Botanical of Iran, Vascular Plant Flora (in Persian). Vol 1-4. Tehran: Tehran University Press; 1975-1979.
14. Assadi M, Maassoumi AA, Khatamsaz M, Mozaffarian V. Flora of Iran. Tehran: Research Institute of Forests and Rangeland Press; 1998-2008.
15. Parsa A. Flora of Iran. Tehran: National Scientific Research Council, Ministry of Science, Culture and Education; 1978-1980.
16. Rechinger KH, ed. Flora Iranica. Akademische Druck–u Verlagsanstalt, Graz; 1963-2009.
17. Davis PH, ed. Flora of Turkey. Edinburgh: Edinburgh University Press; 1965-1985.
18. Townsend CC, Guest E. Flora of Iraq. Baghdad: Minstry of Agriculture and Agrarian Reform; 1966-1985.
19. Mozaffarian V. Dictionary of Iranian Plant Names. 6th ed. Tehran, Iran: Farhang Moaser: 2010.
20. Mosadegh M, Naghibi F, Moazzeni H, Pirani A, Esmaeili S. Ethnobotanical survey of herbal remedies traditionally used in Kohghiluyeh va Boyer Ahmad province of Iran. J Ethnopharmacol. 2012;141:80-95.
21. Ghorbani A. Studies on pharmaceutical ethnobotany in the region of Turkmen Sahra, north of Iran (Part 1): general results. J Ethnopharmacol. 2005;102: 58-68.
22. Miraldi E, Ferri S, Mostaghimi V. Botanical drugs and preparations in the traditional medicine of west Azerbaijan (Iran). J Ethnopharmacol. 2001;75:77-87.

Anti-inflammatory and anti-microbial activities of aqueous leaves extract of *Butea frondosa*

Amit Gupta*, **Sushama R Chaphalkar**

Vidya Pratishthan's School of Biotechnology (Research centre affiliated to Savitribai Phule Pune University), Baramati, District Pune, Maharashtra, India

ARTICLE INFO

Keywords:
Butea frondosa
Anti-inflammatory
Anti-microbial
Hepatitis B vaccine

ABSTRACT

Introduction: *Butea frondosa* has been suggested to be very useful in treating inflammatory diseases but no scientific investigation has been done in such direction. In this study the anti-inflammatory and anti-microbial activities of leaves aqueous extract of *B. frondosa* were determined in infected and non-infected human whole blood against specific vaccine antigen, HBsAg.
Methods: In order to explore the anti-inflammatory and anti-microbial activities of *B. frondosa* (0.5–0 mg/mL; 50 μl), infected (virally) and non infected (control) human whole blood samples were stimulated with hepatitis B vaccine containing surface antigen (HBsAg, 20 μg/mL;10 μl) in order to determined its blood counts and proliferation assay.
Results: Aqueous leaves extract of *B. frondosa* (10 mg/mL; 50 μl) containing HBsAg inhibited the percentage count of monocytes as well as granulocytes population in both cases. In addition, this aqueous extract also reduced its proliferation rate at higher doses.
Conclusion: Aqueous leaves extract of *B. frondosa* possesses both anti-inflammatory and antimicrobial activities and might be used for these purposes.

Implication for health policy/practice/research/medical education:
Butea frondosa has anti-inflammatory and anti-microbial activities and might be used for these purposes.

Introduction

Medicinal plant products can be used as medicines by majority of cultures all around the world (e.g. Indian and Chinese medicines) and provide a source of new drugs to protect human beings against several diseases (1,2). These activities are due to the presence of various primary (carbohydrates, protein, lipids, etc) and secondary (flavonoids, glycosides, terpenoids, saponin, phenolics, etc) metabolites present in medicinal plants (3). According to the World Health Organization (WHO) more than 80% of the world's population still uses or relies on various traditional medicines from plant products against various infectious diseases, as one of their primary health care needs. Meanwhile, the majority of new drugs (70%) introduced in all over the world are derived from natural products, primarily from plants. Studying medicinal plants helps to understand their properties with reference to toxicity and protect humans and animals from natural poisons (1,4). There are approximately 5 lakh plant species occurring worldwide of which only 1% has phytochemically been explored with a great prospective for discovering novel bioactive compounds (1,2).

Butea frondosa (commonly known as palas; family *Fabaceae*), is a medicinal plant growing all over India with various medicinal purposes i.e. flowers (for fever, thirst and diarrhea); decoction of bark (for bleeding piles); paste seeds (for skin diseases, edema and eye diseases) (5,6). In contrast, palasonin (alkaloid) extracted from the seeds show anthelmintic effect especially in roundworm infestations (e.g. *Ascaris lumbricoides*). Recently, new alkaloids, namely butrin and isobutrin have been reported in flowers of *B. frondosa* (7,8). In view of this, a small amount of work has been done with respect to immunopharmacological activities. In this study, we focused on aqueous extracts of *B. frondosa* leaves for determining their anti-inflammatory and anti-microbial activities in infected and non-infected whole human blood against specific vaccine antigen (HBsAg).

***Corresponding author:** Dr. Amit Gupta, Assistant Professor, Department of Immunology and Virology, Vidya Pratishthan's School of Biotechnology, Baramati, Pin code 413133, District Pune, Maharashtra India.
Email: amitgupta@vsbt.res.in

Materials and methods

Collection of fresh leaves of *B. frondosa*

Fresh leaves of *B. frondosa* were collected from the udyan of Vidya Pratishthan's School of Biotechnology during the month of August 2015. They were then dried in a shady area and prepared in finely powdered form.

Phytochemical investigation

Five grams of above powder was macerated with mortar and pestle and then dissolved in phosphate buffered saline (PBS) (pH 7.2; 50 mL). The aqueous extracts were filtered and used to determine the presence of secondary metabolites. The phytochemical investigation of the aqueous extracts was carried out as per standard methods and revealed qualitatively the presence of phenolic compounds, flavonoids (by alkaline reagent test), saponin (by foam test), terpenoids (by acetic anhydride test) and glycosides. In addition, thin layer chromatography of the aqueous extract was performed using n butanol: acetic acid: water (5:3:2). The observed spots were then visualized using anisaldehyde-sulphuric acid reagent.

Human blood samples and estimation of lymphocytes, monocytes and granulocytes count using flow cytometer

Immunopharmacological studies were done using non-infected and infected EDTA anti-coagulant human blood samples (2-3 mL) collected from Mangal Pathology laboratory, Baramati.

To determine the effect of aqueous extracts of *B. frondosa* on whole human blood with various doses (0.5 to 30 mg/mL, 100 μL), pertaining to lymphocytes, monocytes and granulocytes count, were suspended in a stream of fluid using flow cytometry. In this study, EDTA infected and non-infected bloods (50 μL) were divided into two separate sets i.e. each exposed to various doses of aqueous extracts of *B. frondosa*. The samples were then incubated at 37°C for 2 hours. After centrifugation, the supernatant was separated out and washed with PBS. Finally, the pellets were dissolved in PBS and observed through flow cytometry. Data acquisition of 10 000 events representing different phenotypes was analyzed using CellQuest software (9,10).

Lymphocyte proliferation assay

Lymphocytes (10^6 cells/mL) of infected and non-infected samples of whole human blood were plated in 96-well flat = bottom plates (or tissue culture flasks) and incubated in the presence of hepatitis B vaccine (HBsAg, 20 μg/mL; 10 μL) along with serial dilutions of aqueous extracts of *B. frondosa* (0.5-10 mg/mL, 50 μL) at 37°C for 48 hours. After incubation, the 96-well flat-bottom plates were centrifugated (at 3000 rpm for 8 minutes). The supernatant (100 μL) was discarded and then added to an equal volume of fresh medium. The cells were then treated with 20 μL of MTT solution (5 mg/mL) and incubated for 4 hours. Again, the 96-well flat-bottom plates were spinned or centrifuged at 1500 rpm for 4 minutes with discarding the supernatant. 100 μL of DMSO solution was then added to the formazon crystals and the absorbance at 570 nm was measured using ELISA Reader (11,12).

Statistical analysis

One-way analysis of variance (ANOVA) tests (Bonferroni multiple comparison tests) were performed. All values were mentioned as mean ± standard error (SE).

Results

Effect of *B. frondosa* on human blood counts

The effect of aqueous extracts of *B. frondosa* on infected and non-infected whole human blood, pertaining to lymphocytes, monocytes and granulocytes count using HBsAg, was shown in Figure 1. As seen in both cases and at higher doses (10 mg/mL, 100 μL), there was an increase of the monocytes as well as granulocytes count as compared to the control, but at the same time an increase in the number of lymphocytes. From the data obtained, it appears that aqueous extracts of *B. frondosa* have anti-inflammatory as well as anti-microbial activities.

Effect of *B. frondosa* on lymphocyte proliferation assay

The effect of aqueous extracts of *B. frondosa* (0.5 to 10 mg/mL, 50 μL) on proliferation assay using human lysed infected and non-infected whole human blood along with HBsAg was shown in Figure 2. The results show that the aqueous extracts at higher doses (10 mg/mL, 50 μL) caused a decline in the proliferation rate as compared to the control. Overall the data obtained may confirm the inflammatory as well as anti-microbial activities of the aqueous extracts of *B. frondosa*.

Discussion

In recent times, focus on medicinal plant research (e.g. *B. frondosa*) has increased all over the world and a large body of evidence has collected to show immense potential of this medicinal plant used by various traditional systems. This study probably for the first time reveals the aqueous leaves extract of *B. frondosa* for its anti-inflammatory and antimicrobial activities. These activities were evaluated using whole human blood (infected and non-infected) and tested against hepatitis B vaccine containing surface antigen (HBsAg) pertaining to whole human blood counts (lymphocytes, monocytes and granulocytes count) and proliferation assay. The results showed that *B. frondosa* can decrease the count of monocytes as well as granulocytes including proliferation rate (at higher doses and in both cases i.e. infected and non-infected whole blood containing HBsAg). The significant anti-inflammatory and antimicrobial activities shown by the aqueous leaves extract of *B. frondosa* may be linked to flavonoids, terpenoids, glycosides and phenolics found qualitatively in the phytochemical screening. It is well known that flavonoids have inhibitory effects on enzymes and production of chemical mediators and phenolics and terpenoids can interfere with several components of the inflammatory cascade.

The findings of the current study were confirmed through

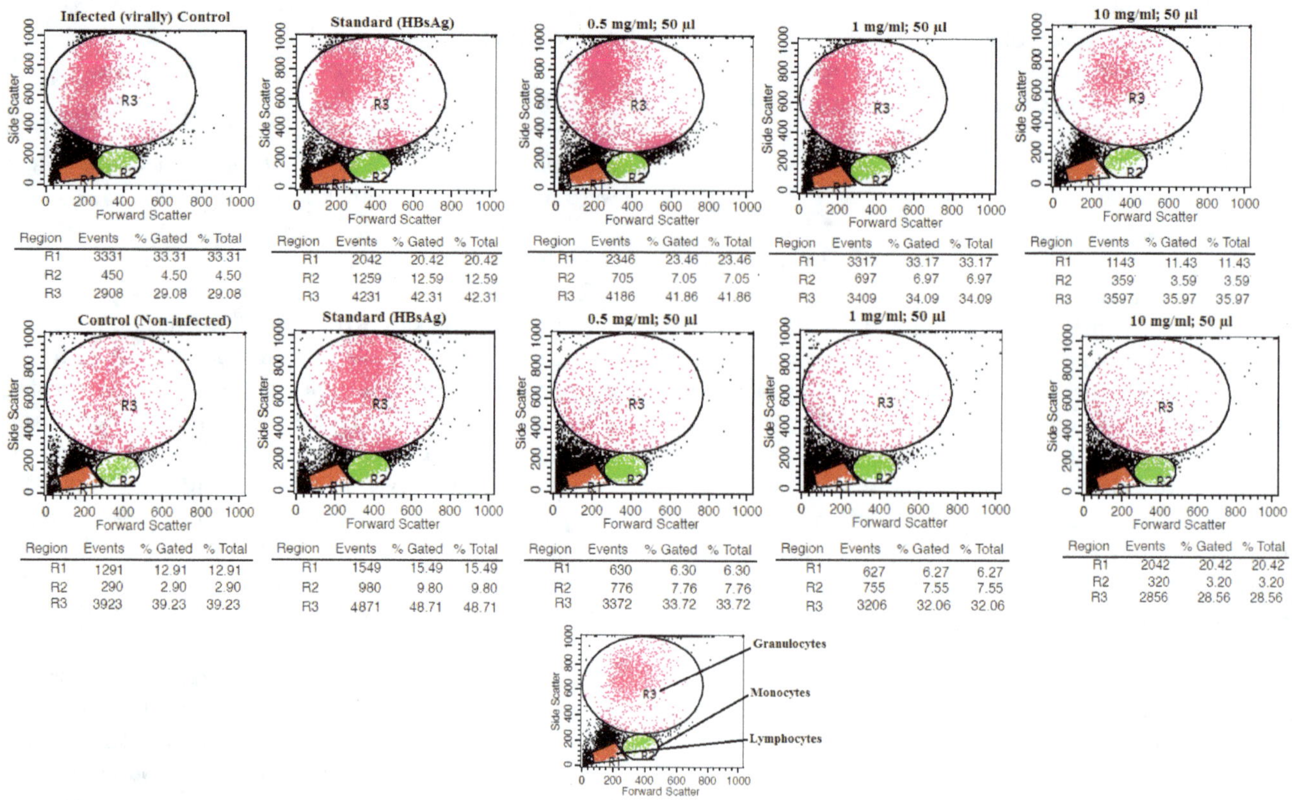

Figure 1. Effect of aqueous leaves extract of *Butea frondosa* on human whole blood (infected and non-infected) using flow cytometry i.e. forward scatter (FSC) and side scatter (SSC). Data acquisition of 10 000 events and fraction or separation of cell populations representing forward and side scatter using Cell quest software. R1, R2 and R3 denote lymphocytes, monocytes and granulocytes count.

flow cytometry and they provide some information related to the immune system. Nowadays the use of flow cytometry has grown qualitatively and quantitatively to determine the total cellular immune response against various antigens (13,14). The flow cytometric results obtained from the present study clearly indicate that aqueous leaves extract of *B. frondosa* have a declining effect in monocytes and granulocytes count (at higher doses and in both cases i.e. infected and non infected blood) stimulated with HBsAg, as compared to the control. The data represents that *B. frondosa* have anti-inflammatory as well as anti-microbial activities.

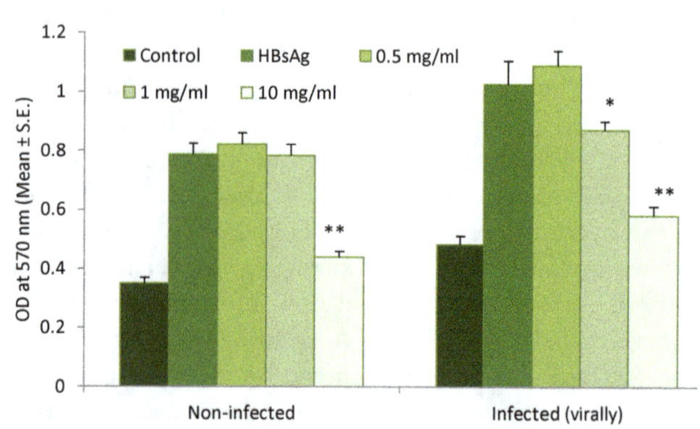

Figure 2. Effect of aqueous leaves extract of *Butea frondosa* on human whole blood using HBsAg. Lysed whole human blood (10^6 cells/mL, 100 µL) were cultured in triplicates in 96-well tissue culture plate along with various doses of aqueous leaves extract (0.5-10 mg/mL; 50 µL) in complete RPMI 1640 medium in presence of HBsAg (20 µg/mL; 10 µL). Proliferation was measured by MTT assay. Values are expressed as mean ± SE. The absorbance at 570 nm was measured using ELISA reader.

To estimate anti-proliferative activity of aqueous leaves extract of *B. frondosa* further immunopharmacological studies were done by lysing whole human blood (infected and non-infected) and lymphocyte proliferation assay using HBsAg. The capacity of aqueous leaves extract is to inhibit T cell immunity with respect to HBsAg (specific antigen). This can be shown by the reduction of lymphocyte proliferation response. The results indicate that the aqueous leaves extract of *B. frondosa* could significantly decrease the activation potential of T cells in lysed whole human blood. Overall, the data suggests that the aqueous leaves extract of *B. frondosa* show anti-inflammatory as well as anti-microbial activities.

Conclusion

This study suggests that the aqueous leaves extract of *B. frondosa* significantly inhibits the production of monocytes as well as granulocytes count including proliferation in both infected and non infected whole human blood. Further investigations of the aqueous leaves extract should be done through in vivo assessment for immunopharmacological studies in mice models with identification of the major active components responsible for anti-microbial and anti-inflammatory activities.

Acknowledgements

We would also like to thank Dr. Gandhi and Mr. Shekhar for providing infected (virally) and non-infected samples from Mangal Pathology laboratory, Baramati, Maharashtra, India.

Authors' contributions

Both the authors designed the study, wrote the protocol and interpreted the data. Both the authors read and approved the final manuscript.

Conflict of interests

Authors declare that they have no competing interests.

Ethical considerations

Ethical issues (including plagiarism, misconduct, data fabrication, falsification, double publication or submission and redundancy) were completely observed by authors.

Funding/Support

We are highly thankful to our organization i.e. Vidya Pratishthan's for conducting these immunological studies.

References

1. Maciel MA, Pinto AC, Veiga VF Jr, Grynberg NF, Echevarria A. Medicinal plants: the need for multidisciplinary scientific studies. Quim Nova. 2002;25(3):429-438.
2. Gupta A, Khamkar PR, Chaphalkar SR. Review on medicinal plants to target and inhibit the epidermal growth factor receptor signaling in cancer and tissue repair therapy. International Journal of Advances in Pharmacy, Biology and Chemistry. 2014;3(1):210-213.
3. Gupta A, Khamkar PR, Chaphalkar SR. Applications and uses of active ingredients from medicinal plants. Indian Journal of Novel Drug Delivery. 2014;6(2): 106-111.
4. Scartezzini P, Speroni E. Review on some plants of Indian traditional medicine with antioxidant activity. J Ethnopharmacol. 2000;71(1-2):23-43.
5. Ramachandran S, Sridhar Y, Sam SK, et al. Aphrodisiac activity of Butea frondosa Koen. ex Roxb. extract in male rats. Phytomedicine. 2004;11(2-3):165-168.
6. Dixit P, Prakash T, Karki R, Kotresha D. Anti-obese activity of Butea monosperma (Lam) bark extract in experimentally induced obese rats. Indian J Exp Biol. 2012;50(7):476-483.
7. Sujith K, Ronald C, Darwin, Roosewelt C. Antidiabetic activity of methanolic extract of Butea frondosa leaves with its possible mechanism of action. Asian Journal of Pharmaceutical and Clinical Research. 2011;4(3): 93-98.
8. Banji D, Banji O, Shanthmurthy M, Singh M. Antidiarrhoeal activity of the alcoholic extract of the leaves of *Butea frondosa* Koen. ex Rox. Indian J Pharm Sci. 2010;72(2):238-240.
9. Gupta A, Shah AP, Chaphalkar SR Immunopharmacological exploration of proteases from Catharanthus roseus on virally infected human whole blood. J Dis Glob Health. 2016;6(1):36-42.
10. Gupta A, Shah AP, Chaphalkar SR. Flow cytometric preliminary evaluation of immunosuppressive and cytotoxic effect of Catharanthus roseus on human whole blood. Journal of International research in Medical and Pharmaceutical Sciences. 2016;8(1):11-16
11. Gupta A, Chaphalkar SR. Immunopharmacological screening of aqueous root extract of Santalum album. J HerbMed Pharmacol. 2016;5(1):7-11.
12. Gupta A, Khajuria A, Singh J, Suri KA. Adjuvant effect of biopolymeric fraction from *Picrorhiza kurroa* to promote both Th1 and Th2 immune responses. Journal of Progressive Research in Biology. 2015;1(1):7-16.
13. Gupta A, Chaphalkar SR. Immunotoxicological studies of leaves aqueous extract of Tobacco plant (Nicotiana tabacum) using flow cytometer. Journal of International Research in Medical and Pharmaceutical Sciences. 2015;5(4):191-198.
14. Gupta A, Chaphalkar SR. Flow cytometric evaluation of anti-proliferative and anti-inflammatory activity of plant viruses: TMV tobacco plant. Journal of International Research in Medical and Pharmaceutical Sciences. 2015;5(4):169-175.

Antioxidative and hepatoprotective effects of hydroalcoholic extract of *Artemisia absinthium* L. in rat

Ali Mohammadian[1], Shirin Moradkhani[2], Sara Ataei[3], Tavakol Heidary Shayesteh[4], Mahsa Sedaghat[3], Nejat Kheiripour[1,5], Akram Ranjbar[4*]

[1]Student Research Center, Hamadan University of Medical Sciences, Hamadan, Iran
[2]Department of Pharmacogenosy, School of Pharmacy, Hamadan University of Medical Sciences, Hamadan, Iran
[3]Department of Clinical Pharmacy, School of Pharmacy, Hamadan University of Medical Sciences, Hamadan, Iran
[4]Department of Toxicology and Pharmacology, School of Pharmacy, Hamadan University of Medical Sciences, Hamadan, Iran
[5]Department of Biochemistry, Hamadan University of Medical Sciences, Hamadan, Iran

ARTICLE INFO

Keywords:
Artemisia
Oxidative toxic stress
ALT
AST
Rat

ABSTRACT

Introduction: *Artemisia absinthium* L. (AA) is a large, diverse genus of the family Asteraceae. AA has long been used as customary herbal medicine in world for the treatment of gastric pain, cardiac stimulation, improvement of memory and for the restoration of declined mental function. The aim of present study was to evaluate the hepatoprotective effects of AA on some factors reflecting the development of oxidative toxic stress in plasma.

Methods: Twenty male rats were equally divided in to 4 groups (5 rats each). Group I acted as control (received normal salin). Treatment groups were II, III and IV which were given *Artemisia* 10, 50 and 100 mg/kg/day respectively only by gavage for 24 hours. After treatment, blood specimens were collected. Liver enzymes such as aspartate aminotransferase (AST) and alanine aminotransferase (ALT) with total antioxidant power (TAP) and total thiol groups (TTG) concentrations were measured.

Results: Levels of ALT, AST and TTG were decreased in the group II compared to the control (group I). ALT and AST in 50 mg/kg group was observed compared with control group. Also, TTG increased in *Artemisia* 50 mg/kg group compared to control group.

Conclusion: Results suggests that alcoholic extract of *Artemisia* can ameliorate liver toxicity in rats through reducing the serum levels of ALT, AST, and oxidative damage.

Implication for health policy/practice/research/medical education:
Artemisia absinthium is able to ameliorate liver toxicity by reducing oxidative damage and might be beneficial in patients using toxic agents.

Introduction

An imbalance between endogenous antioxidant defense system and reactive oxygen species (ROS) level in the body causes oxidative stress, which is associated with overproduction of free radicals from various liver disorders, such as alcoholic liver damage, non-alcoholic fatty liver disease and drug-induced liver injury (1,2). The liver is an important target of the toxicity of drugs and xenobiotics (3). Recently, natural agents with improved effectiveness and safety profiles as a therapy for liver disease have been extensively sought because the administration of drugs sometimes meets with limited therapeutic success and is usually associated with serious complications, especially the long-term use (4,5). ROS derived from many sources influence macromolecules in the liver result in hepatotoxicity (6). In general, ROS can be scavenged by detoxifying systems within the body, such as glutathione, glutathione peroxidase, and catalase (7). However, quantities of ROS that overwhelm the capacity of the body's defence system lead to a disturbance of homoeostasis in ROS production and antioxidant defence. Which in turn eventually damages biological molecules and key cellular components and processes such as lipid peroxidation, enzyme inactivation, and oxidative DNA damage (8). Dietary antioxidant

***Corresponding author:** Akram Ranjbar; Faculty of Pharmacy, Hamadan University of Medical Sciences, Hamadan, Iran. Email: a.ranjbar@umsha.ac.ir supplementation may help to restore this balance eventually inhibition of hepatotoxicity (9,10). Therefore, plant products or alternative medicines that could limit ROS-mediated injuries are essentially needed to protect aid in the protection the liver from against all types of possible damage (11,12). *Artemisia* is a large, diverse genus of the family Asteraceae. *Artemisia absinthium* (AA), which is also known as 'sweet wormwood' and 'Qinghao' has traditionally been used in traditional Chinese medicine for treatment of fever and chills (13). In particular, *Artemisia* and its derivatives have been used clinically in the treatment of drug-resistant malaria while they were reported to have several bioactive functions including antitumor and anti-inflammatory activities (14-16). In addition, coumarins, flavonoids, and other terpenoids constituents present in AA are also reported to have significant pharmacological activities such as antitumor and antibacterial activities that contribute to the therapeutic effects of the herb (17,18). The aim of the present study was to evaluate the hepatoprotective effects of AA on some factors reflecting associated with the development of oxidative toxic stress in plasma.

Materials and methods

Chemicals and reagents

Dithiobis-(2-nitrobenzoic acid) (DTNB) and Tris base, 2,4,6-tripyridyl-s-triazine (TPTZ) from Merck Chemical Co. (Tehran) and alanine aminotransferase (ALT) & aspartate aminotransferase (AST) kit from Parsazemon Co. (Tehran) were used in this study.

Plant material and preparation of extract

Aerial parts of the plant AA were procured from herbs stores. The taxonomic identity of the plant material was authenticated by Herbarium Unit of the Faculty of Pharmacy, Hamadan University of Medical Sciences, Hamadan, Iran with a deposition specimen holder (No: 220). The dried aerial parts of the plant were milled to a fine powder using an electric blender. The methanol extract was prepared by extracting 50 g of the powdered plant material using soxhlet apparatus (20 hours). Thereafter, the resulting methanol extract was reduced in vacuo (40°C), freeze dried and stored at 4°C until further used. The yield was 11.69% (w/w).

Animals and treatments

20 Wistar rats (200 ± 20 g) were purchased from the Animal Center of Pastor Institute, Wuhan University, Wuhan, China. They were housed on 12 hours light–dark cycle at 25 ± 2°C in relative humidity of 30%-60%, and maintained on a standard pellet diet and water ad libitum. The study received clearance from the Institutional Animal Ethical Committee of the Hamadan University of Medical Sciences, Hamadan, Iran.

The experimental animals were divided into 4 equal groups: Group I acted as control (received nothing). Treatment groups were II, III and IV which were respectively given *Artemisia* 10, 50 and 100 mg/kg/day by gavage for 24 hours (Group I (control), while group II was given Artemisia (10 mg/kg/day). Animals of groups III received only Artemisia (50 mg/kg/day). Group IV was given Artemisia (100 mg/kg/day) with gavage for 24 hours. After treatment, blood specimens were collected.

Serum biochemical analysis

Blood specimens were collected from the abdominal aorta. After centrifuging at 3000 g for 15 minutes, the serum was separated and stored in -80°C. The serum levels of AST and alanine transaminase ALT were determined by using autoanalyzer.

Determination of antioxidative biomarkers

Assay of total antioxidant power

Total antioxidant power (TAP) was measured by ferric reducing ability of plasma (FRAP) method. This method is based on the ability of plasma in reducing Fe^{3+} to Fe^{2+} in the presence of TPTZ. The reaction of Fe^{2+} and TPTZ gives a complex with a blue color and maximum absorbance in 593 nm (19).

Assay of total thiol groups

To evaluate the plasma total thiol groups (TTG), DTNB was used as a reagent. DTNB reacts with thiol molecules and creates a yellow complex which has good absorbance at 412 nm in spectrophotometer (20).

Statistical analysis

All experiments were done in triplicate and results were reported as mean ± SEM (n = 5). The data were analyzed by one-way analysis of variance (ANOVA). Statistically significant effects were further analyzed. Means were also compared using Tukey's multiple range tests. Statistical significance was determined at $P < 0.05$.

Results

Table 1 shows the mean ± SE of variables related to either oxidative stress or liver function in the animals tests. A significant increase ($P = 0.041$) in TTG was observed in the group II as compared to control group (group I). ALT of animals-treated with *Artemisia* 50 mg/kg were significantly ($P = 0.046$) lower than that of control group. Levels of ALT in the group II 50 mg/kg *Artemisia* were significantly ($P = 0.046$) lower than those of the control group (group I). Also, 50 mg/kg *Artemisia*, reduced AST, with respect to the control group ($P = 0.035$). No significant differences were observed in the TAP between the groups.

Discussion

This study was aimed to evaluate the hepatoprotective effects of AA on some factors reflecting the development of oxidative toxic stress in plasma. Administration of hydroalcoholic extract of AA would improved the liver

Table 1. Liver function and antioxidative parameters in animal blood test

Groups n = 5	TAP (umol/ml) Mean ± SE	TTG (nmol/ml) Mean ± SE	ALT (U/ml) Mean ± SE	AST (U/ml) Mean ± SE
Control	2.1 ± 0.02	0.12 ± 0.02	24.5 ± 3.8	52.6 ± 13
Artemisia 10 mg/kg	2.4 ± 0.3	0.14 ± 0.02	22.4 ± 2.1	37.1 ± 8.8
Artemisia 50 mg/kg	2.8 ± 0.4	0.77 ± 0.07[a]	16.3 ± 1.6[a]	19.2 ± 2.3[a]
Artemisia 100 mg/kg	2.6 ± 0.7	0.28 ± 0.11	17.9 ± 2.3	31.4 ± 7.8

Abbreviations: AST, aspartate aminotransferase; ALT, alanine aminotransferase; TAP, total antioxidant power; TTG, total thiol groups.
[a] Significantly different from control group at $P < 0.05$.

function and the level of oxidative stress parameters such as TTG in blood. Free radicals are the initiators of a redox reaction cascade, which may lead to changes of the chemical structure of biological macromolecules, such as proteins, lipids and DNA, or trouble of human cell metabolism or even tissue injury (21). In vitro and in vivo studies reported the antioxidant capacity of several species of medicinal plants, acting at cellular level, through cell growth stimulation, membrane potential stabilizing or at molecular level, through ROS scavenging, lipid peroxidation, etc. (22). Also, for the evaluation of liver injury serum concentrations of the most commonly used biochemical markers, ALT and AST were determined. Increased levels of these specific hepatic marker enzymes after chemical or immunological intoxication, compared to control rats, indicated considerable hepato-cellular damage and resulting leakage of cytosolic contents into the systemic circulation (23). AA extract seems to be able to preserve the structural integrity of the hepatocellular membrane, as can be seen with the evident reduction of serum ALT and AST activities of pretreated rats in both experimental models. While previous study showed that 80% aqueous-methanolic extract of *A. absinthium* was effective against CCl4-injury at the concentration of 500 mg/kg (24), our results indicated improving liver function in 50 mg/kg of AA. Previous studies showed the reduction of serum ALT and AST levels (25,26). We elucidated the probable mechanisms of hepato-protection investigating further the effects of AA on the liver antioxidant status. The liver is a principal organ involved in generation of ROS induced by drugs and toxic chemicals (27). In this study, our results suggested that AA could exert its antioxidant or radical scavenging activities thus preventing the formation ROS. AA administration was shown to put off decrease TTG concentration in experimental animals. AA by directly scavenging the free radicals and improving liver function in rats may increases in the glutathion (GSH) content in the rat liver (13). The previous studies showed antioxidant properties of AA, too (15). In addition, to more clarify possible mechanisms of hepato-protective activity of AA, future studies are required investigating the molecular and cellular mechanisms in oxidative toxic stress pathways.

Authors' contributions

All authors contributed to the conception of the work, conducting the study and approval of the final version of the manuscript, and agreed for all aspects of the work.

Conflict of interests

The authors declared no competing interests.

Ethical considerations

Ethical issues (including plagiarism, misconduct, data fabrication, falsification, double publication or submission, redundancy) have been completely observed by the authors.

Funding/Support

This study was supported by a grant from Vice Chancellor of Research of Hamadan University of Medical Sciences (Grant No: 9207162136).

References

1. Videla LA, Rodrigo R, Orellana M, et al. Oxidative stress-related parameters in the liver of non-alcoholic fatty liver disease patients. Clin Sci. 2004;106(3):261-268.
2. Kabiri N, Ahangar-Darabi M, Setorki M, Rafieian-Kopaei M. The effect of silymarin on liver injury induced by thioacetamide in rats. J HerbMed Pharmacol. 2013;2(2):29-33.
3. Zhu R, Wang Y, Zhang L, Guo Q. Oxidative stress and liver disease. Hepatol Res. 2012;42(8):741-749.
4. Salama SM, Abdulla MA, Al-Rashdi AS, Ismail S, Alkiyumi SS, Golbabapour S. Hepatoprotective effect of ethanolic extract of Curcuma longa on thioacetamide induced liver cirrhosis in rats. BMC Complement Altern Med. 2013;13(1):56.
5. Zhang A, Sun H, Wang X. Recent advances in natural products from plants for treatment of liver diseases. Eur J Med Chem. 2013;63:570-577.
6. Abdollahi M, Ranjbar A, Shadnia S, Nikfar S, Rezaiee A. Pesticides and oxidative stress: a review. Med Sci Rev. 2004;10(6):141-147.
7. Birben E, Sahiner UM, Sackesen C, Erzurum S, Kalayci O. Oxidative stress and antioxidant defense. World Allergy Organ J. 2012;5(1):9-19.
8. Allen R, Tresini M. Oxidative stress and gene regulation. Free Radic Biol Med. 2000;28(3):463-499.
9. Naik SR, Thakare VN, Patil SR. Protective effect of curcumin on experimentally induced inflammation, hepatotoxicity and cardiotoxicity in rats: evidence

of its antioxidant property. Exp Toxicol Pathol. 2011;63(5):419-431.

10. Mossa AT, Heikal TM, Mohafrash SM, Refaie AA. Antioxidant potential and hepatoprotective activity of origanum majorana leaves extract against oxidative damage and hepatotoxicity induced by pirimiphos-methyl in male mice. J Appl Sci. 2015;15(1):69.
11. Olaleye MT, Rocha BJ. Acetaminophen-induced liver damage in mice: effects of some medicinal plants on the oxidative defense system. Exp Toxicol Pathol. 2008;59(5):319-327.
12. Girish C, Pradhan S. Hepatoprotective activities of picroliv, curcumin, and ellagic acid compared to silymarin on carbon-tetrachloride-induced liver toxicity in mice. J Pharmacol Pharmacother. 2012;3(2):149.
13. Bora KS, Sharma A. Neuroprotective effect of Artemisia absinthium L. on focal ischemia and reperfusion-induced cerebral injury. J Ethnopharmacol. 2010;129(3):403-409.
14. Msaada K, Salem N, Bachrouch O, et al. Chemical composition and antioxidant and antimicrobial activities of wormwood (Artemisia absinthium L.) essential oils and phenolics. J Chem. 2015;3:45-50.
15. Craciunescu O, Constantin D, Gaspar A, Toma L, Utoiu E, Moldovan L. Evaluation of antioxidant and cytoprotective activities of Arnica montana L. and Artemisia absinthium L. ethanolic extracts. Chem Cent J. 2012;6(1):97.
16. Ahmad F, Khan RA, Rasheed S. Study of analgesic and anti-inflammatory activity from plant extracts of Lactuca scariola and Artemisia absinthium. Journal of Islamic Academy of Sciences. 1992;5(2):111-114.
17. Erel SB, Reznicek G, Şenol SG, Yavaşoğulu NÜK, Konyalioğlu S, Zeybek AU. Antimicrobial and antioxidant properties of Artemisia L. species from western anatolia. Turk J Biol. 2012;36:75-84.
18. Singh R, Verma PK, Singh G. Total phenolic, flavonoids and tannin contents in different extracts of Artemisia absinthium. J Intercult Ethnopharmacol. 2012;1(2):101-4.
19. Benzie IF, Strain J. The ferric reducing ability of plasma (FRAP) as a measure of antioxidant power: the FRAP assay. Anal Biochem. 1996;239(1):70-6.
20. Hu M, Dillard C. Plasma SH and GSH measurement. Methods Enzymol. 1994;233(385):87.
21. Halliwell B. Free radicals and antioxidants: updating a personal view. Nutr Rev. 2012;70(5):257-265.
22. Krishnaiah D, Sarbatly R, Nithyanandam R. A review of the antioxidant potential of medicinal plant species. Food and Bioproducts Processing. 2011;89(3):217-33.
23. Poli G. Pathogenesis of liver fibrosis: role of oxidative stress. Mol Aspects Med. 2000;21(3):49-98.
24. Janbaz KH, Gilani AU. Evaluation of the protective potential of Artemisia maritima extract on acetaminophen and CCl4 induced liver damage. J Ethnopharmacol. 1995;47(1):43-47.
25. Gilani AU, Janbaz KH. Preventive and curative effects of Artemisia absinthium on acetaminophen and CCl4 induced hepatotoxicity. Gen Pharmacol. 1995;26(2):309-15.
26. Amat N, Upur H, Blažeković B. In vivo hepatoprotective activity of the aqueous extract of Artemisia absinthium L. against chemically and immunologically induced liver injuries in mice. J Ethnopharmacol. 2010;131(2):478-484.
27. Marí M, Morales A, Colell A, García-Ruiz C, Fernandez-Checa JC. Oxidative stress in nonalcoholic fatty liver disease. Studies on Hepatic Disorders. Springer; 2015:279-308.

In vivo evaluation of antiplasmodial activity of hydroethanolic stem extract of *Baphia pubescens* in *Plasmodium berghei* infected albino mice

Chibueze Peter Ihekwereme*, Chukwuemeka Amaechi Agbata, Kingsley Obinna Chukwueze, Sandra Chinenye Agu

Department of Pharmacology and Toxicology, Faculty of Pharmaceutical Sciences, Nnamdi Azikiwe University, Awka, Nigeria

ARTICLE INFO

Keywords:
Baphia pubescens
Baphia bancoensis
Parasitemia
Antimalaria
Herbs

ABSTRACT

Introduction: Malaria is a global concern especially with the emergence of multidrug resistant strains of *Plasmodium falciparum*. The need exist for newer and effective antimalarial agents. Hydroethanolic stem extract of *Baphia pubescens* has been used for the treatment of malaria in traditional medical settings. This study explores the antimalarial potential of this extract.
Methods: The lethal dose of hydroethanolic stem extracts of *B. pubescens* was determined. Phytochemical screening of the extract was done using standard methods. Experimental animals received graded doses of the extract once daily for 3 days. In vivo antiplasmodial activity was assessed by the Rane's curative test, using *P. berghei* infected mice.
Results: The extract demonstrated a dose-dependent curative activity at the tested doses (100, 200 and 400 mg/kg). Complete (100%) parasite clearance was achieved (on day 4 post-treatment) at 400 mg/kg dose, which is greater than the standard drug used (artemether-lumefantrine). The extract is considered safe since the lethal dose was higher than 5000 mg/kg.
Conclusion: This study demonstrated that hydroethanolic extracts of *B. pubescens* has promising antimalarial activity. This supports the local use of *B. pubescens* as an anti-malarial agent. Further studies need to be done to identify and characterize the active principles/substances in the extract.

Implication for health policy/practice/research/medical education:
This study demonstrates that the stem part of *Baphia pubescens* possesses antimalarial activity. This plant can be explored as a source of a potential lead antimalarial molecule. Secondly, it can be used for the formulation of a standardised antimalarial herbal formula.

Introduction

There is an urgent need to increase efforts in antimalarial drug discovery in order to develop safe and affordable new drugs to counter further spread of the malaria parasite (1). The emergence of resistant strains necessitates the introduction of potent new drugs or drug combinations against malaria. Preferably, new drugs should have novel modes of action or be chemically different from the drugs in current use (2).

Medicinal plants, a validated source of new medicines, have been used in virtually all cultures at one time or the other (3). It remains a source of safe and effective drugs (3). As a rich source for new drug molecules, several important antimalarial medicines in use today were either obtained or derived from them (4). Quinine and artemisinin are natural products from *Cinchona* bark and *Artemisia annua*, respectively.

Baphia pubescens Hook.f (family Leguminosae) is a plant which has been reviewed (5). The plant, also known as *Baphia bancoensis* Aubrev, has been demonstrated to possess anti-inflammatory property. The leaf extract has been reported to possess antinociceptive (analgesic) activity, too (6).

Though, scientific information on the antiplasmodial activities of *B. pubescens* is scarce, ethnomedicinal use indicates the plant might possess antimalarial property.

***Corresponding author:** Chibueze Peter Ihekwereme BPharm., MPharm., PhD; Department of Pharmacology and Toxicology, Faculty of Pharmaceutical Sciences, Nnamdi Azikiwe University, Awka, Nigeria.
Email: cp.ihekwereme@unizik.edu.ng

Furthermore, a number of antimalarial plants also possess anti-inflammatory property. Popular among them are *Azadiracta indica*, and *Artemisia annua* (7-10). In view of its ethnomedicinal use, its anti-inflammatory property, and the incidence of association of anti-inflammatory and antimalarial properties, we decided to screen the plant for antimalarial property. Consequently, this work investigated the in vivo antiplasmodial potential of the stem extract of *B. pubescens.*

Methods

Plant material

Source

Plant parts (including stems) of *B. pubescens* were collected in December 2014 from Ogidi, Idemili North of Anambra State Nigeria, and were authenticated by Mr. Alfred Ozioko of Bioresource Development and Conservation Programme (BDCP) Nsukka, Enugu State, Nigeria. The voucher specimen was deposited in the Herbarium of the Department of Pharmacognosy and Traditional Medicine, Nnamdi Azikiwe University, Awka, Agulu Campus (Herbarium Number PCG-474/A/021).

Preparation of extracts and fractions

The stems were air-dried at room temperature over a 7-week period, after which they were crushed using a dry mechanical mill. The hydroalcoholic extraction solvent used consisted of water and 95% ethanol in the ratio of 30:70, respectively. A quantity (0.3 kg) of the crushed stem fiber was macerated in 1.5 L of the extraction solvent for 72 hours, then filtered (Whatman® no. 1), and the filtrate evaporated to a paste on a thermostatically controlled water bath at 40°C. The extractive value was determined using a volume (1 mL) of filtrate in an evaporating dish (11).

Acute toxicity study and phytochemical screening

Acute toxicity study was done according to a modified method employed by Diet Riech Lorke (12) using albino mice. This method has two phases. In phase 1, groups (n = 3) of animals received oral doses of either 10, 100 or 1000 mg/kg body weight of the extract. In the second phase, another different set of mice were randomized into 3 groups (n = 3) and each group received either 1600, 2900 or 5000 mg/kg of the extract. All animals were monitored for signs of toxicity and mortality. The oral median lethal dose was calculated using the formula: LD50 = √ minimum toxic dose × maximum tolerated dose. Phytochemical screening tests for the extract were also carried out using standard procedures (11,13).

Animals and parasites

Swiss albino mice (15–21 g, 4–6 weeks old) of either sex used for the study were obtained from the animal house of the College of Medicine, University of Nigeria, Enugu, Nigeria. They were housed under standard environmental conditions of temperature (22–29°C) and 12 hours dark–light cycle, and allowed free access to drinking water and standard pellet diet. *P. berghei* (NK 65) was obtained from National Institute for Pharmaceutical Research and Development (NIPRD), Abuja, Nigeria. The experimental protocols used in this study were approved by the Ethics Committee of the Faculty of Pharmaceutical Sciences, Nnamdi Azikiwe University Awka Nigeria.

Drug

Pure samples of artemether and lumefantrine, which served as the positive control drug, were a gracious gift from Pauco Pharmaceuticals, Awka, Nigeria.

Experimental design

Parasite inoculation

All animals were quarantined for 7 days prior to infection. Blood from mice infected with *P. berghei* was used to infect the animals used for the experiment. Standard inoculums of 1×10^7 *P. berghei* infected erythrocytes in 0.2 mL were prepared by diluting infected blood with 0.9% normal saline. Each mouse was inoculated by intra-peritoneal injection with a blood suspension (0.2 mL) containing 1×10^7 parasitized erythrocytes (14). The parasite was maintained by serial passage of blood from infected to non-infected mice on a weekly basis.

Effect of extract on curative test

The evaluation of the curative potential of the extract in Swiss albino mice was done using the methods described by Ryley and Peters (15). Thirty mice were used for the experiments. Infected animals were divided into 5 groups (n = 5) when the level of parasitemia was observed to be > 4%. The extract was tested at 3 dose levels (100, 200, and 400 mg/kg/b.w./day). Three control groups (n = 5) were used namely, normal (uninfected and untreated), positive (infected and treated with 8 mg/kg of a formulation containing 20 mg artemether and 120 mg lumefantrine), and negative (infected and treated with distilled water). All treatments lasted for 3 consecutive days. Blood samples were collected from the tip of the tails of the animals on day 4 and day 7 post-treatment.

Parasitemia monitoring

Parasitemia was monitored using a previously described method (16). Briefly, blood samples were collected from the tip of the tails of the animals on day 4. Thin, blood films were dried, and fixed (for 15 minutes) using methanol, and subsequently stained with 10% Giemsa for 25 minutes. Stained film was washed off using phosphate buffer, pH 7.2 and allowed to dry. The film was immersed in oil and viewed at x100 magnification. The parasitaemia level was determined by counting the number of parasitized erythrocytes out of 100 erythrocytes in random fields of the microscope (17).

Average percentage parasitemia was calculated using the formula:

$$\%\text{Parasitemia} = \frac{\text{Total number of parasitized erythrocytes}}{\text{Total number of erythrocytes counted}} \times 100$$

Average percentage of chemosuppression was calculated

using the formula:

$$\%Suppression=\frac{\text{Parasitemia in negative control-Parasitemia in test group}}{\text{Parasitemia in negative control}}\times 100$$

Data analysis

The results were presented as the mean ± SEM (standard error of mean) for each group of experiments. The test groups were compared with the negative control group using one-way analysis of variance (ANOVA). All data were analyzed at a 95% confidence interval. P-values less than 0.05 were considered statistically significant.

Results

Acute toxicity and phytochemical screening

All the animals survived at 5000 mg/kg per oral test dose. Physical and behavioral observation of the experimental mice revealed no visible signs of acute toxicity such as hair erection, weakness and reduction in their motor and feeding activities. Though, the result of the phytochemical screening showed the presence of alkaloids, flavonoids, cardiac glycosides, tannins, protein and terpenoid. It failed to detect the presence of steroids. The residue after evaporation was 52 g, which is 17.3% yield.

Effect of extract on curative test

On day 4, the extract suppressed parasitemia by 66.00%, 82.69% and 94.23% at 100, 200 and 400 mg/kg doses, respectively (Table 1). Similarly, on day 7 the extract reduced the parasite load by 90%, 96.15% and 100% at 100, 200 and 400 mg/kg doses, respectively (Table 2).

The result showed that 100 mg/kg afforded 66.00% and 90.00% suppression on day 4 and day 7, respectively. At 400 mg/kg, the values were 94.23% (day 4) and 100% (day 7). The positive control had 89.29% (day 4) and 98.21% (day 7).

Table 1. Antiplasmodial effect of hydroethanolic extract of the stem of *B. pubescens* in *P. berghei*-infected mice on day 4

	Dose (mg/kg bw)	Parasite control	
		% Parasitemia	% Suppression
NC	dH_2O	5.4 ± 0.78	0.00
	100	1.7 ± 0.33[a]	66.00
	200	0.9 ± 0.33[a]	82.69
	400	0.3 ± 0.20[a]	94.23
PC	Artemether/lumefantrine	0.6 ± 0.29[a]	89.29

Abbreviations: NC, negative control; PC, positive control.
[a] Statistically significant ($P < 0.01$).

Table 2. Antiplasmodial effect of hydroethanolic extract of the stem of *B. pubescens* in *P. berghei*-infected mice on day 7

	Dose (mg/kg bw)	Parasite control	
		% Parasitemia	% Suppression
NC	dH_2O	7.6 ± 0.29	0.00
	100	0.5 ± 0.15[a]	90.00
	200	0.2 ± 0.12[a]	96.15
	400	0.0 ± 0.00[a]	100.00
PC	Artemether/lumefantrine	0.1 ± 0.10[a]	98.21

Abbreviations: NC, negative control; PC, positive control.
[a] Statistically significant ($P < 0.01$).

Discussion

The result of our study shows that the hydroethanolic stem extract possesses dose-dependent antiplasmodial activity as evident from the parasite clearance test. The result of the curative test at 400 mg/kg is similar to standard drug, artemether-lumefantrine (8 mg/kg/day).

The pharmacological activities of medicinal plants are believed to arise from its constituent phytochemicals. A number of phytochemical groups may be responsible for the observed activity. Alkaloids are popular for their toxicity against cells of foreign organisms such as bacteria, viruses and protozoans (to which malaria parasites belong). Quinine is a popular antimalarial alkaloid in current clinical use. Saponins are another group associated with antiprotozoal activity (18,19). The mechanism of action by which saponins work might be through their detergent effect on cell membranes (20). Another mechanism of action could be elevation of red blood cell oxidation or by inhibiting protein synthesis in parasite (2). The LD_{50} of the hydroethanolic stem extract suggest the plant is safe for human consumption.

Conclusion

The result of this study shows that the stem extract of *B. pubescens* possesses antimalarial activity. No adverse effect was noticed when the extract was orally administered, alluding that the extract is not acutely toxic when administered to mice through this route. This supports its use in ethnomedicine in the treatment of malaria. Furthermore, it demonstrates its potential as a source of an antimalarial drug molecule. However, the findings are only preliminary, therefore, confirmatory studies, followed by isolation and characterization of the active antimalarial compound(s) responsible for the observed curative activity are recommended.

Authors' contributions

CAA introduced the concept and designed the work. KOC did laboratory experiments and captured data. CAA, KOC and CPI did data analysis. SCA prepared the initial draft. CPI revised the draft and produced the final manuscript.

Conflict of interests

The authors of the manuscript declare that they have no conflict of interest.

Ethical considerations

Ethical issues (including plagiarism, misconduct, data fabrication, falsification, double publication or submission and redundancy) were completely observed by the authors.

Funding/Support

This project was funded from the personal finances of the

authors.

References

1. Fidock DA, Rosenthal PJ, Croft SL, Brun R, Nwaka S. Antimalarial drug discovery: efficacy models for compound screening. Nat Rev Drug Discov. 2004; 3:509-20.
2. Muregi FW, Ishih A, Miyase T, et al. Antimalarial activity of methanolic extracts from plants used in Kenyan ethnomedicine and their interactions with chloroquine (CQ) against a CQ-tolerant rodent parasite, in mice. J Ethnopharmacol. 2007;111:190-5.
3. Ntie-Kang F, Onguéné PA, Lifongo LL, Ndom JC, Sippl W, Mbaze LM. The potential of anti-malarial compounds derived from African medicinal plants, part II: a pharmacological evaluation of non-alkaloids and non-terpenoids. Malar J. 2014;13:81.
4. Basco LK, Mitaku S, Skaltsounis AL, et al. In vitro activities of furoquinoline and acridone alkaloids against Plasmodium falciparum. Antimicrob Agents Chemother. 1994;1169-71.
5. Anowi CF, Onyekaba T, Utoh-Nedosa U, Obi PE. An investigation into the antipyretic activity of n- hexane extract of the leaves of Baphia pubescens Hook. F (family Leguminosae). J Pharmacogn Phytochem. 2014;3:127–131.
6. Anowi CF, Onyekaba TU, Obi PE, Ezea CC. Anti-Inflammatory, phytochemical and toxicological investigations of ethanol extract of the leaves of Baphia pubescens Hook.F (Family Leguminosae). Asian J Biochem Pharm Res Issue. 2014;2:246-54.
7. Patel MB, Kadakia VM, Mishra SH. Simultaneous estimation of andrographolide and wedelolactone in herbal formulations. Indian J Pharm Sci. 2008; 70:689-93.
8. Chukwujekwu JC, Van Staden J, Smith P. Antibacterial, anti-inflammatory and antimalarial activities of some Nigerian medicinal plants. South African J Bot. 2005;71:316-25.
9. Melillo De Magalhes P, Dupont I, et al. Anti-inflammatory effect and modulation of cytochrome P450 activities by Artemisia annua tea infusions in human intestinal Caco-2 cells. Food Chem. 2012;134:864–871.
10. Patel DK, Dhanabal SP. Development of bioanalytical parameters for standardization of Azadiracta indica. Asian Pacific J Reprod. 2013;2:132-5.
11. Trease G, Evans W. A Textbook of Pharmacognosy. 13th ed. London: Bailliere Tinall Ltd; 1989.
12. Lorke D. A new approach to practical acute toxicity testing. Arch Toxicol. 1983;54:275-87.
13. Richardson PM, Harborne JB. Phytochemical Methods: A Guide to Modern Techniques of Plant Analysis. 2nd ed. Brittonia: Springer; 1990. p. 115.
14. Moll K, Ljungström I, Perlmann H, Scherf A, Wahlgren M. Methods in Malaria Research. Manassas: University Boulevard; 2008.
15. Ryley J, Peters W. The antimalarial activity of some quinone esters. Ann Trop Med Parasitol. 1970;84:209-22.
16. Arrey Tarkang P, Okalebo FA, Ayong LS, Agbor GA, Guantai AN. Anti-malarial activity of a polyherbal product (Nefang) during early and established Plasmodium infection in rodent models. Malar J. 2014;13:456.
17. Toma A, Deyno S, Fikru A, Eyado A, Beale A. In vivo antiplasmodial and toxicological effect of crude ethanol extract of Echinops kebericho traditionally used in treatment of malaria in Ethiopia. Malar J. 2015;14:196.
18. Wallace RJ, Arthaud L, Newbold CJ. Influence of Yucca shidigera extract on ruminal ammonia concentrations and ruminal microorganisms. Appl Environ Microbiol. 1994;60:1762-7.
19. Newbold CJ, el Hassan SM, Wang J, Ortega ME, Wallace RJ. Influence of foliage from African multipurpose trees on activity of rumen protozoa and bacteria. Br J Nutr. 1997;78:237-49.
20. Francis G, Kerem Z, Makkar HP, Becker K. The biological action of saponins in animal systems: a review. Br J Nutr. 2002;88:587-605.

Wound healing effects of *Artemisia sieberi* extract on the second degree burn in mice skin

Jahangir Kaboutari Katadj[1*], Mahmoud Rafieian-Kopaei[2], Hossein Nourani[3], Behnaz Karimi[1]

[1]Department of Basic Sciences, Faculty of Veterinary Medicine, Shahrekord University, Shahrekord, Iran
[2]Medical Plants Research Center, Shahrekord University of Medical Sciences, Shahrekord, Iran
[3]Department of Pathobiology, Faculty of Veterinary Medicine, Ferdowsi University of Mashhad, Mshhad, Iran

ARTICLE INFO

Keywords:
Aremisia sieberi
Second degree burn
Healing

ABSTRACT

Introduction: Previous studies have shown anti-ulcerogenic effects of *Artemisia sieberi (A. sieberi)* on gastric lesions and experimental skin wound, so this study was conducted to evaluate healing effects of *A. sieberi* on the experimental second degree burn in mice skin.
Methods: Ninety adult male mice in 3 groups were used. Second degree burn was made in the dorsum and then silver sulfadiazine (SSD) 1% ointment and *A. sieberi* extract were applied in the positive control and treatment groups respectively, while in the negative control no medication was done. Digital photographs were taken daily for determination of healing percentage. For histopathological assessment, 5 mice of each group on the days 1, 3, 7, 14 & 21 post burn, were chosen and after euthanasia, a full thickness skin flap of the burn was taken and after tissue processing, specimens were stained with Hematoxylin-Eosin (H&E) and examined for granulation tissue, inflammation, re-epithelialization and collagen sediment, also hydroxyproline content of burn was measured. Data were presented as mean ± SE and analyzed by using Kruskal-Wallis and Dunn post huc tests ($P \leq 0.05$).
Results: *A. sieberi* enhanced wound healing via significantly decreased inflammation, increased granulation tissue, hydroxyproline content and healing percentage in comparison to negative control in such a manner which was comparable to standard SSD.
Conclusion: It seems that *A. sieberi* can promote burn healing due to anti-inflammatory, antioxidant, anti-microbial and mitogenic properties of the plant.

Implication for health policy/practice/research/medical education
A. sieberi increased granulation tissue, hydroxyproline content and healing percentage parallel to decreased inflammation which leading to promote burn healing due to anti-inflammatory, antioxidant, anti-microbial and mitogenic properties

Introduction

Burn is a tissue injury due to extreme heat, electrical, radiation, corrosive chemical and friction sources. It is one of the major reasons of death and inability and accounts the fourth cause of injuries worldwide (1). Burns are classified most commonly based on the depth of injury into first degree, second degree, third degree and forth degree. In the second degree burn, injury extends to the superficial/deep dermis. Many of the burn injuries are due to disturbance in the normal protective and physiological functions of skin (2). Cave portraits indicated that burn and its management came back to more than 3500 years ago (3). Various folk remedies particularly herbal medications had been indicated in different civilizations, for example Avicenna recommitted medicinal plant for sore dressing (4). Today there are topical treatments for burn wounds e.g. silver sulfadiazine (SSD), silver impregnated dressings, silver nitrate, mafenide acetate, neomycin, polymyxin B, mupirocin. Although SSD 1% ointment is considered as the gold standard for topical burn treatment, nephrotoxicity, leukopenia, risk of antibiotic resistant and delayed wound healing are considered as its adverse effect (5). So, finding new, efficient therapeutic agents with more safety has always been a great concern (6). Medicinal plants lived long before human being and nowadays, they are prominent source of indigenous products for human health, because of suitable efficacy, less toxicity and side effects than chemical drugs (4,7,8). *Artemisia* species are medicinal plants with a long history of different indications

***Corresponding author:** Dr. Jahangir Kaboutari, Discipline of Pharmacology, Department of Basic Sciences, School of Veterinary Medicine, Shahrekord University, POB 115, Postcode 88186/34141, Shahrekord, Iran.
Email: Kaboutari-j@vet.sku.ac.ir

in the traditional and modern medicine as anti-malaria, anti-pyretic, analgesic, anti-oxidant, anti-inflammatory, anti-hepatitis, anti-ulcerogenic, anti-helminthic, anti-amoebic and anti-hemorrhagic (9-13). Anti-ulcerogenic action of some sesquiterpene lactones of *A. annua* and ethanolic extract of its aerial parts had been shown (14,15). Histopathological and biochemical analysis of *A. Anuua* extract showed that it can hasten healing of experimental dermal injuries (16). Later accelerating effects of ethanolic extract of *A. aucheri* on wound healing and reducing the healing period was reported (17). Also the ability of *A. sieberi* extract to increase thickness of skin layers and collagen fibers have been reported (8). So due to anti-microbial, anti-inflammatory, anti-oxidant and anti-ulcerogenic activity of *Artemisia* species and its suitable effects on the histopathological, histomorphometric and biochemical parameters of the skin and wound healing, this study was conducted to evaluate the effects of *A. sieberi* extract on the healing of second degree burn.

Materials and methods

Plant extraction

Aerial parts of *A. sieberi* were collected from Yazd province in the center of Iran, dried at room temperature, grounded and sieved and then Artemisinin extraction was done by using petroleum ether (8,11).

Animals

Ninety adult male mice (20-25 g) in three experiments were used. Animals were housed under standard laboratory conditions in accordance with the European community guidelines for laboratory animals (12 hours light/dark cycle, ambient temperature of 22±1°C, 60% humidity) and under supervision of the Ethical Committee of the University, while chow pellet and water were freely available. After 1 week of acclimatization, they were divided accidentally into three groups (n=30). Mice were anesthetized with an intra-peritoneal (i.p) injection of 40 mg/kg sodium thiopental (UVB Pharma, Czech Republic). The skin of dorsum was shaved and thoroughly depilated and thereinafter washed with povidone iodine. Burn was made by contact of a round 1 cm diameter metal plate (105°C, 5 seconds, without pressure) and then for prevention of shock, 1 ml of normal saline was injected i.p and each animal was kept in a separate cage. Group one was treated with SSD 1% ointment (King Pharmaceuticals, USA), group two was treated with *A. sieberi* extract but group three was selected as negative control and received no medication. Treatments were done every 12 hours for 21 days.

Histopathological evaluation

The burns were monitored for sign of infection and digital photographs were taken daily and after analysis by using ImageJ software, they were used for measurement of wound area and calculating healing percentage (18): [(area of the first day- area of the second day)/ (area of the first day)]×100.

For histopathological study, 5 mice of each group on the days 1, 3, 7, 14 and 21 post-treatments were chosen randomly and after euthanasia, a full thickness skin flap of the burn was taken and fixed. Tissue processing was done (Autotechnicon tissue processor Citadel 1000, Thermo Shandon, UK), specimens were stained with H&E and examined for tissue granulation, inflammation, re-epithelialization and collagen sediment (19,20). Hydroxyproline content of burn as the index of tissue collagen was measured (21).

Statistical analysis

Data were presented as mean±SD and analyzed by using SPSS version 16.0 (Chicago, IL, USA). Kruskal-Wallis and Dunn post hoc tests were used for data analysis ($P \leq 0.05$).

Results

Healing percentage

Healing percentage of *A. sieberi* and SSD was significantly higher than control on days 7&14 ($P \leq 0.05$), while on day 7, the difference between *A. sieberi* and SSD was not significant ($P > 0.05$; Figure 1).

Inflammation

From day 1 to 21 inflammation score was decreasing, but only on days 3 & 7 in the *A. sieberi* and SSD groups it was significantly lower than control ($P \leq 0.05$), while on the rest of days such a significant difference was not seen ($P > 0.05$; Figure 2).

Granulation tissue

On day 3 granulation tissue of *A. sieberi* and SSD was significantly higher than control ($P \leq 0.05$), while there was no significant difference neither between *A. sieberi* and SSD on day 3, and nor between *A. sieberi* and SSD with control on other days ($P > 0.05$; Figure 3).

Hydroxyproline

Hydroxyproline content of burn as the index of collagen synthesis was measured on day 14. It was significantly

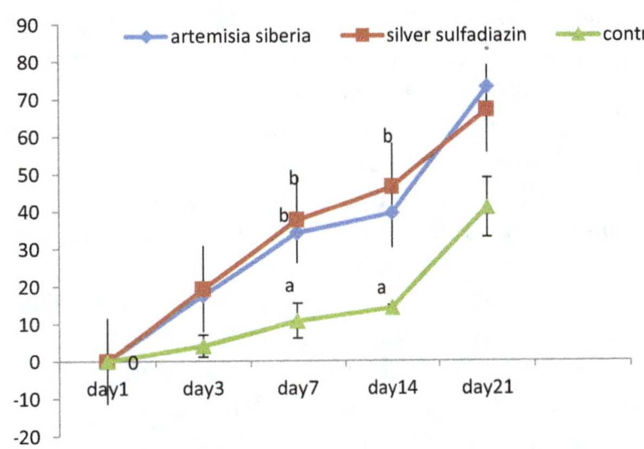

Figure 1. Healing percentage of burn in the silver sulfadiazine (SSD), *Artemisia sieberi* and control groups on sampling days. Different letters indicate significant difference ($P > 0.05$; Dunn test).

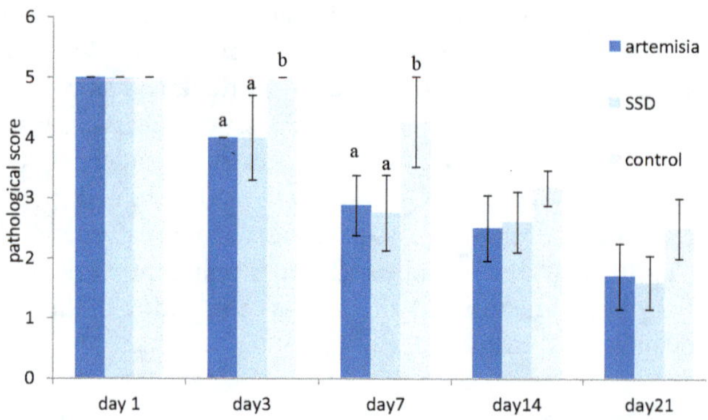

Figure 2. Pathological score of the inflammation of burn in the silver sulfadiazine (SSD), *Artemisia sieberi* and control groups on sampling days. Different letters indicate significant difference ($P > 0.05$; Dunn test).

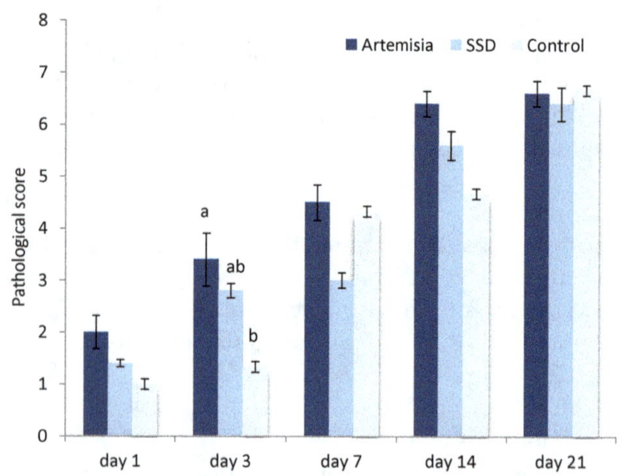

Figure 3. Pathologic score of granulation tissue of burn in the silver sulfadiazine (SSD), *Artemisia sieberi* and control groups on sampling days. Different letters indicate significant difference ($P > 0.05$; Dunn test).

higher in SSD and *A. sieberi* groups than control ($P \leq 0.05$), but the difference between SSD and *A. sieberi*, was not significant ($P > 0.05$; Figure 4).

Histopathological results

Histopathological evaluation of the burn is illustrated in Figure 5. On the day 3,in the *A. sieberi* group, tissue necrosis was seen on the surface of the burn, inflammation was evident and many inflammatory cells especially neutrophils were presented, and despite that regeneration of the epithelium has been stared but it was not complete and number of blood vessels was few (Figure 5A). On the day 7, healing proceed in the *A. sieberi* group, so that epithelial tissue has been regenerated but surface keratinization has not been done and also collagen fibers have been formed (Figure 5B). In the day 21 in the both SSD and *A. sieberi* groups healing has been completed, epithelial and connective tissues were completely regenerated and their structures were seen normally, so that in the SSD group hair follicles were clearly visible. Collagen fibers in the dense bundles and horizontal orientation were seen, numbers of fibrocytes increased

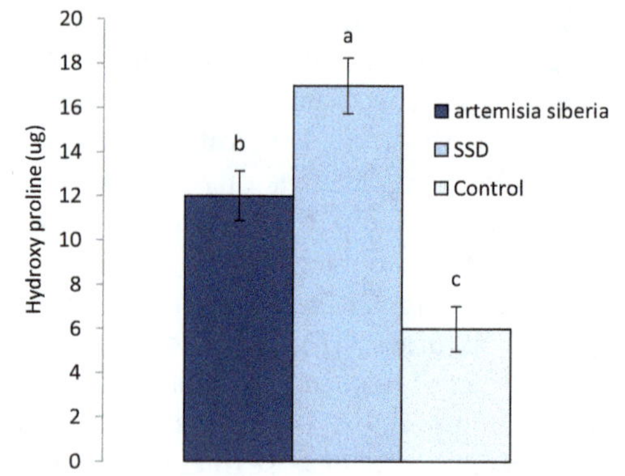

Figure 4. Comparison of hydroxyproline content of burn in the silver sulfadiazine (SSD), *Artemisia sieberi* and control groups on day 14. Different letters indicate significant difference ($P > 0.05$; Dunn test).

and were more than fibroblasts and new vascularization has been decreased (Figure 5C and 5D).

Discussion

Wound healing in the least possible time and decreasing functional and emotional consequences of the burn injuries is the ultimate purpose of burn treatment (5). Form past times abundant plants and derivative products have been used in traditional and modern medicine for wound healing (4,8,22). Burn healing is a complex, time consuming process, which inflammation is the first stage of this process, but overtime it may offend wound area and surrounding tissue and thus hinder healing, so, modulation of inflammation can promote wound healing (6,23). In this study *Artemisia* extract significantly decreased inflammation score on the days 3 & 7. Previously it was shown that almost *Artemisia* genus possess immunosuppressive and anti-inflammatory potential (8,12,14,16). Sesquiterpene lactones including Artemisinin, dehydroleucodine, and flavones e.g. apigenin, crisilineol and 6-methoxytricin are active ingredients of *Artemisia* which seems to exert anti-inflammatory and immunosuppressive activity via interaction with nuclear factor κB (NF-κB) and inhibiting liberation of inflammatory mediators (8,12,14,16,24). Scoparone is another constituent of the plant that inhibits iNOS and COX-2 enzymes which decline release of inflammatory mediators (8,12,16). Additionally plant extract contains phenolic components such as tannin, xanthines, cumarine and flavonoids and micronutrients e.g. copper, zinc & manganese which are potent anti-oxidant and anti-free radicals (8,16). *Artemisia* extract increases superoxide dismutase, catalase and glutathione S-transferase which potentiate the antioxidant capacity against free radicals (8,12,16). Modulation of inflammation and application of antioxidants in the initial days of healing and in the proliferative stage accelerate healing process, so it seems that *Artemisia* plant via impeding lipid peroxidation, lessening the inflammation and collecting and counteracting free radicals help and enhance healing. Burn infection is one of the major complications of the burn which hinders healing and is the principle reason

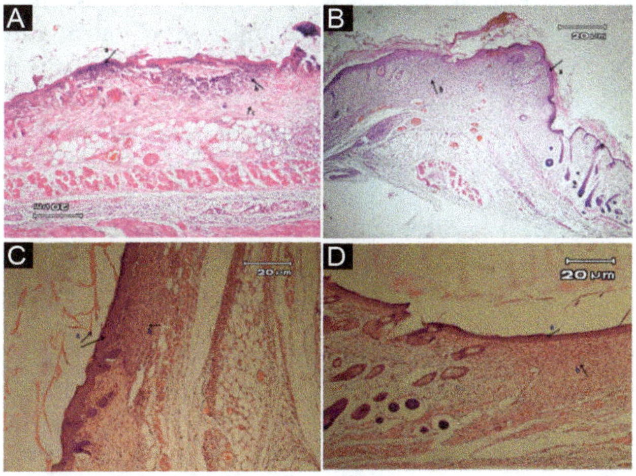

Figure 5. A) Light microscope structure of the burn in the *A. sieberi* group, day 3. Necrotic tissue on the surface and starting of epithelialization (a), tissue inflammation with plenty of neutrophil cells (b), little number of blood vessels (c). **B)** Light microscope structure of the burn in the *A. sieberi* group, day 7. Regeneration of epithelium, without keratinization (a), collagen fiber formation (b). **C)** Light microscope structure of the burn in the *A. sieberi* group day 21. Complete regeneration of epithelium and keratinization (a), suitable arrangement of collagen fibers (b). **D)** Light microscope structure of the burn in the SSD group, day 21. Complete regeneration of epithelium and keratinization, skin structures and hair follicles are seen (a), complete connective tissue and dense collagen fibers on the horizontal surface of the epithelium, vascularization decreased, fibrocytes are more than fibroblasts (b). H&E staining, magnification ×20.

of death in severe burns, therefore decreasing the hazard of burn infection can improve healing (4,6,18). Prior studies have shown that *Artemisia* possesses antibacterial property against bacteria including *Staphylococcus aureus, Streptococcus, Bacillus subtilis, Pseudomonas aeruginosa, Escherichia coli* and dermatophytic infections, which are the most important infectious agents of the burn. These anti-bacterial effects is attributed to the constituents such as verbenol, camphor, cineole, linalool, borneol, cymene, sabinene, α & β thujone and 1,8- cineole in the *Artemisia* plant that may be another mechanism responsible for promotion of wound healing (8,13,25-29). This study indicated that *Artemisia* during days 7&14 significantly improved healing, so that in the day 14 it was significantly better that SSD. Some sesquiterpene lactones of *Artemisia* exhibit antiulcerogenic effects by augmentation of gastric glycoprotein, mucus and prostaglandin synthesis against gastric ulcers (14,15). Later, increasing number of fibroblast, capillary buds, epithelial gap and improving the tensile stability of the wound following application of *A. sieberi* extract was reported (16). Also *A. sieberi* extract significantly increased epidermis, dermis and hypodermis thickness and percentage of collagen fiber in normal skin (8). Intensification of collagen formation and epithelialization can promote healing. During remodeling stage of wound healing, collagen fibers play a vital role to supply strength of the extracellular matrix and support wound and eventually intensifying tensile of the skin (16,18,23). The effects of *Artemisia* on the increment of the hydroxyproline content of burn can be due to the mitogenic characteristic of the plant leading to more collagen synthesis and durability of the healing tissue, improvement of re-epithelialization and establishment of granulation tissue which finally leads to enhancement of healing (8,16).

Conclusion

Artemisia extract promotes burn healing which can be due to antioxidant, anti-inflammatory, anti-microbial and mitogenic properties of the plant leading to modulation of inflammation, prevention of oxidative stress and free radical collecting, prevention of wound infection, amplification of collagen synthesis, re-epithelialization and granulation tissue.

Authors' contributions

JK: research design & manuscript preparation; JK and BK: performing animal experiments; BK, HN and MR: histopathological examinations & statistical analysis

Conflict of interests

The authors of the manuscript declare that they have no conflict of interest.

Ethical considerations

The authors have been entirely regarded ethical issues such as plagiarisms, data assembly, fraud, double publication or submission. All animal experiments had been approved by the ethical committee of the University and carried out according to the International Guide for the Care and Use of Laboratory Animals.

Funding/Support

The authors appreciate Deputy of Research, Shahrekord University, Shahrekord, Iran unselfishly for financial support of the project.

References

1. Peck MD. Epidemiology of burns through the world, part 1: distribution and risk factors. Burns. 2011; 37(3):1087-100.
2. Tintinalli E. Tintinallis Emergency Medicine: A Comprehensive Study Guide. 7th ed. New York: McGraw Hill; 2010.
3. Herndon D. A brief history of acute burn care management. In: Herndon D, ed. Total Burn Care. 1st ed. Edinburgh: Saunders; 2012:1.
4. Akhoondinasab MR, Akhoondinsasab M, Saberi M. Comparison of healing effects of Aleo Vera extract and silver sulfadiazine in burn injuries in experimental rat model. WJPS. 2014;3(1):29-34.
5. Atyiyeh BS, Costalgiola M, Hayek SN, Dibo SA. Effects of silver on burn wound infection control and healing. Burns. 2007;33:139-48.
6. Shakespeare P. Burn wound healing and skin substitutes. Burns. 2001;27:517-22.
7. Kimura Y, Sumiyoshi M, Kawahira K, Sakanaka

M. Effects of ginseng saponins isolated from Red Ginseng roots on burn wound healing in mice. Br J Pharmacol. 2006;148:860-870.

8. Kaboutari J, Haydarnejad MS, Fatahian Dehkordi R, Raeisi Vanani S. Histomorphometric study on the effects of Artemisia sieberi extract in mice skin. J Herb Med Pharmacol. 2015;4(1):20-24.
9. Woodrow CJ, Haynes RK, Krishna S. Artemisinins. Postgrad Med J. 2005;81:71-78.
10. Klayman DL. Qinghaosu (artemisinin): an antimalarial drug from China. Science. 1985;228:1049-1055.
11. Kaboutari J, Arab HA, Ebrahimi K, Rahbari S. Prophylactic and therapeutic effects of a novel granulated formulation of Artemisia extract on broiler coccidiosis. Trop Anim Health Prod. 2014;46:43-48.
12. Yin Y, Gong FY, Wu XX, Sun Y, Li YH, Chen T, et al. Anti-inflammatory and immunosuppressive effects of flavones isolated from Artemisia vestita. J Ethnopharma. 2008;120:1-6.
13. Ul-Haq I, Mannan A, Ahmed I, Hussain I, Jamil M, Mirza B. Antibacterial activity and brine shrimp toxicity of Artemisia dubia extract. Pak J Bot. 2012; 44(4):1487-1490.
14. Foglio MA, Cirrea Dias P, Antonio MA, Possenti A, Rodrigues RA, et al. Anti-ulcerogenicactivity of some sesquiterpene lactones isolated from Artemisia annua. Planta Med. 2002;68(6):515-518.
15. Dias PC, Foglio MA, Possenti A, Nogueira DC, de Carvalho JE. Aniulcerogenic activity of crude ethanol extract and some fractions obtained from aerial parts of Artemisia annua L. Phytotherapy Res. 2001;15:670-675.
16. Derakhshanfar A, Oloumi MM, Kabootari J, Arab H. Histopathological and biomechanical study on the effect of Artemisia sieberi extract on experimental skin wound healing in rat. Iran J Vet Surg. 2006;1(1):36-42.
17. Âllahtavakoli M, ÂrabBanissad F, Mahmoudi M, Jafari Naveh HR, Tavakolian V, Kamli M, et al. Effect of hydro-alcoholic extract of Artemisia aucheri on healing of skin wound in rat. J Mazandaran Uni Med Sci 2010;20:70-76.
18. Khorasani G, Hosseinimehr SJ, Azadbakht M, Zamani A, Mahdavi MR. Aleo vera versus silver sulfadiazine creams for second degree burns: a randomized controlled study. Surg Today. 2009;9:587-591.
19. Gal P, Kilik R, Mokry M, Vidinsky B, Vasilenko T, Mozes S, et al. Simple method of open skin wound healing model in corticosteroid-treated and diabetic rats: standardization of semi-quantitative and quantitative histological assessments. Vet Med. 2008;53(12):652-659.
20. Simonetti O, Cirioni O, Lucarini G, Orlando F, Ghiselli R, Silvestri C, et al. Tigecycline accelerates staphylococcal-infected burn wound healing through matrix metalloproteinase-9 modulation. Antimicrob Chemother. 2012;67:191-201.
21. Woessner JF. The determination of hydroxyproline in tissue and protein samples containing small proportions of this amino acid. Arch Biochem Biophys. 1961;93:440-447.
22. Jiaprakash B, Chandramohan D, Narasimba R. Burn wound healing activity of Euphorbia hirta. Ancient Sci life. 2006;25(3-4):16-18.
23. Artlett CM. Inflammosomes in wound healing and fibrosis. J Pathol. 2013;229:157-167.
24. Guardia T, Juarez A, Guerreiro E, Guzman J, Pelzer L. Anti-inflammatory activity and effect on gastric acid secretion of dehydroleucodine isolated from Artemisia douglasiana. J Ethnopharmacol. 2003;88(2):195-198.
25. Ramezani M, Fazli-Bazzaz BS, Saghif-Khadem F. Antimicrobial activity of four Artemisia species of Iran. Fitoterapia. 2004;75:201-203.
26. Setzer WN, Vogler B, Schmidt JM, Leahy JG, Rives R. Antimicrobial activity of Artemisia douglasiana leaf essential oil. Fitoterapia. 2004;75(2):192-200.
27. Farzaneh M, Ghorbani-Ghouzhdi H, Ghorbani M, Hadian J. Composition and antifungal activity of essential oil of Artemisia sieberi on soil-borne phytopathogens. Pak J Biol Sci. 2006;9(10):1979-1982.
28. Jan G, Khan MA, Jan F. Medicinal value of the Asteraceae of DirKohistan Valley, NWFP, Pakistan. Ethno Leaflets. 2009;13:1205-1215.
29. Vahdani M, Faridi P, Zarshenas MM, Javadpour S, Abolhassanzadeh Z, Moradi N, et al. Major compounds and antimicrobial activity of essential oils from five Iranian endemic medicinal plants. Pharmacognosy J. 2011;3(22):48-53.

Analysis of fatty acid composition of two selected *Phlomis* species

Samaneh Zafari-Shayan[1,2], **Shirin Moradkhani**[1,2*], **Dara Dastan**[1,2]

[1]Medicinal Plants and Natural Products Research Center, Hamadan University of Medical sciences, Hamadan, Iran
[2]Department of Pharmacognosy and Pharmaceutical Biotechnology, School of Pharmacy, Hamadan University of Medical sciences, Hamadan, Iran

ARTICLE INFO

Keywords:
Phlomis bruguieri
Phlomis olivieri
fatty acid
GC-MS
Derivatization

ABSTRACT

Introduction: *Phlomis bruguieri* and *Phlomis olivieri* are two species of genus *Phlomis*, growing in Iran. Different species of this genus have shown various biological activities and also contain a wide range of compounds. It has been proved that both species increase sunflower oil stability and inhibit its oxidation. The aim of this study was to analyze fatty acid composition of these two species, of which *P. olivieri* is endemic in Iran and yet there is no report on their fatty acid composition.
Methods: Aerial parts of two plants were collected, hexane extracts were prepared through soxhlet extraction and concentrated by recovering the solvent, derivatization was performed and then gas chromatography-mass spectrometry (GC-MS) was done for detecting fatty acids.
Results: Both plants contained saturated and unsaturated fatty acids. In hexane extract of *P. bruguieri* 10 fatty acids were identified and 9-octadecenoic acid, 6-octadecynoic acid and hexadecanoic acid were found in high concentrations. *P. olivieri* also contained 8 fatty acids of which 9-octadecanoic acid, 12,15-otadecadiynoic acid and 7-hexadecenoic acid were detected in high concentrations.
Conclusion: Two investigated plants are common in 3 fatty acids and in both of them octadecenoic acid is found in the highest amount. Unsaturated fatty acids have higher amount than the saturated fatty acids in both plants. This study opens new frontiers and applications of *P. bruguieri* and *P. olivieri* due to various bioactive components, especially for pharmaceutical applications.

Implication for health policy/practice/research/medical education:
Unsaturated fatty acids have been used in prevention of heart disease, inflammation and in enhancing immunity. Some fatty acids have been recognized in *Phlomis* species including linoleic acid, octadecadienoic acid, elaidic acid, Oleic acid, lauric acid, hexadecanoic acid, pentadecanoic acid and stearic acid. This study opens new frontiers and applications of *P. bruguieri* and *P. olivieri* due to various bioactive components for pharmaceutical applications.

Introduction

Phlomis, a large genus of family *Lamiaceae*, consists of more than 100 species, distributed in Euro-Asia and North Africa (1). A survey in 2010 estimated that 31 species of *Phlomis* exist in Iran and they are mainly distributed in provinces such as Azerbaijan, Fars, Gilan, Hamadan, Isfahan, Kurdistan and Mazandaran, 10 of the species seem to be endemic of Iran (2,3).
Some *Phlomis* species are used in Iranian traditional medicine as stimulant, tonic, carminative, analgesic, anti-hemorrhoid, anti-inflammation and anti-diarrhea. Other folk applications are treatment of wounds, respiratory tract disorders and appetizer (4-6).
Besides conventional usages, *Phlomis* species have been shown to possess antidiabetic (1,7), antiulcerogenic (8), antimicrobial (9), anti-inflammatory, antinociceptive (10), antimutagenic (11) and free radical scavenging properties (12).
Plants belonging to the genus *Phlomis* have been shown to contain different classes of glycosides comprising diterpenoids, iridoids, phenylpropanoids, phenylethanoids and flavonoids (4).
So far connection between reported properties and some compounds have been identified. For example many of the phenylpropanoids showed significant biological activities such as cytotoxic, cytostatic, anti-inflammatory, immunosuppressant and antimicrobial properties (4). High cytotoxic activity of *P. lanceolata* is due to the presence of heavy triterpenes and lipophilic compounds (5). Free radical scavenging activity of *P. caucasica* is probably

***Corresponding author:** Shirin Moradkhani,
Email: shirin.moradkhani@yahoo.com

related to flavonoids (13).

Different species of genus *Phlomis* are categorized into 4 chemotypes, based on main components of essential oil: 1. first chemotype is rich in sesquiterpenes, 2. second chemotype is rich in monoterpenes and sesquiterpenes, 3. main components of third chemotype are fatty acids, aliphatic compounds and alcohol, 4. the last chemotype is rich in fatty acids, terpenes, aliphatic compounds and alcohol (14). Based on this category fatty acids are considered as chemotaxonomic factors in genus *Phlomis*, therefore identification of these compounds is important.

Recently fatty acids have attracted a great attention from different aspects including food industry, diagnosis and even treatment of several disorders (15).

Fatty acids are carboxylic acids coupled with an aliphatic chain, which may be saturated or unsaturated, and this point makes differences in their properties. Monounsaturated and polyunsaturated fatty acids have been used in lowering the risk of heart disease, against inflammation and in enhancing immunity or immune system (15). Studies have shown that dietary omega-3 fatty acids, which exist in fish or fish oil specially eicosapentaenoic acid (EPA), docosahexaenoic acid (DHA) and α-linolenic acid, significantly reduced all-cause mortality, myocardial infarction, cardiac and sudden death or stroke (16).

Recent studies have revealed new pharmacological properties of some of fatty acids, for example Linolenic acid which is necessary for the maintenance of growth. It is a potent inhibitor of cyclooxygenase-2 (COX-2) and catalyses biosynthesis of prostaglandins (15).

So far some fatty acids have been recognized in *Phlomis* species including linoleic acid, oleic acid and lauric acid (17). Hexadecanoic acid has been recognized in *P. herba-venti* as well (18). *P. bracteosa* is another species of genus *Phlomis* which has been investigated for fatty acid composition, not only saturated fatty acids like pentadecanoic acid and stearic acid, but also unsaturated fatty acids like octadecadienoic acid and elaidic acid have been reported in this plant (15).

In this study we are going to analyze fatty acid composition of two *Phlomis* species, *P. olivieri* and *P. bruguieri* by GC-MS. *P. olivieri*, which is an endemic species of Iran, has been evaluated for its antinociceptive effects (19). Its phytochemicals has been assessed (20) and its essential oil components (21) have been reported before. About *P. bruguieri*, composition of essential oil (22) and antimicrobial activity (23) have been investigated and also positive effect of this plant on enhancing a herbal oil, sunflower oil, has been approved (24). Yet there is no report of fatty acid composition in these two species, which is the subject of the present study.

Materials and Methods

Plant material

Aerial parts of *P. bruguieri* and *P. olivieri* were collected during the flowering stage from the mountains of Hamadan province of Iran. Voucher specimens (No: 73,81) were deposited in Department of Pharmacognosy, School of Pharmacy, Hamadan University of Medical Sciences, Hamadan, Iran.

Extraction of the oils and derivatization of fatty acids

About 20 g of powdered material of aerial parts of two selected plants (*P. bruguieri* and *P. olivieri*) were extracted with 750 mL n-hexane for eight hours through soxhlet extraction apparatus. The extracts were concentrated by recovering the solvent using rotary evaporator. The next step was derivatization of the fatty acids in order to make them volatile to be capable of being analyzed with gas chromatography-mass spectrometry (GC-MS). Methylation is the most general method of converting non-volatile fatty acids into volatile fatty acids methyl esters. This method of derivatization was performed with BF3-methanol as derivatizing agent. Derivatization was performed according to the AOAC standard reference method. To a known amount of sample was added 10 mL sodium hydroxide solution in methanol (2%), sealed and heated in boiling water for 10 minutes. The hydrolyzed sample was cooled and added 4.36 mL of boron trifluoride solution in methanol. The solution was then sealed and heated in boiling water bath for 2-3 minutes and cooled. To the esterified solution was added 3 mL hexane and then added 2 mL saturated sodium chloride solution (300 g/L) and shaked. Finally 1 g sodium sulfate as a humectant was added and centrifuged for 2-5 minutes in 2500 round per minutes. The hexane extract was filtered through 0.45 μm membrane filter and injected 1 μL to GC-MS using auto injector system (15).

Chromatographic separation of fatty acid methyl esters

A gas chromatograph to a mass spectrometer equipped with an auto-sampler and an auto-injector was used. Helium was used as carrier gas. All chromatographic separations were performed on a capillary column (HP-5MS) having specifications: length; 30 m, i.d.; 250 μm, thickness; 0.250 μm. Other GC-MS conditions were: ion source temperature (EI); 250°C, interface temperature; 240°C, pressure; 100 KPa, solvent cut time; 1.8 minutes. 1 μL of sample was injected into the GC column. Injector was operated in a split mode with a split ratio of 1:20. Injection temperature was 50°C. The column temperature program started at 50°C for 1 minute. The temperature was raised to 175°C at the rate of 2.5°C/min and hold for 5 minutes. Then the temperature was increased to 220°C at the rate of 2.5°C/min and kept constant for 3 minutes. Total elution time was 77 minutes. MS scanning was performed from *m/z* 85 to *m/z* 380. GC-MS solutions software provided by the supplier was used to control the system and to acquire the data. Identification of the compounds was carried out by comparing the mass spectra obtained with those of standard mass spectra from the NIST library.

Results

Tables 1 and 2 summarize the results obtained from GC-MS analysis of hexane extract of two selected species of *Phlomis*. Fatty acids were the main portion of extracts,

Table 1. Quantitative results of fatty acid methyl esters of *Phlomis bruguieri* oil

No.	Name	Concentration %
1	9-Octadecenoic acid, elaidic acid, methyl ester (C18:1)	56.79
2	6-Octadecynoic acid, methyl ester (C18:1)	17.98
3	Hexadecanoic acid, palmitic acid, methyl ester (C16:0)	12.96
4	9-cis,11-trans-octadecadienoic acid, methyl ester (C18:2)	6.07
5	12,15-Octadecadiynoic acid, methyl ester (C18:2)	2.57
6	Nonahexacontanoic acid, methyl ester (C69:0)	1.70
7	11-Hexadecenoic acid, methyl ester (C 16:1)	1.19
9	Z-8-methyl-9-tetradecenoic acid, methyl ester (C15:1)	0.37
10	9-Octadecenoic acid, oleic acid, methyl ester (C18:1)	0.35

Table 2. Quantitative results of fatty acid methyl esters of *Phlomis olivieri* oil

No.	Name	Concentration %
1	9-octadecenoic acid, Oleic acid, methyl ester (C18:1)	47.86
2	12,15-Octadecadiynoic acid, methyl ester (C18:2)	15.25
3	(Z)-7-Hexadecenoic acid, methyl ester (C16:1)	13.47
4	Hexadecanoic acid, methyl ester (C16:0)	13.15
5	cis-11-Eicosenoic acid, methyl ester (C20:1)	7.40
6	6-cis,9-cis,11-trans-octadecatrienoic acid, methyl ester (C19:3)	2.87

which constituted 83.30% of total extract in *P. bruguieri* and 52.68% of total extract in *P. olivieri*. In both plants, saturated and unsaturated fatty acids were identified. Palmitic acid and nonahexacontanoic acid were two saturated fatty acids recognized in *P. bruguieri*. Palmitic acid was also detected in *P. olivieri*, as the only saturated fatty acid recognized in this plant. Octadecanoic acid was found in plants in high concentration, 56.41% in *P. bruguieri* and 44.43% in *P. olivieri*. Palmitic acid was another fatty acid, which was common in the investigated species.

12,15-Octadecadiynoic acid was the third common fatty acid in two plants. Oleic acid was a monounsaturated fatty acid which was found in both plant species. Also other unsaturated fatty acids were detected in both plants (Tables 1 and 2).

Discussion

Considering the beneficial effects of naturally occurring unsaturated fatty acids in diet, there is a great interest on investigation of fatty acid profile of plant species, which was the aim of the present study. Two selected species of *Phlomis* including *P. bruguieri* and *P. olivieri* were extracted with hexane. The hexane extracts were full of fatty acids. The derivatization was done according to the AOAC standard reference method. The volatile fatty acids were injected to GC/MS apparatus. Both investigated species had large amounts of fatty acids in their hexane extracts (83.3%, 52.68% of total extracts). Both investigated species contained saturated and unsaturated fatty acids. Unsaturated fatty acids were higher amount than saturated ones in both species. Three fatty acids are common in these two species, including palmitic acid, 12,15-octadecadiyenoic acid and 9-octadecenoic acid. Palmitic acid has been identified in other species of genus *Phlomis* as well, for example *P. harba-venti* (18) and *P. bracteosa* (15). This saturated fatty acids have been reported from *Leucas aspera* (25) and Vitex negundo (26). Antioxidant, hypocholesterolemic, nematicide, pesticide, antiandrogenic flavor, hemolytic and 5-alpha reductase inhibitory effects are the properties attributed to palmitic acid (26). Oleic acid has shown anti-inflammatory, antiandrogenic, cancer preventive, dermatitigenic, hypocholestrolemic, 5-alpha reductase inhibitory, anemiagenic, insectifuge and flavor activities (27). In a study investigating the effects of methanolic extract of a plant called *Leucas aspera* on inhibiting Naja naja venom enzymes, it was found that 9-cis,11-trans-octadecadienoic acid, detected in *P. bruguieri*, and other unsaturated fatty acids found in *Leucas aspera* would help in maintaining the cell integrity which in turn prevented the distribution of venom components from the bite site (28). The compound E-8-methyl-9-tetradecen-1-ol acetate, found in *P. olivieri*, has a special activity in insect pheromone (29).

In sum, this study opens new frontiers and applications of *P. bruguieri* and *P. olivieri* due to various bioactive components for pharmaceutical and pharmacological applications.

Acknowledgments

This article is part of the thesis of Samaneh Zafari Shayan for the fulfillment of Pharm. D. degree in School of Pharmacy, Hamadan University of Medical Sciences, Hamadan, Iran. The authors are grateful to deputy of vice chancellor of research and technology for financial supports.

Authors' contributions

SM and DD were the supervisor and advisor of the thesis project, respectively. All read and confirmed the manuscript.

Conflict of interests

The authors declare that there is no conflict of interest.

Ethical considerations

Ethical issues (including plagiarism, misconduct, data

fabrication, falsification, double publication or submission, redundancy) have been completely observed by the authors.

Funding/ Support
This study was financially supported by deputy of vice chancellor of research and technology, Hamadan University of Medical Sciences, Hamadan, Iran.

References

1. Jabeen B, Riaz N, Saleem M, et al. Isolation of natural compounds from Phlomis stewartii showing a-glucosidase inhibitory activity. Phytochemistry. 2013;96:443–8.
2. Morteza-Semnani K, Saeedi M. The essential oil composition of Phlomis bruguieri Desf. from Iran. Flavour Frag J. 2005;20:344–6.
3. Li MX, Shang XF, Jia ZP, Zang RX. Phytochemical and biological studies of plants from the genus Phlomis. Chem Biodivers. 2010;7:283-301.
4. Ullah R, Al-Zeghayer YS, Haider S. Immunomodulatory potential of Phlomis bracteosa. Afr J Pharm Pharmacol. 2011;5(15):1811-12.
5. Soltani-Nasab F, Asgarpanah J, Majdzadeh M, Ostad SN. Investigating the effect of Phlomis lanceolata Boiss and Hohen on cancer cell lines. Acta Medica Iranica. 2014;52(5):333-6.
6. Ulukanli Z, Akkaya A. Antibacterial activities of Marrubium catariifolium and Phlomis pungens var. Hirta grown wild in Eastern Anatolia, Turkey. Int J Agric Biol. 2011;13:105-9.
7. Sarkhail P, Rahmanipour S, Fadyevatan S, et al. Antidiabetic effect of Phlomisanisodonta: effects on hepatic cell lipid peroxidation and antioxidant enzymes in experimental diabetes. Pharmacol Res. 2007;56:261-6.
8. Gurbuz I, Ustun O, Yesilada E, Sezik E, Kutsal O. Anti-ulcerogenic activity of some plants used as folk remedy in Turkey. J Ethnopharmacol. 2003;88:93-7.
9. Demirci F, Cuven K, Demirci B, Dadandi MY, Baser KH. Antibacterial activity of two Phlomis essential oil against food pathogens. J food Cont. 2008;19:1159-64.
10. Wang QS, Yang L, Cui WY, Chen L, Jiang YH. Anti-inflammatoryandantinociceptiveactivitisofmethanol extract from aerial part of Phlomis younghusbandii Mukerjee. PLoS One. 2014;9(3):89149.
11. Turker AU, Yildirm AB. Evaluation of antibacterial and antitumor activities of some Turkish Endemic Plants. Trop J Pharm Res. 2013;12(6):1003-10.
12. Gu H, Gu X, Xu Q, Kang WY. Antioxidant activity in vitro and hepatoprotective effect of Phlomis maximowiczii in vivo. Afr J Tradit Complement Altern Med. 2014;11(3):46-52.
13. Delazar A, Sabzevari A, Mojarrab M, et al. Free-radical-scavenging principles from Phlomis caucasica. J Nat Med. 2008;62:464–6.
14. Amor I, Bounaker J, Sgaier MB, et al. Phytochemistry and biological activities of Phlomis species. J Ethnopharmacol. 2009;125:183-203.
15. AbdElslam M, Ullah N, Ali R, Hussain J. Analysis of the fatty acid composition of Phlomis bracteosa oil by gas chromatography-mass spectrometer. Life Sci. 2013;10(7s):959-62.
16. Wang Ch, S Harris W, Chung M, et al. 3 Fatty acids from fish or fish-oil supplements, but not α-linolenic acid, benefit cardiovascular disease outcomes in primary- and secondary-prevention studies: a systematic review. Am J Clin Nutr. 2006;84:5-17.
17. Li MX, Shang XF, Jia ZP, Zhang RX. Phytochemical and biological studies of plants from the genus Phlomis. Chem Biodivers. 2010;7:283-301.
18. Morteza-Semnani K, Azadbakht M, Goodarzi A. The essential oils composition of Phlomisherba-ventiL. leaves and flowers of Iranian origin. Flavour Frag J. 2004;19:29-31.
19. Sarkhail P, Abdollahi M, Shafiee A. Antinociceptive effect of Phlomisolivieri Benth., Phlomisanisodonta Boiss. And Phlomis persica Boiss. total extracts. Pharmacol Res. 2003;48:263-6.
20. Zardoost MR, Gheibi S. Extraction and identification of flavonoid in Phlomis olivieri Benth. Iran J Org Chem. 2011;3(4):751-3.
21. Sarkhail P, Amin G, Shafiee A. Composition of the essential oil of Phlomis olivieri Benth from north of Iran. Daru. 2006;14(2):71-4.
22. Morteza-Semnani K, Saeedi M. The essential oil composition of Phlomis bruguieri Desf. from Iran. Flavour Frag J. 2005;20:344-6.
23. Morteza-semnani K, Saeedi M, Mahdavi MR, Rahimi F. Antimicrobial studies on extract of three species of Phlomis. Pharm Biol. 2006; 44(6):426-9.
24. Morteza-Semnani K, SaeediM, Shahani S. Antioxidant activity of the methanolic extracts of some species of Phlomis and Stachys on sunflower oil. Afr J Biotechnol. 2006;5(24):2428-32.
25. Gopi K, Renu K, Jayaraman G. Inhibition of Najanaja venom enzymes by the methanolic extract of Leucas aspera and its chemical profile by GC-MS. Tox Rep. 2014;1:667-73.
26. Kumar PP, Kumaravel S, Lalitha C. Screening of antioxidant activity, total phenolics and GC-MS study of Vitexnegundo. Afr J Biochem Res. 2010;4(7):191-5.
27. Lakshmi PT, Rajalakshmi P. Identification of phyto-components and its biological activities of Aloe vera through the Gas chromatography-Mass spectrometry. IRJP. 2011;2(5):247-9.
28. Gopi K, Renu K, Jayaraman G. Inhibition of Naja naja venom enzymes by the methanolic extract of Leucas aspera and its chemical profile by GC-MS. Tox Rep. 2014;1:667-73.
29. RamalakshmiS, MuthuchelianK. Analysis of bioactive constituents from the leaves of Mallotustetracoccus (ROXB.) KURZ, by gas chromatography-mass spectrometry. IJPSR. 2011;2(9):1449-54.

Overview of medicinal plants used for cardiovascular system disorders and diseases in ethnobotany of different areas in Iran

Babak Baharvand-Ahmadi[1], **Mahmoud Bahmani**[2*], **Zohreh Eftekhari**[3], **Mahyar Jelodari**[4], **Mahmoud Mirhoseini**[5]

[1]Razi Herbal Medicines Research Center & Madani Heart Hospital, Lorestan University of Medical Sciences, Khorramabad, Iran
[2]Food and Beverages Safety Research Center, Urmia University of Medical Sciences, Urmia, Iran
[3]Production and Research Complex, Pasteur Institute of Iran, Tehran, Iran
[4]Faculty of Veterinary, University of Urmia, Urmia, Iran
[5]Medical Plants Research Center, Shahrekord University of Medical Sciences, Shahrekord, Iran

ARTICLE INFO

Keywords:
Cardiovascular disorders
Hypertension
Hyperlipidemia
Diabetes
Herbs
Iran

ABSTRACT

Background and Aims: Today, cardiovascular diseases are the prominent cause of death in industrialized countries which include a variety of diseases such as hypertension, hyperlipidemia, thromboembolism, coronary heart disease, heart failure, etc. Recent research findings have shown that not only the extent of cultivation and production of medicinal plants have not been reduced, but also day-to-day production and consumption have increased. In traditional botanical knowledge, herbal medicines are used for the treatment of cardiovascular disorders. In this study, we sought to gather and report medicinal plants used to treat these diseases in different regions of Iran.

Methods: The articles published about ethnobotanical study of cardiovascular diseases in various regions of Iran, such as Arasbaran, Sistan, Kashan, Kerman, Isfahan Mobarakeh, Lorestan and Ilam were prepared and summarized.

Results: The results of ethnobotanical studies of various regions of Iran, such as Arasbaran, Sistan, Kashan, Kerman, Isfahan Mobarakeh, Lorestan and Ilam were gathered. The results showed that sumac plants, barberry, yarrow, wild cucumber, horsetail, Eastern grape, hawthorn, wild rose, spinach, jujube, buckwheat, chamomile, chicory, thistle, Mary peas, nightshade, verbena, sorrel , cherry, citrullus colocynthis, Peganum harmala, sesame and so many other plants are used for the treatment of cardiovascular diseases and disorders.

Conclusion: Herbal medicines are used effectively for some cardiovascular diseases. Rigorous training of patients to take precautions and drug interactions into account and to avoid the arbitrary use of medicinal plants is very important.

Implication for health policy/practice/research/medical education:
Medicinal plants are used effectively for some cardiovascular diseases. Cautious about drug interactions and side effects of medicinal plants is very important.

Introduction

Studies show that cardiovascular diseases are currently the leading cause of death in industrialized countries. Documented reports indicate that cardiovascular diseases in the United States led to death of 950 000 people in 1998 and spending of 118 billion dollars (1). Cardiovascular diseases include a broad range of diseases, including hypertension, hyperlipidemia, thromboembolism, coronary heart disease, heart failure, etc (2-4). Hyperlipidemia is a predisposing factor for many diseases that can cause complications such as atherosclerosis, hypertension, increased risk of stroke and fatty liver (5,6). Hypertension is the most common disorder and is known as a risk factor for the diagnosis of myocardial infarction, stroke, peripheral vascular disease, and a major factor in the development of cardiovascular disease and mortality (7-9). Pathophysi-

***Corresponding author:** Dr. Mahmoud Bahmani; Food and Beverages Safety Research Center, Urmia University of Medical Sciences, Urmia, Iran.
Email: mahmood.bahmani@yahoo.com

ological disorders such as type 2 diabetes occur due to impaired insulin secretion, insulin resistance, and overproduction of glucose by the liver (10). The usage of natural herbs increased because of beneficial effects of herbs and easier return to nature in comparison to chemical drugs (11-22). In some countries, 80% of the drugs supplied to the pharmaceutical market have natural origin, so that now 90% of people in these countries use herbal medicines (23-34). Recent research findings have shown that not only the extent of cultivation and production of medicinal plants have not been reduced, but also day-to-day production and consumption have increased (35-42). In traditional botanical knowledge, herbal medicines are used for the treatment of cardiovascular disorders. In this study, we tried to gather medicinal plants used to treat these diseases in different parts of Iran.

Methods

The articles published about ethnobotanical study of cardiovascular diseases in various regions of Iran, such as Arasbaran, Sistan, Kashan, Kerman, Isfahan Mobarakeh, Lorestan and Ilam were prepared and summarized.

Results

The findings on native medicinal plants used for the treatment of cardiovascular disorders in different areas of Iran including Arasbaran, Sistan, Kazeroon, Kashan, Kerman, Isfahan (Mobarakeh), Ilam and Lorestan are respectively summarized in Tables 1 to 8.

Conclusion

The herbal medicines can be beneficial for some heart diseases. Rigorous training of patients to take precautions and drug interactions into account and to avoid the arbitrary use of medicinal plants is very important (34).

Along with the increased use of herbal medicines, useful information about the interactions of these supplements and medications should be given to the patients to prevent the complications resulting from their interactions that are sometimes very critical. There are many plants that have therapeutic effects, may prevent cardiovascular diseases, and influence hypolipidemia, blood pressure and heart failure through antioxidant, anti-clotting, hypotensive, anti-atherosclerosis, heart rate-regulating and vasodilating properties (6,7). The plants may also have a negative impact on the performance of the heart and blood vessels, including the development of arrhythmia, blood pressure and similar effects on the sympathetic nervous currents that cause interference in the activity of the heart.

Authors' contributions

All the authors contributed in design and preparation

Table 1. Medicinal plants used in the treatment of cardiovascular diseases in Arasbaran (43)

Scientific name	Family Name	Persian Name	Organ Used	Treatment Effect
Cotinus coggygria	Anacardiaceae	Derakht Par	Leaf	Astringent
Rhus coriaria L.	Anacardiaceae	Sumagh	Leaf and Fruit	Blood purification
Berberis vulgaris L.	Berberidaceae	Zereshk	Fruit	Reduction of blood pressure
Achillea millefolium L.	Compositae	Boomadarn	Flowering branches	Reduction of blood pressure
Ecbalium elaterium L.	Cucurbitaceae	Khiare Vahshi	Fruit	Reduction of blood pressure
Juniperus communis	Cupressaceae	Pirou	Fruit	Blood purification
Equisetum arvense	Equisetaceae	Dom Asb	Aerial	Diabetes
Ribes orientale	Grossulariaceae	Ghalesh Anghour	Fruit	Regulation of blood pressure, removal of bile
Polypodium vulgare	Polypodiaceae	Besfij	Rhizome	Removal of bile, fat digestion and fat reduction
Portulaca olraca	Portulaceae	Khorfeh	Aerial	Blood purification
Crataegus monogyna	Rosaceae	Zalzalak	Flower and Leaf	Nourishing of the heart, regulation of heart rate and blood pressure
Rosa canina	Rosaceae	Nastaran Vahshi	Flower and Leaf	Blood purification
Fragaria vesca L.	Rosaceae	Tootfarangi Vahshi	Leaf, rhizome and Fruit	Nourishing of the heart, treatment of anemia
Rubus caesius L.	Rosaceae	Tameshk	Fruit and Leaf	Astringent, anti-diabetic, tonic and blood purification
Taxus baccata L.	Taxaceae	Sorkhedar	Leaf	Reduction of blood pressure

Table 2. Medicinal herbs used in the treatment of cardiovascular diseases in Sistan (44)

Scientific name	Family Name	Persian Name	Organ Used	Treatment Effect
Capparis spinosa L.	Capparidaceae	Koor	Root	Treatment of anemia
Eucalyptus camaldulensis Dehnh.	Myrtaceae	Moort	Leaf	Astringent
Nigella sativa L.	Ranunculaceae	Siah Daneh	Fruit	Treatment of blood fat, blood pressure, diabetes
Suaeda aegyptiaca	Chenopodiaceae	Esfenaj	Leaf	Treatment of anemia, blood purifier
Zizyphus jujube	Rhamnaceae	Annab	Fruit	Blood purifier

Table 3. Medicinal plants used in the treatment of cardiovascular diseases in Kazeroon (45)

Scientific name	Family Name	Persian Name	Organ Used	Treatment Effect
Anthemis austro-iranica	Asteraceae	Babooneh	Aerial	Cardiac tonic
Cichorium intybus L.	Asteraceae	Kasni	Aerial	Blood purifier and cardiac tonic
Silybum marianum	Asteraceae	Kharmaryam	Fruit and leaf	Lowering of blood pressure
Capsella bursa-pastoris	Brassicaceae	Kiseh Keshish	Leaf and stem	Astringent
Teucrium polium L.	Lamiaceae	Maryam Nokhodi	Leaf	Diabetes, blood fat
Melilotus indicus	Papilionaceae	Shabdar	Leaf	Increase in venous blood
Prosopis farcta	Papilionaceae	Jagjege	Fruit	Anti-atherosclerosis
Portulaca oleracea L.	Portulacaceae	Khorfe	Aerial	Blood purification
Rosa canina L.	Rosaceae	Nastaran	Flower	Astringent
Solanum nigrum L.	Solanaceae	Tajrizi	Fruit and leaf	Diabetes and blood fat
Verbena officinalis L.	Verbenaceae	Shahpasand	Fruit and leaf	Blood fat

Table 4. Medicinal plants used in the treatment of cardiovascular disease in Kashan (46)

Scientific name	Family Name	Persian Name	Organ Used	Treatment Effect
Anthemis gayana Boiss.	-	Babooneh	Leaf and flower	Treatment of blocked arteries
Rumex conglomerates Murr	-	Torshak	Leaf and stem	Blood purification

Table 5. Medicinal plants used in the treatment of cardiovascular disease in Kerman (47)

Scientific name	Family Name	Persian Name	Organ Used	Treatment Effect
Berberis integerrima	Berberidaceae	Zereshk	Fruit	Blood purification
Cerasus vulgaris	Rosaceae	Albaloo	Fruit	Reduction in blood fat
Citrullus colocynthis	Cucurbitaceae	Hendevane Aboljahl	Fruit	Diabetes
Coriandrum sativum	Apiaceae	Ghashniz	Fruit	Reduction in blood fat Hypoglycemic effect
Hordeumvulgare	Poaceae	Joo	Fruit	Hypoglycemic effect
Peganumharmala	Zygophyllaceae	Esfand	Seed	Hypoglycemic effect
Sesamun indicum	Pedaliaceae	Konjed	Seed	Reduction in blood fat

Table 6. Medicinal plants used in the treatment of cardiovascular disease in Mobarakeh, Isfahan (48)

Scientific name	Family Name	Persian Name	Organ Used	Treatment Effect
Gundelia tournefortii L	Asteracea	Kangar	Leaf	Reduction in blood fat
Ziziphus jujuba(L) H.Karst	Rhamnaceae	Annab	Fruit	Blood purification
Mentha spicata L	Lamiaceae	Nana	Leaf	Reduction in blood fat
Cichorium intybus L	Asteraceae	Kasni	Aerial	Blood purification
Rumex crispus L.	Polygonaceae	Torshak	Fruit	Reduction in blood fat
Arctium minus Hill.	Asteraceae	Baba Adam	Root	Blood purification
Anethum graveolens L.	Apiaceae	Shavid	Leaf	Reduction in blood fat
Zingiber officinale Roscoe	Zingiberaceae	Zanjebil	Leaf	Reduction in blood fat
Trigonella foenum-graecum L.	Papilionaceae	Shanbalileh	Leaf and Seed	Reduction in blood fat
Senna alexandrina Mill	Papilionaceae	Sana	Leaf	Reduction in blood fat
Rumex crispus L.	Polygonaceae	Torshak	Leaf	Reduction in blood pressure
Ziziphus jujuba(L) H.Karst	Rhamnaceae	Annab	Fruit	Reduction in blood pressure
Olea europaea L	Oleaceae	Zeytoon	Fruit	Reduction in blood pressure

Table 7. Medicinal plants used in the treatment of cardiovascular disease in Ilam (49)

Scientific name	Family	Persian name	Organ used	Treatment effect
Anethum graveolens	Umbelliferae	Shevid	All parts of Plant	Reduction in blood fat
Cichorium intybus	Asteraceae	Kasni	Root	Reduction in blood fat
Lactuca sativa	Compositae	Kahoo	Leaf	Reduction in blood fat
Malva neglecta	Malvaceae	Panirak	Leaf and Stem	Blood purification
Nectaro scordeum tripedale N. coelzi	Alliaceae	Piaz Lorestani	Aerial	Treatment of hypolipidemia
Ocimum bacilicum	Laminaceae	Reyhan	Leaf	Reduction in blood fat

Table 8. Medicinal plants used in the treatment of cardiovascular disease in Lorestan (50)

Scientific name	Family	Persian Name	Organ Used	Treatment Effect
Citrullus colocynthis (L.) Schrad.	Cucurbitaceae	Henzel	Fruit	Diabetes
Crataegus pontica C. Koch.	Rosaceae	Zalzalk	Fruit	Blood pressure
Glycyrrhiza glabra L. var. *glabra*		Shirin Bayan	Root and flower	Diabetes
Gundelia tournefortii L.	Asteraceae	Kangar	Leaf and stem	Diabetes
Nerium oleander L.	Apocynaceae	Khar Zahre	Leaf and flower	Cardiac tonic
Paliurus spina-christi Miller.	Rhamnaceae	Darg dar	Fruit	Blood pressure
Prosopis farcta	Mimosaceae	Kohorak	Fruit	Diabetes
Quercus brantii	Fagaceae	Baloot	Fruit	Diabetes
Rheum ribes L.	Polygonaceae	Rivas	Stem	Blood pressure
Ulmus glabra Hudson.		Vazm	Leaf	Cardiac disorders and arrhythmias
Olea europea	Oleaceae	Zeitoon	Leaf and seed	Blood fat control
Urtica dioica	Urticaceae	Ghazane	Leaf and branches	Reduction in blood fat
Vitis vinifera	Vitaceae	Angour	Fruit	Reduction in blood fat
Morus alba	Moraceae	Toot	Fruit	Reduction in glycemia
Berberis integrima	Berberidaceae	Zereshk	Leaf and stem	Treatment of diabetes
Pistacia atlantica	Anacardiaceae	Boneh	Juice	Treatment of glycemia
Capparis spinosa	Capparaceae	Hendevne Aboljahl	Fruit and leaf	Reduction in glycemia
Urtica dioica	Urticaceae	Ghazane	Branches	Reduction in glycemia
Valeriana officinalis L	Valerianaceae	Sonboleteib	Fruit	Reduction in glycemia
Melilotus officinalis	Leguminosae	Yonje	Flower, Leaf and Stem	Reduction Blood Glucose
Nectaroscordeum tripedale *Nectaroscordeum coelzi*	Amaryllidaceae	Piaze Lorestani	Branches	Reduction in blood pressure
Falcaria vulgaris	Apiaceae	Gazayaghi	Leaf, flower and Stem	Reduction in blood pressure
Smyrnium cordifolium	Umbelliferae	Andool	Seed	Reduction in blood pressure
Crocus hasskenechtii	Iridaceae	Zaferan	Root	Reduction in blood pressure
Berberis integrima	Berberidaceae	Zereshk	Leaf and Stem	Reduction in blood pressure
Ziziphus spina-christi *Ziziphus nummularia*	Rhamnaceae	Sedr	Flower, leaf and Fruit	Reduction in blood pressure
Allium ursinum	Liliaceae	Sir	Bulb	Reduction in blood pressure
Tragapogon caricifolius	Compositae	Shang	All parts of plant	Reduction in blood pressure
Anethum graveolens	Umbelliferae	Shevid	All parts of plant	Reduction in blood pressure
Amygdalus scoparia	Rosaceae	Badam	Fruit	Reduction in blood pressure

of the data, read and confirmed the final version of the manuscript.

Conflict of interests
The authors declared no competing interests.

Ethical considerations
Ethical issues (including plagiarism, misconduct, data fabrication, falsification, double publication or submission, redundancy) have been completely observed by the authors.

Funding/Support
None.

References
1. Eisenberg DM, David RB, Ettner SL. Trends in alternative medicine use in the United States, 1990–1997: results of a follow-up national survey. JAMA 1998;280:1569-1575.
2. Obesity: preventing and managing the global epidemic. Report of a WHO consultation. World Health Organ Tech Rep Ser. 2000;894:1-253.

3. Khosravi-Boroujeni H, Sarrafzadegan N, Mohammadifard N, Sajjadi F, Maghroun M, Asgari S, et al. White rice consumption and CVD risk factors among Iranian population. J Health Popul Nutr. 2013;31(2):252-261.
4. Sadeghi M, Khosravi-Boroujeni H, Sarrafzadegan N, Asgary S, Roohafza H, Gharipour M, et al. Cheese consumption in relation to cardiovascular risk factors among Iranian adults- IHHP Study. Nutr Res Pract. 2014;8(3):336-41.
5. Tajfard M, Ghayour Mobarhan M, Rahimi HR, Mouhebati M, Esmaeily H, et al. Anxiety, depression, coronary artery disease and diabetes mellitus; an association study in ghaem hospital, Iran. Iran Red Crescent Med J. 2014;16(9):e14589.
6. Asgary S, Rafieian-Kopaei M, Shamsi F, Najafi S, Sahebkar A. Biochemical and histopathological study of the anti-hyperglycemic and anti-hyperlipidemic effects of cornelian cherry (Cornus mas L.) in alloxan-induced diabetic rats. J Complement Integr Med. 2014;11(2):63-9.
7. Baradaran A, Nasri H, Rafieian-Kopaei M. Oxidative stress and hypertension: Possibility of hypertension therapy with antioxidants. J Res Med Sci. 2014;19(4):358-67.
8. Vasan RS, Beiser A, Seshadri S, Larson MG, Kannel WB, et al. Residual lifetime risk for developing hypertension in middle-aged women and men: the Framingham Heart Study. JAMA 2002;287:1003-1010.
9. Asgary S, Sahebkar A, Afshani M, Keshvari M. Haghjooyjavanmard Sh, Rafieian-Kopaei M. Clinical evaluation of blood pressure lowering, endothelial function improving, hypolipidemic and anti-inflammatory effects of pomegranate juice in hypertensive subjects. Phytother Res. 2014;28(2):193-199.
10. Rafieian-Kopaei M, Behradmanesh S, Kheiri S, Nasri H. Association of serum uric acid with level of blood pressure in type 2 diabetic patients. Iran J Kidney Dis. 2014;8(2):152-154.
11. Bahmani M, Shirzad HA, Majlesi M, Shahinfard N, Rafieian-Kopaei M. A review study on analgesic applications of Iranian medicinal plants. Asian Pac J Trop Med. 2014;7(Suppl 1):43-53.
12. Bahmani M, Farkhondeh T, Sadighara P. The anti-parasitic effects of Nicotina tabacum on leeches, Comp Clin Pathol. 2012;21(3):357-359.
13. Bahmani M, Karamati SA, Banihabib EKh, Saki K. Comparison of effect of nicotine and levamisole and ivermectin on mortality of leech. Asian Pac J Trop Dis. 2014;4(Suppl 1):477-480.
14. Delfan B, Bahmani M, Rafieian-Kopaei M, Delfan M, Saki K. A review study on ethnobotanical study of medicinal plants used in relief of toothache in Lorestan Province, Iran. Asian Pac J Trop Dis. 2014; 4(Suppl 2):879-884.
15. Bahmani M, Banihabib EK. Comparative assessment of the anti-annelida (Limnatis nilotica) activity of Nicotine with Niclosamide. Global Veterinaria. 2013; 10(2):153-157.
16. Amirmohammadi M, Khajoenia SH, Bahmani M, Rafieian-Kopaei M, Eftekhari Z, Qorbani M. In vivo evaluation of antiparasitic effects of Artemisia abrotanum and Salvia officinalis extracts on Syphacia obvelata, Aspiculoris tetrapetra and Hymenolepis nana parasites. Asian Pac J Trop Dis. 2014;4(Suppl 1): 250-254.
17. Bahmani M, Eftekhari Z. An ethnoveterinary study of medicinal plants in treatment of diseases and syndromes of herd dog in southern regions of Ilam province, Iran. Comp Clin Path. 2012;22:403-407.
18. Eftekhari Z, Bahmani M, Mohsenzadegan A, Gholami-Ahangaran M, Abbasi J, Alighazi N. Evaluating the anti-leech (Limnatis nilotica) activity of methanolic extract of Allium sativum L. compared with levamisole and metronidazole. Comp Clin Path. 2012;21:1219-1222.
19. Bahmani M, Abbasi J, Mohsenzadegan A, Sadeghian S, Gholami-Ahangaran M. Allium sativum L.: the antiammature leech (Limnatis nilotica) activity compared to Niclosomide. Comp Clin Path. 2013;22:165-168.
20. Sarrafchi A, Bahmani M, Shirzad H, Rafieian-Kopaei M. Oxidative stress and Parkinson's disease: New hopes in treatment with herbal antioxidants. Curr Pharm Des. 2015 Nov 12.
21. Gholami-Ahangaran M, Bahmani M, Zia-Jahromi N. Comparative and evaluation of anti-leech (Limnatis Nilotica) effect of Olive (Olea Europaea L.) with levamisol and tiabendazole. Asian Pac J Trop Dis. 2012;2(1):S101-S103.
22. Bahmani M, Golshahi H, Mohsenzadegan A, Ghollami-Ahangarani M, Ghasemi E. Comparative assessment of the anti-Limnatis nilotica activities of Zingiber officinale methanolic extract with levamisole. Comp Clin Pathol. 2013;22(4):667-670.
23. Forouzan S, Bahmani M, Parsaei P, Mohsenzadegan A, Gholami-Ahangaran M. Anti-parasitic activites of Zingiber officinale methanolic extract on Limnatis nilotica. Glob Vet. 2012;9(2):144-148.
24. Gholami-Ahangaran M, Bahmani M, Zia-Jahrom N. In vitro antileech effects of Vitis vinifera L., niclosamide and ivermectin on mature and immature forms of leech Limnatis nilotica. Glob Vet. 2012;8: 229-232.
25. Bahmani M, Zargaran A, Rafieian-Kopaei M. Identification of medicinal plants of Urmia for treatment of gastrointestinal disorders. Rev Bras Farmacogn. 2014;24(4):468-448.
26. Bahmani M, Banihabib EK, Rafieian-Kopaei M, Gholami-Ahangaran M. Comparison of disinfection activities of nicotine with copper sulphate in water containing Limnatis nilotica. Kafkas Univ Vet Fak

Derg. 2015;21(1):9-11.

27. Delfan B, Bahmani M, Eftekhari Z, Jelodari M, Saki K, Mohammadi T. Effective herbs on the wound and skin disorders: a ethnobotanical study in Lorestan province, west of Iran. Asian Pac J Trop Dis. 2014; 4(Suppl 2):938-942.
28. Bahmani M, Saki K, Rafieian-Kopaei M, Karamati SA, Eftekhari Z, Jelodari M. The most common herbal medicines affecting Sarcomastigophora branches: a review study. Asian Pac J Trop Med. 2014;7(Suppl 1): 14-21.
29. Asadi-Samani M, Bahmani M, Rafieian-Kopaei M. The chemical composition, botanical characteristic and biological activities of Borago officinalis: a review. Asian Pac J Trop Med. 2014;7(Suppl 1):22-28.
30. Bahmani M, Zargaran A, Rafieian-Kopaei M, Saki M. Ethnobotanical study of medicinal plants used in the management of diabetes mellitus in the Urmia, Northwest Iran. Asian Pac J Trop Med. 2014;7(Suppl 1):348-354.
31. Delfan B, Bahmani M, Hassanzadazar H, Saki K, Rafieian-Kopaei M. Identification of medicinal plants affecting on headaches and migraines in Lorestan Province, West of Iran. Asian Pac J Trop Med. 2014; 7(Suppl 1): 376-379.
32. Bahmani M, Rafieian-Kopaei M, Hassanzadazar H, Saki K, Karamati SA, Delfan B. A review on most important herbal and synthetic antihelmintic drugs. Asian Pac J Trop Med. 2014;7(Suppl 1):29-33.
33. Saki K, Bahmani M, Rafieian-Kopaei M. The effect of most important medicinal plants on two important psychiatric disorders (anxiety and depression)-a review. Asian Pac J Trop Med. 2014;7(Suppl 1):34-42.
34. Sewell RD, Rafieian-Kopaei M. The history and ups and downs of herbal medicine usage. J HerbMed Pharmacol. 2014;3(1):1-3.
35. Asadbeigi M, Mohammadi T, Rafieian-Kopaei M, Saki K, Bahmani M, Delfan B. Traditional effects of medicinal plants in the treatment of respiratory diseases and disorders: an ethnobotanical study in the Urmia. Asian Pac J Trop Med. 2014;7(Suppl 1): S364-S368.
36. Karamati SA, Hassanzadazar H, Bahmani M, Rafieian-Kopaei M. Herbal and chemical drugs effective on malaria. Asian Pac J Trop Dis. 2014; 4(Suppl 2):599-601.
37. Bahmani M, Rafieian-Kopaei M, Jeloudari M, Eftekhari Z, Delfan B, Zargaran A, et al. A review of the health effects and uses of drugs of plant licorice (Glycyrrhiza glabra L.) in Iran. Asian Pac J Trop Dis. 2014; 4(Suppl 2):847-849.
38. Saki K, Bahmani M, Rafieian-Kopaei M, Hassanzadazar H, Dehghan K, Bahmani F, et al. The most common native medicinal plants used for psychiatric and neurological disorders in Urmia city, northwest of Iran. Asian Pac J Trop Dis. 2014;4(Suppl 2):895-901.
39. Bahmani M, Karamati SA, Hassanzadazar H, Forouzan SH, Rafieian-Kopaei M, Kazemi-Ghoshchi B, et al. Ethnobotanic study of medicinal plants in Urmia city: identification and traditional using of antiparasites plants. Asian Pac J Trop Dis. 2014;4(Suppl 2):906-910.
40. Shaygannia E, Bahmani M, Zamanzad B, Rafieian-Kopaei M. A Review Study on Punica granatum L. J Evid Based Complementary Altern Med. 2015 Jul 30. pii: 2156587215598039.
41. Bahmani M, Rafieian M, Baradaran A, Rafieian S, Rafieian-kopaei M. Nephrotoxicity and hepatotoxicity evaluation of Crocus sativus stigmas in neonates of nursing mice. J Nephropathol. 2014;3(2):81-85.
42. Bahmani M, Eftekhari Z, Saki K, Fazeli-Moghadam E, Jelodari M, Rafieian-Kopaei M. Obesity phytotherapy: review of native herbs used in traditional medicine for obesity. J Evid Based Complementary Altern Med. 2015 Aug 12. pii: 2156587215599105.
43. Zolfaghari A, Adeli A, Mozafarian V, Babaei S, Habibi-Bibalan G. Identification of medicinal plants and indigenous knowledge of local people Arasbaran. J Med Arum Plants. 2013;28(3):534-550.
44. Ranmanesh M, Najafi SH, Yousefi M. Ethnobotanical study of Medicinal Plants of Sistan region. J Herbal Drugs. 2010;2:61-68.
45. Dolatkhahi M, Ghorbani-Nahoji M, Mehrafarin E, Amininezhad GR, Dolatkhahi E. Ethnobotanical study of medicinal plants of Kazeroun: identification, transmittal and traditional uses. J Med Plants. 2013;11(2), 45: 163-178.
46. Abbasi SH, Afsharzadeh S, Mohajeri A. Ethnobotanical study of medicinal plants in Natanz region (Kashan), Iran. J Herbal Drugs. 2012; 3(3):157-166.
47. Sharififar F, Kouhpayeh A, Motaghi MM, Amir-Khosravi A, Pou-Mohseninasab A. The reviews ethnobotany of medicinal plants city of Sirjan, Kerman Province. J Herbal Drugs. 2010;3:19-28.
48. Mardaninejad SH, Vazirpour M. Ethnobotany of Medicinal Plants by Mobarake people(Isfahan). J Herbal Drugs. 2013;3(2):111-129.
49. Ghasemi Pirbalouti A, Momeni M, Bahmani M. Ethnobotanical study of medicinal plants used by kurd tribe in dehloran and abdanan districts, ilam province, Iran. Afr J Tradit Complement Altern Med. 2013;10(2):368-385.
50. Delfan B, Saki K, Bahmani M, Rangsaz N, Delfan M, Mohseni N, et al. A study on anti-diabetic and anti-hypertension herbs used in Lorestan province, Iran. J Herbmed Pharmacol. 2014;3(2):71-76.

Effects of date palm pollen on fertility and development of reproductive system in female Balb/C mice

Fazeleh Moshfegh[1], Javad Baharara[2*], Farideh Namvar[3], Saeedeh Zafar-Balanezhad[1], Elaheh Amini[4], Lobat Jafarzadeh[5]

[1]Department of Biology, Mashhad Branch, Islamic Azad University, Mashhad, Iran
[2]Research Center for Animal Development Applied Biology, Mashhad Branch, Islamic Azad University, Mashhad, Iran
[3]Department of Medicine, Mashhad Branch, Islamic Azad University, Mashhad, Iran
[4]Department of Animal Biology, Faculty of Biological Sciences, Kharazmi University, Tehran, Iran
[5]Medical Plants Research Center, Shahrekord University of Medical Sciences, Shahrekord, Iran

ARTICLE INFO

Keywords:
Palm pollen
Fertility
Balb/C

ABSTRACT

Introduction: The *Phoenix dactylifera* or date palm pollen (DPP) is widely used for male infertility in traditional medicine. The aim of this study was to evaluate the effect of DPP on fertility and development of female reproductive system in Balb/C mice.
Methods: Ten groups were assigned to 2 control and 8 experimental groups. On the control groups 1 and 2 no treatment was conducted, but in the control group 2, after 10 days the mice were mated. In experimental groups 1 and 2, the animals received DPP (100 and 200 mg/kg, respectively) by oral administration for 10 days. In experimental groups 3 and 4 percentage of mating was evaluated after 10 days. Experimental groups 5 and 6 received DPP during gestation. Embryos were removed to evaluate ovaries histology. For experimental groups 7 and 8, DPP was administered until 21th day after birth. The offspring ovaries were removed to evaluate histological parameters. The levels of sexual hormones were also measured.
Results: Several parameters of ovaries in offspring, including mass index, diameter of ovaries, number of primary and secondary graph follicles and corpora luteal, percentage of mating, body mass index and Crown rump (CR) of embryos, diameter of ovary, basic sexual cell number in embryos, and mass index increased in experimental groups in comparison to the controls. However, luteinizing hormone (LH) and follicle-stimulating hormone (FSH) in the experimental groups were not significantly different from those in control groups ($P>0.05$), while estrogen and progesterone considerably increased in experimental groups ($P<0.05$).
Conclusion: Results of our investigation propose that DPP can create an appropriate situation for oogenesis and maintain efficient fertility in female mice which it may be considered as useful nutraceuticals for potentiation of fertility in future human studies.

Implication for health policy/practice/research/medical education:
Date palm is effective in elevation of fertility rate in male subjects and might be used for potentiating fertility rate in females. Isolation of date palm bioactive compounds is recommended.

Introduction

Infertility is referred to the state in which a couple wanting children cannot conceive after 12 months of unprotected intercourse (1). Infertility is a complicated disorder that could lead to significant medical, psychosocial and economic consequences (2). By World Health Organization (WHO) estimates, 8%–12% of couples worldwide experience difficulty conceiving a child (3), making 50-80 million individuals face challenges in becoming an integrated family (4). In most developing countries, approximately 10% of all women's visits to doctors are due to childlessness-related problems (5). Why a couple is not able to conceive, or may not be able to conceive without medical intervention could be due to a variety of reasons (6). Reproductive alterations, such as infertility, could be attributed to environmental toxic agents (7). Daily use of antioxidants and some vitamins can protect sperm DNA against free radicals and also

***Corresponding author:** Javad Baharara; Professor, Department of Biology, Research Center for Animal Developmental Applied Biology, Mashhad Branch, Islamic Azad University, Mashhad, Iran,
Email: baharara78@gmail.com

increase blood-testis barrier stability (8).

Historically, medicinal plants were considered as the only form of health care to which majority of populations had immediate access (9). By WHO reports, 70%-80% of the people worldwide trust in traditional medicine as primary health care (2). Over 50% of all modern clinical drugs are natural product-derived and therefore natural products contribute greatly to developing drugs (10).

Herbs should be taken with adequate knowledge about the toxicity, purity, dosage, appropriate solvent for extraction, and adverse effects (11). Plant-derived chemicals may be used to treat sexual dysfunction and they can improve sex potentials (12).

Date palm (*Phoenix dactylifera* L.), one of the oldest cultivated plants, could be used as a shade for a person to sit or for other small plants to grow in. *P. dactylifera* is thought to have origin in crops cultivated in desert and semi-desert regions (13).

Suspension of *P. dactylifera* date palm pollen (DPP) is a herbal mixture widely used as a folk remedy for treatment of male infertility in traditional medicine. The male flowers of date palm are eaten as a fresh vegetable to improve fertility. Egyptian scientists have already demonstrated the gonad stimulating potency of DPP. Pollen grains of date palm were used to strengthen women's fertility in ancient Egypt (14). *P. dactylifera* is a tree species belonging to the family Arecaceae. All species of this genus are dioecious, with male and female flowers growing on separate trees (15).

In North Africa and Middle East *P. dactylifera* is a staple food that can be produced easily in unfavorable natural conditions (16). For centuries, *P. dactylifera* has been used in the Middle East as a tonic main food. *P. dactylifera* is also an alleged aphrodisiac and symbol of fertility. The Arab believe that date pollen juice increases the possibility of pregnancy. Many studies have shown that pollen contains estrogen-like hormones. Phytochemical studies have demonstrated the presence of sterols, oestrone-like compounds and steroidal saponin glycoside in DPP grains (17). Date is an old fruit crop which has been cultivated in North Africa and the Middle East for about 5000 years. Dates grow in extremely hot and dry climates, and to some extent tolerate salty and alkaline soils (18). Dates contain vitamin C, and vitamins B1 and B2, nicotinic acid and vitamin A. In addition 23 different amino acids have been observed in date's proteins, many of which are absent in most fruits (19).

Recent studies indicate that the aqueous extracts of date have potent antioxidant activity. The antioxidant activity of date is attributed to the wide range of phenolic compounds including p-coumaric, ferulic acid, sinapic acids, flavonoids, and procyanidins (20).

Objectives

In the present study, the effect of DPP on fertility and development of reproductive system in female Balb/C mice was investigated.

Materials and methods

Balb/C mice were obtained from animal house of Razi Institute, Mashhad and kept under 12-hour light/dark cycle and temperature of 22 ± 2°C. Standard pellet food and distilled water were freely available to the mice. The animals were acclimatized to the laboratory conditions for one week till the start of the experiments. Two doses, 100 and 200 mg/kg, of drug were selected. The animals were divided into 10 groups of 10 each (8 experimental and 2 control groups).

Control groups

Control 1 received no drug. After 10 days the mice were deeply anesthetized with anesthetic ether and sacrificed. Histological changes in ovary were measured.

Control 2 received no drug. After 10 days the mice were mated overnight at a 3:1 ratio of female and male, respectively.

Experimental groups

Experimental groups 1 and 2: Animals treated once daily by oral administration of 100 and 200 mg/kg of the drug under study. Body weight (BW) DPP suspension was given via drinking water for 10 days. The weight of the ovary was also determined, and after tissue processing, their histology were studied by light microscope.

Experimental groups 3 and 4: Animals treated once daily by oral administration of 100 and 200 mg/kg. BW DPP suspension was given via drinking water for 10 days. Then percentage of mating was determined.

Experimental groups 5 and 6: Animals in these groups received DPP via drinking water during gestation at doses of 100 and 200 mg/kg. After 18 days, embryos were removed from uterus. The ovary of embryos was studied by light microscope.

Experimental groups 7 and 8: Animals received 100 and 200 mg/kg DPP via drinking water during gestation and lactation until day 21 after birth. The ovary of embryos was removed after sexually maturation and fixed in Bouin's solution. By preparing serial tissue sections, structural changes in ovary were studied.

Statistical analysis

Data were presented as mean±SD by statistical software of *GraphPad InStat* V2.01. Statistical analysis was by one-way analysis of variance (ANOVA) and the comparison between the control and experimental groups was done by Tukey-Kramer test.

Results

Regarding the obtained results, both ovary mass index and diameter significantly increased in experimental groups 1 and 2 in comparison with the control group ($P<0.05$, $P<0.01$, respectively). The remarkable differences have been observed in BW (g) in animals of the groups treated with DPP (Table 1).

The obtained results demonstrated that DPP caused a considerable enhancement of the mean number of primary, secondary and graph follicles and corpora luteal when compared to the corresponding variables in the control group (Table 2, Figure 1).

In the studied groups, both luteinizing hormone (LH) and follicle-stimulating hormone (FSH) showed no considerable difference compared to the control group ($P>0.05$). On the other hand, for estrogen and progesterone, a significant enhancement was observed in the studied groups ($P<0.05$; Table 3).

Also, a significant increase was observed for both mass index and CR of embryos in treated mice in contrast to control group ($P<0.001$; Table 4).

The comparative evaluation between control and experimental groups revealed that consumption of DPP suspensions leads to significant increase in diameter of embryos ovary ($P<0.05$; Table 4).

The basic sexual cells count in female embryos obviously increased in experimental groups when compared to the control group ($P<0.01$; Table 4).

A significant increase was seen in the number of primary, secondary and graph follicles and corpora luteal in ovary of female offspring as compared to control group (Table 5; Figure 1).

Based on our findings, a significant increase in offspring ovary mass index and diameter were observed in animals of the groups treated with DPP as compared to the control group ($P<0.01$; Table 6).

The comparative evaluation between control and experimental groups revealed that consumption of DPP suspensions led to a significant increase in percentage of mating ($P<0.05$; Table 7).

Discussion

We conducted this study to investigate the efficacy of palm pollen suspensions at different concentrations on female infertility.

Results obtained in this study showed that the DPP leads to significant increase in the serum values of estrogen and progesterone whereas the serum values of LH and FSH in the experimental groups have shown no significant difference compared to the controls. Moshtsghi et al showed that the serum density of LH and FSH in the experimental group was not significantly different compared to the control group. The groups in which values of 200 and 400 mg/kg DPP were administered showed remarkable increase in estrogen and progesterone. Also in this study, it was suggested that DPP contains flavonoid and alkaloid compounds that have estrogenic activity (21). Based on obtained results in the present study it can be concluded that the DPP significantly increases the number of ovarian follicles (primary, secondary and graph) and corpora luteal. Previous studies have shown that date palm contains estradiol and flavonoid (22). An experimental study on black seed (*Nigella sativa*) showed that hydro-alcoholic extract of black seed led to a significant increase in ovaries weight and follicles number. According to the findings in the study on *N. sativa*, it was suggested that the presence of linoleic acid in *N. sativa* stimulates several molecular pathways and consequently increases oogenesis (23). Our obtained results confirmed that consumption of DPP suspensions during gestation led to considerable impacts on development of reproductive system in mice. In conclusion, present study showed that both basic sexual cells count and ovary diameter in female

Table 1. Effect of date palm pollen (DPP) on ovary mass index (mi), ovary diameter (mm) and Body mass (g)[a]

	Ovary mass index (mi)	Ovary diameter (mm)	Body mass (g)
C 1	0.024 ± 0.002	2.98 ± 3.06	29.6 ± 2.10
E 1	0.812 ± 2.57	5.04 ± 3.06	33.06 ± 2.07
E 2	1.05 ± 0.018	5.06 ± 7.32	35.8 ± 2.03
Value	$P<0.05$	$P<0.01$	$P<0.05$

Abbreviations: C 1, Control 1; E 1, Experimental group 1; E 2, Experimental group 2.
[a]Values have been shown as mean ± SD.

Table 2. Effect of date palm pollen on ovarian follicles (primary, secondary and graph) and corpora luteal

	Primary follicle	Secondary follicle	Graafian follicle	Corpora lutea
C 1	7.25 ± 3	5.51 ± 1.7	1.38 ± 0.52	4.2 ± 1.3
E 1	16 ± 3.53	8 ± 1.58	2.8 ± 0.83	8.4 ± 2.7
E 2	19.2 ± 7.32	1.2 ± 3.7	3.4 ± 1.14	10.8 ± 2.58
Value	$P<0.05$	$P<0.05$	$P<0.05$	$P<0.05$

Abbreviations: C 1, Control 1; E 1, Experimental group 1; E 2, Experimental group 2.

Table 3. Effect of date palm pollen (DPP) on the serum values of LH, FSH, estrogen and progesterone

	Serum density of LH (mlu/ml)	Serum density of FSH (mlu/ml)	Serum density of estrogens hormones (pg/ml)	Serum density of progesterone hormones (g/ml)
C 1	0.132 ± 0.026	0.584 ± 0.054	4.1 ± 0.91	49.5 ± 14.59
E 1	0.132 ± 0.022	0.594 ± 0.042	10.6 ± 1.15	66.3 ± 5.66
E 2	0.131 ± 0.011	0.594 ± 0.78	11.6 ± 1.60	68.5 ± 7.63
Value	$P>0.05$	$P>0.05$	$P<0.001$	$P<0.05$

Abbreviations: C 1, Control 1; E 1, Experimental group 1; E 2, Experimental group 2.

Table 4. Effect of date palm pollen (DPP) on embryos weight (g)

	Weight embryos (g)	CR (mm)	Diameter of embryos ovary (μm)	Basic sexual cells of female embryos
C 2	0.66 ± 0.053	16.11 ± 1.1	173.8 ± 9.35	17.6 ± 6.58
E 5	1.25 ± 1.31	21.3 ± 1.73	179.4 ± 6.01	48 ± 10.79
E 6	1.11 ± 0.17	24.55 ± 1.76	178.82 ± 7.88	39 ± 4.94
Value	$P < 0.001$	$P < 0.001$	$P < 0.05$	$P < 0.01$

Abbreviations: CR (mm), diameter of embryos ovaries (μm) and basic sexual cells count of male embryo; C 2, Control 2; E 5, Experimental group 5; E 6, Experimental group 6.

Table 5. Effect of date palm pollen (DPP) on number of offspring primary, secondary and graph follicle and corpora luteal

	No. of offspring primary follicle	No. of offspring secondary follicle	No. of offspring Graf follicle	No. of offspring corpora lutea
C 2	5.68 ± 1.14	6.65 ± 1.8	1.84 ± 0.54	5.1 ± 2.3
E 7	16.8 ± 1.58	7.4 ± 0.82	2.4 ± 1.14	8.4 ± 2.3
E 8	17 ± 6.76	10.6 ± 3.43	2.8 ± 1	10.2 ± 4.43
Value	$P < 0.001$	$P < 0.05$	$P < 0.01$	$P < 0.001$

Abbreviations: C 2, Control 2; E 7, Experimental group 7; E 8, Experimental group 8.

Table 6. Effect of date palm pollen (DPP) on offspring ovary weight (g) and diameter (mm)

	Offsprig ovary weight (g)	Offsprig ovary diameter (mm)
C 2	0.022±0.001	2.89±0.52
E 7	0.027±0.003	4.46±0.61
E 8	0.024±0.008	4.18±0.78
Value	$P < 0.01$	$P < 0.01$

Abbreviations: C 2, Control 2; E 7, Experimental group 7; E 8, Experimental group 8.

Table 7. Effect of date palm pollen (DPP) on percentage of mating

	Percentage of mating
C 2	40±0.63
E 3	75±3.4
E 4	75±3.6
Value	$P < 0.05$

Abbreviations: C 2, Control 2; E 3, Experimental group 3; E 4, Experimental group 4.

embryos increased in experimental groups as compared to the control group. Also according to our findings, it can be concluded that use of DPP suspension during gestation and lactation increases oogenesis in offspring significantly. DPP contains cytochrome p450 enzyme and like-estrogen compounds. Cytochrome p450 enzyme is able to transfer cholesterol to progesterone and increase progesterone hormone. Like-estrogen compounds also increase estrogen hormone (21). These compounds that exist in DPP transfer to embryos and offspring via lactate and placenta and affect reproductive system in adult mice. Finally, our study showed that DPP possesses facilitative

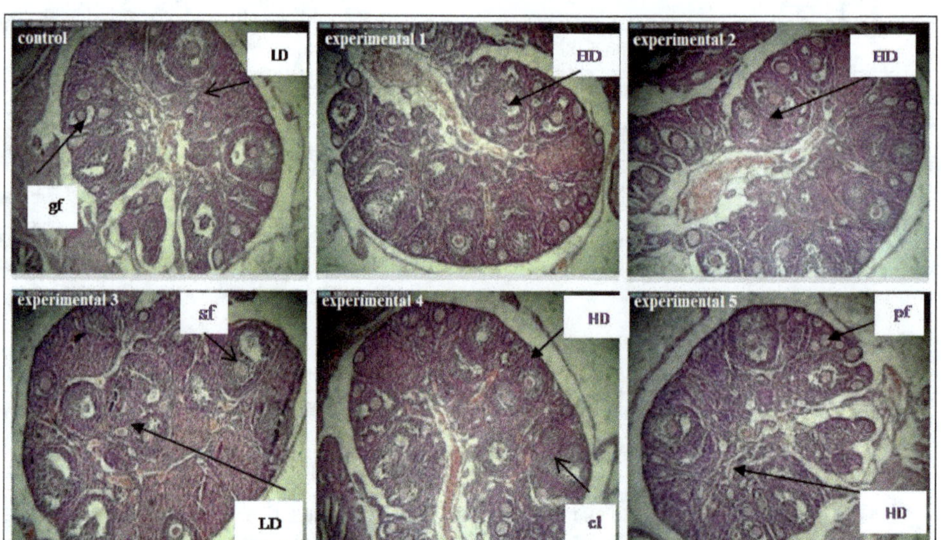

Figure 1. Effect of date palm pollen on density of follicles in control and various experimental groups (×100, H&E); ovary in treated groups shows increased number of follicles; LD: low density; HD: high density; Pf: primary follicle; sf: secondary follicle; gf: graph follicle; cl: corpora luteal.

effects that increase sexual arousal and percentage of mating. In another study, Abedi et al examined the aphrodisiac activity of aqueous extract of *P. dactylifera* pollen grain on the sexual behavior in male rats. They demonstrated that the aqueous extract of *P. dactylifera* pollen grain improved sexual behavior in male rats. The improved sexual appetitive behavior in male rats may be attributed to the alkaloids, saponins, and or flavonoids because these phytochemicals have engorgement, androgen enhancing properties (12).

Conclusion

According to the findings of this study, it can be concluded that the DPP suspension (at 100 and 200 mg/kg BW) for 10 days improves sperm quality, enhances fertility in female adult mice and also causes a positive effect on reproductive system in female emberyos. These effects may be explained by the chemical composition of the plant. Therefore, it may be useful to improve infertility problems.

Acknowledgments

This study was obtained from an MSc thesis funded by Department of Animal Biology, Islamic Azad University, Mashhad Branch, Iran. We thank the individuals and organizations who participated in this research.

Authors' contributions

Design and Supervision: JB and FM; Data Collection and/or Processing: FM and LJ; Literature Search: FN and SZB; Writing: FM and EA; Critical Reviews: JB, FN, AND SZB.

Conflict of interests

The authors declared no competing interests.

Ethical considerations

Ethical issues (including plagiarism, misconduct, data fabrication, falsification, double publication or submission, redundancy) have been completely observed by the authors.

Funding/Support

This research was financially supported by vice chancellor scientific research of Mashhad Branch, Islamic Azad University

References

1. Seshagiri P. Molecular insights into the causes of male infertility. J Biosci. 2001;26(4):429-435.
2. Parandi R, Yousofvand N, Ghorbani R. The enhancing effects of alcoholic extract of Nigella sativa seed on fertility potential, plasma gonadotropins and testosterone in male rats. Iranian Journal of Reproductive Medicine. 2012; 10(4):355-362.
3. Aboulghar M. The importance of fertility treatment in the developing world. Int J Gynaecol Obstet. 2005;112:1174-1176.
4. Roupa Z, Polikandrioti M, Sotiropoulou P, et al. Causes of infertility in women at reproductive age. Health Science Journal. 2009;3(2):80-87.
5. Wiersema NJ, Drukker AJ, Mai BT, Giang HN, Nguyen TN, Lambalk CB. Consequences of infertility in developing countries: results of a questionnaire and interview survey in the South of Vietnam. J Transl Med. 2006;4:54.
6. Gaware VM, Parjane SK, Merekar Abhijit N, et al. Female infertility and its treatment by alternative medicine: a review. J Chem Pharm Res. 2009;1(1):148-162.
7. Tchernitchin AN, Gaete L, Bustamante R, Báez A. Effect of prenatal exposure to lead onestrogen action in the prepubertal rat uterus. International Scholarly Research Network. 2011;2011:1-8.
8. Khaki A, Fathiazad F, Nouri M, et al. Evaluation of androgenic activity of alliumcepa on spermatogenesis in the rat. Folia Morphol (Warsz). 2009;68(1):45-51.
9. Adaay M, Mattar A. Effect of aqueous and ethanolic extracts of tribulusterrestris, phoenix dactylifera and nasturtium officinale mixture on some reproductive parameters in male mice. Journal of Baghdad for Science. 2012;9(4):640-650.
10. Deka MC, Kalita JC, Sarma GC. Traditional use of fertility inducing plants used by the herbal practitioners in some parts of the state Assam, N E India, a survey report. International Journal of Science and Advanced Technology. 2011;1(6):133-142.
11. Nwangwa EK. Antifertility effects of ethanolic extract of xylopiaaethiopica on male reproductive organ of Wistar rats. American Journal of Medicine and Medical Sciences. 2012;2(1): 12-15
12. Abedi A, Parviz M, Karimian SM, Sadeghipour Rodsari HR. Aphrodisiac activity of aqueous extract of Phoenix dactylifera pollen in male rats. Advances in Sexual Medicine. 2013;3:28-34.
13. Dada M, Nwawe CN, Okere RA, Uwubanmwen IO. Potentials of date palm tree to the Nigerian economy. World Journal of Agricultural Sciences. 2012;8 (3):309-315.
14. Bahmanpour S, Talaei T, Vojdani Z, et al. Effect of phoenix dactylifera pollen on sperm parameters and reproductive system of adult male rats. Iranian Journal of Medical Sciences. 2006;31(4):208-212.
15. Kgazal M, Salbi M, Salbi MI, Alsaadawi IS, Fattah FA. Bisexuality in date palm in Iraq. Journal of Islamic Academy of Sciences. 1990;3(2):131-133.
16. Organic Farming in the Tropics and Subtropics. Naturland e.V.; 2002.
17. Faleh B. Effect of palm pollen grains extracs(Phoenixdactylifera L) on spermatogenic activity of male rabbits. Basrah Journal of Agricultural Sciences.2006;5(1-2):1-10.

18. Chao C, Krueger R. The Date Palm (Phoenix dactylifera L.): Overview of Biology, Uses, and Cultivation. Hort Science. 2007;;42(5):1077-1082.
19. Sulieman AM, Abd Elhafise IA, Abdelrahim AM. Comparative study on five Sudanese date (Phoenix dactylifera L.) fruit cultivars. Food and Nutrition Sciences. 2012;3:1245-1251.
20. Bastway Ahmed M, Hasona NA, Selemain AH. Protective effects of extract from dates (Phoenix Dactylifera L.) and ascorbic acid on thioacetamide-induced hepatotoxicity in rats. Iran J Pharm Res. 2008;7(3):193-201.
21. Moshtaghi A, Johari H, Shariati M, Amiri J. Effects of phoenix dactylifera on serum concentration of estrogen, progesterone and gonadotropins in adult female rats. Journal of Rafsanjan University of Medical Sciences. 2010;9(2):117-124.
22. Robert R, Krueger R. The date palm (Phoenix dactylifera L.): overview of biology, uses, and cultivation. Hort Science. 2007;24(5):1077-1082.
23. Modaresi M, Poor-Naji N. The effect of black seed (Nigella sativa) hydro-alcoholic extract on breeding factors in female mice. Journal of Shahrekord University of Medical Sciences. 2012;13(6):63-70.

Virucidal potential of *Prosopis spicigera* and *Mangifera indica* on human peripheral blood mononuclear cells

Amit Gupta[1*], **Sushama R Chaphalkar**[2]

[1]Department of Immunology and Virology, Vidya Pratishthan's School of Biotechnology (VSBT, Research Centre affiliated to Savitribai Phule Pune University), Baramati-413133, Maharashtra, India
[2]Department of Microbiology, Vidya Pratishthan Arts, Science and Commerce College, Baramati-413133, Maharashtra, India

ARTICLE INFO

Keywords:
Mangifera indica
Prosopis spicigera
Anti-microbial
PBMC

ABSTRACT

Introduction: The treatment of viral infections with the available antiviral drugs is not free of side effects. Therefore, in the present study, our group focused on antiviral activity against Newcastle disease (NDV) and IBD viruses using medicinal plants especially leaves of *Prosopis spicigera* and *Mangifera indica*.
Methods: Different medicinal plant products especially leaves of *P. spicigera* and *M. indica* were tested in the form of aqueous leaves extracts (0.5- 30 mg/mL; 50 μL) for anti-microbial activities on human peripheral blood mononuclear cells (PBMC) pertaining to determine their proliferation rate (cytotoxicity assay), tumor necrosis factor alpha (TNFα) production and CD14 monocyte surface marker.
Results: Three medicinal plant aqueous extracts showed significant antimicrobial activity against PBMC at higher doses with respect to decline in proliferation assay, TNFα production and CD14 monocyte surface marker as compared to control.
Conclusion: Aqueous leaves extract of *P. spicigera* and *M. indica* showed antimicrobial activities and might be useful for the treatment of various viral diseases.

Implication for health policy/practice/research/medical education:
Prosopis spicigera and *Mangifera indica* (aqueous leaves extract) demonstrated a significant decrease in proliferation, TNFα production including CD14 surface marker against NDV/IBD which may indicate antiviral properties of these components.

Introduction

Medicinal plant products have a long traditional history with respect to their medicinal properties and uses. The major advantage of these medicinal plants over synthetic drugs is low side effects (1,2). In this regard, there is an increasing trend in the field of immunopharmacology for discovering novel drugs based on various herbal formulations. Plants synthesize a variety of phytochemicals most of which are extractable with various immunopharmacological activities (3,4). So, medicinal plant products proved to be a major resort for the treatment of animal and human diseases (3,4).

Mangifera indica (Mango; family *Anacardiaceae*) and *Prosopis spicigera* (Shami, family *Fabaceae*) showed number of medicinal properties e.g. anti-inflammatory, antioxidant, anti-asthma, etc. In addition, leaves of *M. indica* are used traditionally in India especially in weddings and religious ceremonies (5-7).

Newcastle disease (NDV) remains a constant threat or problem for poultry farm worldwide, strains of NDV (*Paramyxoviridae* family and *Avulavirus*, genus) contain one serotype and are also known as *avian paramyxovirus* serotype-1 (APMV-1). NDV (pleomorphic in shape, single-stranded, non-segmented and negative sense RNA viruses) is reported to infect birds and thus has a wide host range. Low virulent NDV typically produce subclinical disease with some morbidity, whereas virulent isolates can result in rapid and high mortality of birds (8).

One of the highly contagious diseases in chickens is IBD (*birnaviridae*; RNA viruses family) manifested by inflammation and successive atrophy of bursa of Fabricus (birds) including various degrees of nephroso-nephritis and immunosuppression. Clinically, IBD disease is seen only in those chickens that are older than 3 weeks (9). Recently, treatments are not available for NDV and IBD. However, vaccination is an effective method to control this disease

***Corresponding author:** Amit Gupta,
Emails: amitvsbt@gmail.com; amitgupta@vsbt.res.in

but it does not provide any protection. Thus there is a need to search for those medicinal plant products which are able to restrict the load of NDV and IBD diseases in poultry animals. In the present study, therefore, we focused on antiviral activity against NDV and IBD using medicinal plant products especially leaves of *Prosopis spicigera* and *Mangifera indica.*

Materials and Methods

Collection and preparation of plant material

Fresh plant leaves (From *P. spicigera* and *M. indica*) were obtained from Nakshatra garden of Vidya Pratishthan's School of Biotechnology in Baramati region, Maharashtra, India. These medicinal plants were washed and air dried (away from direct sunlight). Leaves of these medicinal plants were crushed in mortar and pestle to prepare fine powder.

Estimation of secondary metabolites (qualitative and quantitative)

Secondary metabolites of fresh plant leaves were determined qualitatively in the aqueous leaves extract of *P. spicigera* and *M. indica.* Different assays were performed qualitatively in order to determine the presence of secondary metabolites and showed qualitatively the presence of flavonoids (alkaline reagent test); terpenoids (acetic anhydride test) and phenolic compounds (ferric chloride test).

Virus sample collection (IBD and NDV)

Poultry suspected disease samples of NDV and IBD were collected aseptically from suspected birds including Baramati poultry farm and the study was conducted under Biovillage programme scheme, Vidya Pratishthan's School of Biotechnology, Baramati, India.

For NDV collection, dead birds underwent postmortem examinations on them concurrent infections were determined through various laboratory tests. Briefly, pooled tissues (lung, spleen, intestine etc.) were properly minced and dissolved in phosphate buffered saline (PBS) containing penicillin and streptomycin. Then, the samples were cleared by centrifugation at 3000 rpm for 10 minutes and the supernatant was collected and determined haemagglutination (HA) test for detection of NDV. Thereafter, 0.2 ml of supernatant was directly injected into the allantoic cavity route of embryonated (9-11 day old) chicken eggs that were totally pathogenic free (Venkys India Ltd). These chicken eggs (big sized embryos) were selected for inoculation and observed at regular time intervals to examine or determine embryo motility rate. After death, fluid of amnio-allantoic cavity was harvested and identified the presence of virus which was determined through haemagglutination (HA, 128) titre (8).

Similarly, IBDVs were processed by using chicken embryo fibroblast cell culture (9). Briefly, bursal sample was macerated into small pieces using mortar and pestle and finally dissolved in PBS containing penicillin and streptomycin. The samples were incubated for 1 hour and shacked every 5 minutes. After incubation, the supernatant was inoculated into sterile blood agar media for bacteriological sterility and was incubated at 37°C for 24 hours. This sterile suspension (bacteriologically) was used as inoculums for isolation of virus.

Proliferation assay and TNF alpha production

Fresh anti-coagulant (EDTA) human whole blood samples were collected (Mangal Pathology Laboratory, Maharashtra, India) and the human PBMC was separated by means of density gradient centrifugation and then cultured (10^5 cells/well) in 96 well plate for 48 h incubation with variable doses of aqueous leaves extracts (0.5–30 mg/mL, 50 µL) of *Prosopis spicigera* and *Mangifera indica* along with NDV (1:80 dilution, 10 µL) or IBD (1:100 dilution, 10 µL). Thereafter, the plates (96 well) were centrifuged at 2600 rpm for 12 minutes at 4°C and then the supernatant (after centrifuging) was collected for estimation of TNF alpha production and then equal volume of fresh complete medium was added into the 96-well plates. Again, the plates were incubated for another 4 hours along with MTT (5 mg/mL, 10 µL). Afterwards, the plates were centrifuged and the supernatant was collected and finally dispersed or dissolved in dimethyl sulphoxide (DMSO) solution. The optical density was measured at 570 nm (8,9). In addition, measurement of TNF alpha production from PBMC cell culture supernatant of *P. spicigera* and *M. indica* (exposed to NDV and IBD virus) was carried out using conventional ELISA kits and reagents (BD Biosciences, according to the manufacturer's instructions (10).

CD14 monocyte surface marker

In another set of experiment, human PBMC were cultured with variable concentrations of aqueous leaves extract of *Prosopis spicigera* and *Mangifera indica* along with or without NDV (1:80 dilution, 10 µL) or IBD (1:100 dilution, 10 µL) for 48 hours in 96-well plates. After incubation, treated and non-treated PBMC samples of *Prosopis spicigera and Mangifera indica* were collected and stained with CD14 FITC (5 µL) monoclonal antibody. The samples were then incubated (at room temperature), lysed (red cell lysis buffer containing ammonium chloride, potassium bicarbonate and EDTA) and washed with PBS (pH, 7.2). The resulting stained cell pellet was resuspended in 500 µL of PBS and run on a FACS Calibur flow cytometer (11).

Statistical analysis

All values were mentioned as mean ± S.E. Data were analysed by one-way analysis of variance (ANOVA) test (Bonferroni multiple comparison test).

Results

Proliferation assay

The effect of aqueous leaves extract on PBMC proliferation assay using NDV and IBD is shown in Figure 1. The results showed that aqueous leaves extract at higher doses significantly inhibited the PBMC proliferation assay as compared to control. NDV and IBD used as standard and there was significant increase in proliferation as compared

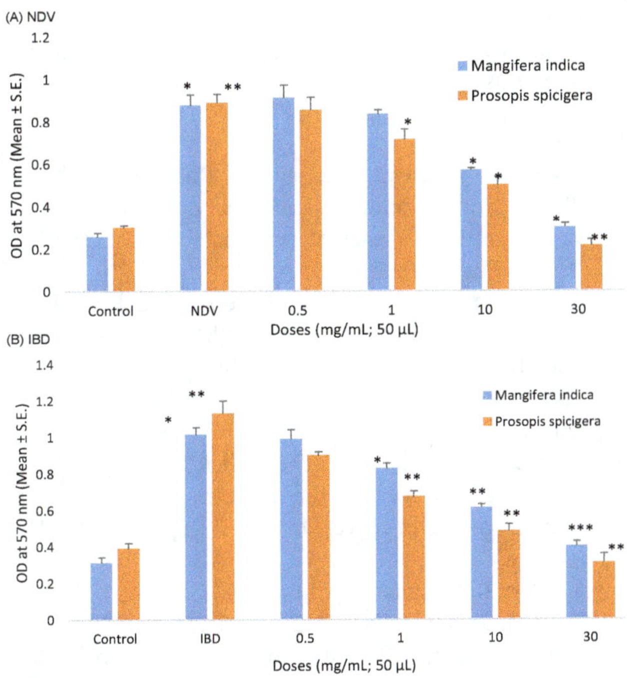

Figure 1. PBMC proliferation assay. Human PBMC (10^5 cells/well) were cultured with NDV or IBD along with variable doses of aqueous leaves extract or NDV/IBD alone. After 48 hours, proliferation was measured by MTT assay. The results are presented as mean ± SE. *$P < 0.05$, **$P < 0.01$, ***$P < 0.001$ as compared to control.

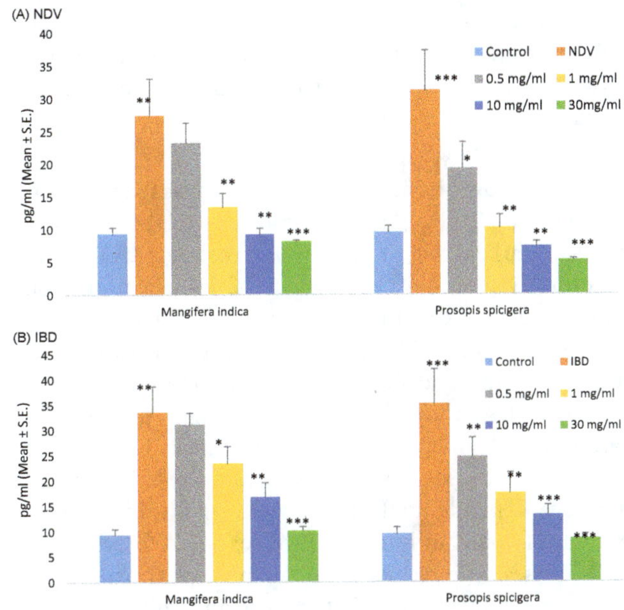

Figure 2. TNF alpha production from human PBMC cell culture supernatant. Human PBMC (10^5 cells/well) were cultured with NDV or IBD along with variable doses of aqueous leaves extract or NDV/IBD alone. After 48 hours, supernatant was collected for the estimation of Th1 cytokine (TNF alpha). Values are expressed as mean ± SE. *$P < 0.05$, **$P < 0.01$, ***$P < 0.001$ as compared to control.

to control.

TNF alpha production

The effect of aqueous leaves extract on TNF alpha production from PBMC cell culture supernatant (using NDV and IBD) is shown in Figure 2. The results showed that aqueous leaves extract at higher doses significantly inhibited TNF alpha production as compared to control.

CD14 monocyte surface marker

The effect of aqueous leaves extract on CD14 monocyte surface marker using NDV and IBD is shown in Figure 3. At higher doses, aqueous extract significantly inhibited CD14 monocyte surface marker as compared to control.

Discussion

The objective of our present work was to examine the antiviral activities of medicinal plants especially *P. spicigera* and *M. indica* against NDV and IBD. As per the literature, numerous medicinal plant products were reported and showed antiviral properties against number of viruses. In this study, our group analyzed anti-viral activities of aqueous leaves extract of *P. spicigera* and *M. indica*. In the initial screening of these medicinal plants, our group used aqueous leaves extract and determined their anti-inflammatory activities against hepatitis B surface antigen (12). It was easier to screen many pathogenic samples i.e. NDV and IBD. In this study, treatment of aqueous leaves extract on human PBMC, which is exposed with NDV and/or IBD in two different sets of experiments, showed anti-

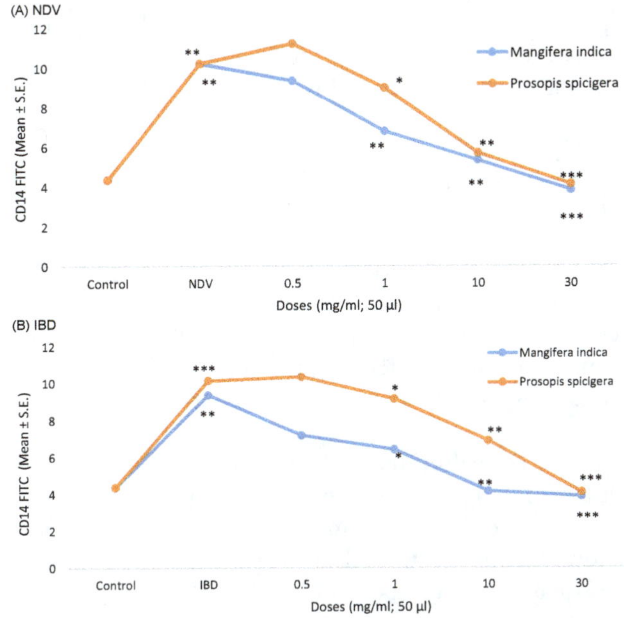

Figure 3. CD14 monocyte surface marker. Flow cytometric analysis of aqueous leaves extract (0.5–30 mg/mL; 50 μL) extracted from *Mangifera indica* and *Prosopis spicigera* for determine its effect (CD14, monocyte surface marker) in human PBMC against NDV and IBD. Data acquisition of 10000 events and fraction or separation of cell populations representing different phenotypes analysed using cell quest software. Values are expressed as mean ± SE. *$P < 0.05$, **$P < 0.01$, ***$P < 0.001$.

viral properties because of rapid decline in proliferation rate at higher doses. In addition, NDV and IBD viruses were not able to mutate with the medicinal plants because of the presence of secondary metabolites (terpenoids, flavonoids, saponin and phenolics). There is only one major difference on the basis of phytochemical investigation, glycosides are absent in *P. spicigera* and alkaloids in *M. indica*.

For these studies, basic parameters were selected i.e. proliferation assay, TNF alpha production and CD14 monocyte surface marker, that are totally interconnected with our immune system and provide general information about aqueous leaves extract of *P. spicigera and M. indica*. In this regard, NDV and IBD are two important viruses related to poultry farm and showed enhancement in the number of monocytes count (CD14 surface marker), proliferation rate and TNF alpha production. The results indicate that aqueous leaves extracts of *P. spicigera* and *M. indica* have a dosage-dependent effect and could significantly reduce the CD14 count in human PBMC exposed to NDV and IBD viruses. The results of our immunopharmacological studies on human PBMC after exposing with NDV and IBD suggested that the aqueous leaves extracts had anti-viral effects on human PBMC.

Currently, TNF alpha inhibitors from natural origins are generally used for the treatment of various inflammatory disorders. Enhancement of TNF alpha is totally associated with diabetes, arthritis etc (13). Currently, only protein based drugs are available for the clinical inhibition of TNF alpha activity. So, overall results indicated that aqueous leaves extract of *Prosopis spicigera* and *Mangifera indica* had anti-viral activities against NDV and IBD.

Conclusion

These studies suggest that aqueous leaves extract of *Prosopis spicigera* and *Mangifera indica* significantly inhibits proliferation rate, TNF alpha production and CD14 monocyte surface marker. Further investigations of the aqueous leaves extract should be done through in vivo assessment for immunopharmacological (anti-viral) studies in mice models with identification of the major active candidates responsible for anti-microbial activities.

Authors' contributions

Dr Gupta designed the study, wrote the protocol and interpreted the data. Dr Gupta anchored the field of the study, gathered the initial data and performed preliminary data analysis. Dr Gupta and Dr Chaphalkar managed the literature searches and produced the initial draft. Both the authors read and approved the final manuscript.

Conflict of interests

The authors declared no competing interests.

Ethical considerations

Ethical issues (including plagiarism, misconduct, data fabrication, falsification, double publication or submission and redundancy) were completely observed by authors.

Funding/Support

This research was financially supported by our organization (in house project).

References

1. Negi CS, Nautiyal S, Dasila L, Rao KS, Maikhuri RK. Ethnomedicinal plant uses in a small tribal community in a part of central Himalaya, India. J Hum Ecol. 2002;14(1):23.
2. Gupta A, Khamkar PR, Chaphalkar SR. Review on medicinal plants to target and inhibit the epidermal growth factor receptor signaling in cancer and tissue repair therapy. Int J Adv Pharm Biol Chem. 2014;3(1):210- 13.
3. Gupta A, Khamkar PR, Chaphalkar SR. Applications and uses of active ingredients from medicinal plants. Indian Journal of Novel Drug Delivery. 2014;6(2):106 -11.
4. Chopra RN, Nayar SL, Chopra IC. Glossary of Indian medicinal plants. New Delhi, India: CSIR; 2002.
5. Gupta A, Chaphalkar SR. Flow cytometric analysis of crude saponin from the leaves of Mangifera indica and Anthocephalus cadamba for its anti-inflammatory activity. Eur J Biomed Pharm Sci. 2015;2(2):163-73
6. Gupta A, Chaphalkar SR. Immunopharmacological activity of saponin from Terminalia Arjuna and Prosopis spicigera. J Pharm Rep. 2015;1(1):1-4.
7. Gupta A, Chaphalkar SR. Cytotoxic and immunosuppressive activity of terpenoids from Prosopis spicigera, Mimusops elengi and Terminalia arjuna. International Journal of Universal Pharmacy and Biosciences 2016;5(1):32-9
8. Gupta A, Chaphalkar SR. Immunopharmacological activity of Zingiber officinale on human peripheral blood mononuclear cells. Asian Journal of Medical and Pharmaceutical Researches 2015;5(2):13-7.
9. Gupta A, Chaphalkar SR. Inhibitory potential of aqueous leaves extract of Messua ferrea and Mimusops elengi on antigen specific immune response using human whole blood. Asian Journal of Medical and Pharmaceutical Researches. 2015;5(3):22-6.
10. Gupta A, Khajuria A, Singh J, Singh S, Suri KA, Qazi GN. Immunological adjuvant effect of Boswellia serrata (BOS 2000) on specific antibody and cellular response to ovalbumin in mice. Int Immunopharm. 2011;11(8):968-975.
11. Gupta A, Chaphalkar SR. Inhibitory potential of aqueous extract of Ficus benghalensis on human peripheral blood mononuclear cells. J Pharma Res. 2014;3(11):250-3.
12. Gupta A, Chaphalkar SR. Potential immunosuppressive and anti-inflammatory activity of aqueous extract of Mangifera indica. Adv Herb Med. 2015;1(4):47–54.
13. Khajuria A, Gupta A, Singh S, et al. RLJ-NE-299A: A new plant based vaccine adjuvant. Vaccine. 2007;25:2706-15.

Permissions

All chapters in this book were first published in JHP, by Shahrekord University of Medical Sciences; hereby published with permission under the Creative Commons Attribution License or equivalent. Every chapter published in this book has been scrutinized by our experts. Their significance has been extensively debated. The topics covered herein carry significant findings which will fuel the growth of the discipline. They may even be implemented as practical applications or may be referred to as a beginning point for another development.

The contributors of this book come from diverse backgrounds, making this book a truly international effort. This book will bring forth new frontiers with its revolutionizing research information and detailed analysis of the nascent developments around the world.

We would like to thank all the contributing authors for lending their expertise to make the book truly unique. They have played a crucial role in the development of this book. Without their invaluable contributions this book wouldn't have been possible. They have made vital efforts to compile up to date information on the varied aspects of this subject to make this book a valuable addition to the collection of many professionals and students.

This book was conceptualized with the vision of imparting up-to-date information and advanced data in this field. To ensure the same, a matchless editorial board was set up. Every individual on the board went through rigorous rounds of assessment to prove their worth. After which they invested a large part of their time researching and compiling the most relevant data for our readers.

The editorial board has been involved in producing this book since its inception. They have spent rigorous hours researching and exploring the diverse topics which have resulted in the successful publishing of this book. They have passed on their knowledge of decades through this book. To expedite this challenging task, the publisher supported the team at every step. A small team of assistant editors was also appointed to further simplify the editing procedure and attain best results for the readers.

Apart from the editorial board, the designing team has also invested a significant amount of their time in understanding the subject and creating the most relevant covers. They scrutinized every image to scout for the most suitable representation of the subject and create an appropriate cover for the book.

The publishing team has been an ardent support to the editorial, designing and production team. Their endless efforts to recruit the best for this project, has resulted in the accomplishment of this book. They are a veteran in the field of academics and their pool of knowledge is as vast as their experience in printing. Their expertise and guidance has proved useful at every step. Their uncompromising quality standards have made this book an exceptional effort. Their encouragement from time to time has been an inspiration for everyone.

The publisher and the editorial board hope that this book will prove to be a valuable piece of knowledge for researchers, students, practitioners and scholars across the globe.

List of Contributors

Majid Tabbakhian, Mohammad Ali Shahtalebi and Ehsan Salehi
Department of Pharmaceutics, School of Pharmacy and Pharmaceutical Sciences, Isfahan University of Medical Science, Isfahan, Iran

Mahtab Keshvari
Isfahan Cardiovascular Research Center, Isfahan Cardiovascular Research Institute, Isfahan University of Medical Sciences, Isfahan, Iran

Narges Askarian Dehkordi, Rezvan Meshkate and Mahbube Kiyani
Department of Immunology, Shahrekord University of Medical Sciences, Shahrekord, Iran

Hedayatollah Shirzad and Behnam Zamanzad
Cell and Molecular, Research Center, Shahrekord University of Medical Sciences, Shahrekord, Iran

Loghman Salimzadeh
Medical Plants Research Center, Shahrekord University of Medical Sciences, Shahrekord, Iran

Mahdi Khozaei and Rahman Emamzadeh
Department of Biology, University of Isfahan, Isfahan, Iran

Fatemeh Ghorbani
Department of Science, Islamic Azad University, Olom Tahghighat Branch, Tehran, Iran

Gashtasb Mardani
Medical Plants Research Center, Shahrekord University of Medical Sciences, Shahrekord, Iran

Mehrdad Modaresi
Biology Faculty, Khorasgan (Isfahan) Branch, Islamic Azad University, Isfahan, Iran

Hormat Khorrami
Payam-e-Noor University, Isfahan Center, Isfahan, Iran

Majid Asadi-Samani
Medical Plants Research Center, Shahrekord University of Medical Sciences, Shahrekord, Iran

Navid Mazroi Arani
Food and Hygiene Control Laboratory, Deputy of Food and Drug, Kashan University of Medical Sciences, Kashan, Iran

Reza Sharafati Chaleshtori
Research Center for Biochemistry and Nutrition in Metabolic Diseases, Kashan University of Medical Sciences, Kashan, Iran

Mahmoud Rafieian-kopaei
Medical Plants Research Center, Shahrekord University of Medical Sciences, Shahrekord, Iran

Nima Jafarpoor and Saeid Abbasi-Maleki
Department of Pharmacology, Urmia Branch, Islamic Azad University, Urmia, Iran

Majid Asadi-Samani
Medical Plants Research Center, Shahrekord University of Medical Sciences, Shahrekord, Iran

Mir Hadi Khayatnouri
Department of Pharmacology, Tabriz Branch, Islamic Azad University, Tabriz, Iran

Marziyeh Abolhasani and Abbas Doosti
Department of Biology, Islamic Azad University, Shahrekord Branch, Shahrekord, Iran

Morteza Hashemzadeh-Chaleshtori and Hossein Teimori
Cellular and Molecular Research Center, Shahrekord University of Medical Sciences, Shahrekord, Iran

Nematolah Amini Sarteshnizi
Department of Biology, University of Mohaghegh Ardabili, Ardabil, Iran

Mostafa Gholami-Arjenaki
Clinical Biochemistry Research Center, Shahrekord University of Medical Sciences, Shahrekord, Iran

Parivash Rahimi
Department of Biology, Faculty of Sciences, Isfahan University, Isfahan, Iran

Sedigheh Asgary
Isfahan Cardiovascular Research Center, Isfahan Cardiovascular Research Institute, Isfahan University of Medical Sciences, Isfahan, Iran

Najmeh Kabiri
Shahrekord University of Medical Sciences, Shahrekord, Iran

Wesam Kooti, Maryam Moradi, Sara Ali-Akbari and Naim Sharafi-Ahvazi
Member of Student Research Committee, Kurdistan University of Medical Sciences, Sanandaj, Iran

Majid Asadi-Samani
Medical Plants Research Center, Shahrekord University of Medical Sciences, Shahrekord, Iran

Damoon Ashtary-Larky
Member of Student Research Committee, Ahvaz Jundishapur University of Medical Sciences, Ahvaz, Iran

Bahram Delfan and Mahmoud Bahmani
Razi Herbal Medicines Research Center, Lorestan University of Medical Sciences, Khorramabad, Iran

Kourosh Saki
Shahid Beheshti University of Medical Sciences, Tehran, Iran

Nader Rangsaz
Faculty of Veterinary Medicine, Islamic Azad University, Shahrekord Branch, Shahrekord, Iran

Mohammad Delfan
Deputy for Food and Drug, Lorestan University of Medical Sciences, Khorramabad, Iran

Nima Mohseni
Faculty of Veterinary Medicine, Islamic Azad University, Karaj Branch, Karaj, Iran

Hedayatollah Shirzad
Medical Plants Research Center, Shahrekord University of Medical Sciences, Shahrekord, Iran

Zahra Babaeian
Deputy of Research and Technology, Ministry of Health and Medical Education, Tehran, Iran

Hassan Moghim, Simin Taghipoor, Najmeh Shahinfard, Soleiman Kheiri and Zahra Heydari
Medical Plants Research Center, Shahrekord University of Medical Sciences, Shahrekord, Iran

Samira Rafieian
Pharmaceutical Faculty, Isfahan University of Medical Sciences, Isfahan, Iran

Khodadad Pirali Kheirabadi
Department of pathobiology, Faculty of Veterinary Medicine, Shahrekord University, Shahrekord, Iran

Siavash Saei Dehkordi
Department of Food Hygiene and Quality Control, Faculty of Veterinary Medicine, Shahrekord University, Shahrekord, Iran

Parviz Kheibari
Faculty of Veterinary Medicine, Shahrekord University, Shahrekord, Iran

Hossein Nazarli and Ali Ahmadi
Department of Agronomy and Plant Breeding, University College of Agriculture and Natural Resources, University of Tehran, Karaj, Iran

Javad Hadian
Medicinal Plants and Drugs Research Institute, University College of Agriculture, University of Shahid Beheshti, Tehran, Iran

Abofazl Khoshdel
Clinical Biochemistry Research Center, Shahrekord University of Medical Sciences, Shahrekord, Iran

Fatemeh Famuri, Masoud Lotfizadeh and Karam-Ali Kasiri
Medical Plants Research Center, Shahrekord University of Medical Sciences, Shahrekord, Iran

Elham keivani
Student Research Committee, Shahrekord University of Medical Sciences, Shahrekord, Iran

Mortaza Rafieian
Isfahan Governor Office, Isfahan, Iran

Nasrollah Ghassemi-Dehkordi and Mustafa Ghanadian
Department of Pharmacognosy, School of Pharmacy, Isfahan University of Medical Sciences, Isfahan, Iran

Sajjad Arabha
Isfahan Pharmaceutical Sciences Research center, Isfahan University of Medical Sciences, Isfahan, Iran

Mehrdad Modaresi
Biology Faculty, Khorasgan (Isfahan) Branch, Islamic Azad University, Isfahan, Iran

Arezoo Pouriyanzadeh
Payam-e-Noor University, Isfahan Center, Isfahan, Iran

Majid Asadi-Samani
Medical Plants Research Center, Shahrekord University of Medical Sciences, Shahrekord, Iran

Jahangir Kaboutari and Rahmat allah Fatahian Dehkordi
Department of Basic Sciences, Faculty of Veterinary Medicine, Shahrekord University, Shahrekord, Iran

Mohammad Saeed Haydarnejad and Sedigheh Raeisi Vanani
Department of Biology, Faculty of Basic Sciences, Shahrekord University, Shahrekord, Iran

Reza Habibipour
Department of Microbiology, Faculty of Basic Sciences, Hamedan Branch, Islamic Azad University, Hamedan, Iran

Mohsen Rajabi
Young Researchers and Elite Club, Hamadan Branch, Islamic Azad University, Hamadan, Iran

Javad Baharara
Research Center for Animal Development Applied Biology & Department of Biology, Mashhad Branch, Islamic Azad University, Mashhad, Iran

Elaheh Amini
Department of Animal Biology, Faculty of Biological Sciences, Kharazmi University, Tehran, Iran

Farzaneh Salek-Abdollahi and Najme Nikdel
Faculty of Biological Science, Mashhad Branch, Islamic Azad University, Mashhad, Iran

Majid Asadi-Samani
Medical Plants Research Center, Shahrekord University of Medical Sciences, Shahrekord, Iran

Farzaneh Salek Abdollahi
MSC Student, Department of Biology, Faculty of Sciences, Mashhad Branch, Islamic Azad University, Mashhad, Iran

Javad Baharara
PhD. Research Center for Animal Development Applied Biology, Mashhad Branch, Islamic Azad University, Mashhad, Iran

Khadijeh NejadShahrokhabadi
PhD, Department of Biology, Faculty of Sciences, Islamic Azad University, Mashhad Branch, Mashhad, Iran

Farideh Namvar
Ph.D. Institute of Tropical Forestry and Forest Products (INTROP), University Putra Malaysia, UPM Serdang, Selangor 43400, Malaysia

Elaheh Amini
Department of Animal Biology, Faculty of Biological Sciences, Kharazmi University, Tehran, Iran

Mehdi Ghasemi, Mahdi Ayyari and Abdolali Shojaeiyan
Department of Horticulture Science, Tarbiat Modares University, Tehran, Iran

Aghafakhr Mirlohi
Department of Agronomy and Plant Breeding, Isfahan University of Technology, Isfahan, Iran

Ali Karimi
Faculty of Paramedicine, Shahrekord University of Medical Science, Shahrekord, Iran

Mohammad-Taghi Moradi
PhD student, Medical Plants Research Center, Shahrekord University of Medical Science, Shahrekord, Iran

Hassan Moghim, Simin Taghipoor and Ramin Panahi
Medical Plants Research Center, Shahrekord University of Medical Sciences, Shahrekord, Iran

Najmeh Shahinfard
Department of E-learning in Medical Education, Virtual School, Tehran University of Medical Sciences, Tehran, Iran

Soleiman Kheiri
Social Health Determinants Research Center, Shahrekord University of Medical Sciences, Shahrekord, Iran

Nader Pestechian and Somayeh Abedi-Madiseh
Department of Medical Mycoparasitology, School of Medicine, Isfahan University of Medical Sciences, Isfahan, Iran

Mustafa Ghanadian
Pharmaceutical Sciences Research Center, Isfahan University of Medical Sciences, Isfahan, Iran
Pharmacognosy Department, Isfahan Faculty of Pharmacy, Isfahan University of Medical Sciences, Isfahan, Iran

Mehdi Nateghpour
Department of Medical Parasitology and Mycology, School of Public Health, Tehran University of Medical Sciences, Tehran, Iran

Mohammad Mustakim Billah, Kashfia Nawrin and Mohammed Sahek Ullah Jabed
Department of Pharmaceutical Sciences, North South University, Bangladesh

Kh Tanvir Ahmed
Mylan School of Pharmacy, Duquesne University, USA

Md. Nasidul Islam
Department of Pharmacy, East West University, Bangladesh

Md. Main Uddin
Department of Clinical Pharmacy and Pharmacology, University of Dhaka, Bangladesh

Amir-Hosein Barati and Faezeh Fazeli
School of Physical Education and Sport Science, Shahid Rajaee Teacher Training University, Tehran, Iran

Mehdi Lotfipour
Department of Sport Physiology, School of Physical Education and Sport Science, Shahid Rajaee Teacher Training University, Tehran, Iran

Lila Alizadeh and Kolsoum Beyranvand
Razi Herbal Medicines Research Center, Lorestan University of Medical Sciences, Korramabad, Iran

Reza Karamian, Ali Mohammadian and Esfandiar Hassanimoghadam
Razi Herbal Medicines Research Center, Lorestan University of Medical Sciences, Korramabad, Iran
Agriculture and Natural Resources Research Center, Korramabad, Iran

Nargess Abdali
Razi Herbal Medicines Research Center, Lorestan University of Medical Sciences, Korramabad, Iran
Student Research Committee, Lorestan University of Medical Sciences, Khorramabad, Iran

Mahtab Keshvari
Isfahan Cardiovascular Research Center, Cardiovascular Research Institute, Isfahan University of medical Sciences, Isfahan, Iran

Seyed Masih Hosseini
Medical Plants Research Center, Shahrekord University of Medical Sciences, Shahrekord, Iran

Amit Gupta
Department of Immunology, Vidya Pratishthan's School of Biotechnology, Baramati, District Pune, Maharashtra India

Sushama R Chaphalkar
Director, Vidya Pratishthan's School of Biotechnology, Baramati, District Pune, Maharashtra India

Hassan Moghim, Simin Taghipoor, Najmeh Shahinfard and Hamideh Khabbazi
Medical Plants Research Center, Shahrekord University of Medical Sciences, Shahrekord, Iran

Soleiman kheiri
Social Health Determinants Research Center, Shahrekord University of Medical Sciences, Shahrekord, Iran

Mohammad Reza Khazdair
Pharmaciutical Research Center and Department of Physiology School of Medicine, Mashhad University of Medical Sciences, Mashhad, Iran

Mohammad Hossein Boskabady
Neurogenic Inflammation Research Centre and Department of Physiology, School of Medicine, Mashhad University of Medical Sciences, Mashhad, Iran

Mona Mohamadi and Simin Taghipur
Clinical Biochemistry Research Center, Shahrekord University of Medical Sciences, Shahrekord, Iran

Bahman Khalili
Cellular and Molecular Research Center, Shahrekord University of Medical Sciences, Shahrekord, Iran

Fatemeh Drees
Medical Plants Research Center, Shahrekord University of Medical Sciences, Shahrekord, Iran

Wesam Kooti and Naim Sharafi-Ahvazi
Member of Student Research Committee, Kurdistan University of Medical Sciences, Sanandaj, Iran

Maryam Ghasemi-boroon, Mahmoud Harizi and Reza Afrisham
Member of Student Research Committee, Ahvaz Jundishapur University of Medical Sciences, Ahvaz, Iran

Mehri Ghafourian
Health Research Institute, Research Center of Thalassemia & Hemoglobinopathy, Department of Immunology, Ahvaz Jundishapur University of Medical Sciences, Ahvaz, Iran

Majid Asadi-Samani
Medical Plants Research Center, Shahrekord University of Medical Sciences, Shahrekord, Iran

Naser Mirazi
Department of Biology, Faculty of Basic Sciences, Bu-Ali Sina University, Hamedan, Iran

Maryam Rezaei and Mahmoud Mirhoseini
Medical Plants Research Center, Shahrekord University of Medical Sciences, Shahrekord, Iran

Acharya Balkrishna
University of Patanjali, Haridwar, Uttarakhand 249402, India
Patanjali Natural Coloroma Pvt Ltd, Haridwar, Uttarakhand 249404, India

Hemanth Kumar Manikyam, Vinay K Sharma and Niti Sharma
Patanjali Natural Coloroma Pvt Ltd, Haridwar, Uttarakhand 249404, India

Dimitris P. Makris
School of Environment, University of the Aegean, Mitr. Ioakim Street, Myrina - 81400, Lemnos, Greece

Ioanna Karagiorgou
School of Environment, University of the Aegean, Mitr. Ioakim Street, Myrina - 81400, Lemnos, Greece
Department of Food Technology, Technological Educational Institute (T.E.I.) of Thessaly, N. Temponera Street, Karditsa - 43100, Greece

Stavros Lalas
Department of Food Technology, Technological Educational Institute (T.E.I.) of Thessaly, N. Temponera Street, Karditsa - 43100, Greece

Spyros Grigorakis
Food Quality & Chemistry of Natural Products, Mediterranean Agronomic Institute of Chania (M.A.I.Ch.), International Centre for Advanced Mediterranean Agronomic Studies (CIHEAM), Chania-73100, Greece

Habib-allah Mohammadi and Seyed-Ebrahim Sajjadi
Department of Pharmacognosy, School of Pharmacy, Isfahan University of Medical Sciences, Isfahan, Iran

Mostafa Noroozi
Isfahan Center for Research of Agricultural Science and Natural Resources, Isfahan, Iran

Mahmoud Mirhosseini
Medical Plants Research Center, Shahrekord University of Medical Sciences, Shahrekord, Iran

Amit Gupta and Sushama R Chaphalkar
Vidya Pratishthan's School of Biotechnology (Research centre affiliated to Savitribai Phule Pune University), Baramati, District Pune, Maharashtra, India

Ali Mohammadian
Student Research Center, Hamadan University of Medical Sciences, Hamadan, Iran

Shirin Moradkhani
Department of Pharmacogenosy, School of Pharmacy, Hamadan University of Medical Sciences, Hamadan, Iran

Sara Ataei and Mahsa Sedaghat
Department of Clinical Pharmacy, School of Pharmacy, Hamadan University of Medical Sciences, Hamadan, Iran

Tavakol Heidary Shayesteh and Akram Ranjbar
Department of Toxicology and Pharmacology, School of Pharmacy, Hamadan University of Medical Sciences, Hamadan, Iran

Nejat Kheiripour
Student Research Center, Hamadan University of Medical Sciences, Hamadan, Iran
Department of Biochemistry, Hamadan University of Medical Sciences, Hamadan, Iran

Chibueze Peter Ihekwereme, Chukwuemeka Amaechi Agbata, Kingsley Obinna Chukwueze and Sandra Chinenye Agu
Department of Pharmacology and Toxicology, Faculty of Pharmaceutical Sciences, Nnamdi Azikiwe University, Awka, Nigeria

Jahangir Kaboutari Katadj and Behnaz Karimi
Department of Basic Sciences, Faculty of Veterinary Medicine, Shahrekord University, Shahrekord, Iran

Mahmoud Rafieian-Kopaei
Medical Plants Research Center, Shahrekord University of Medical Sciences, Shahrekord, Iran

Hossein Nourani
Department of Pathobiology, Faculty of Veterinary Medicine, Ferdowsi University of Mashhad, Mshhad, Iran

Samaneh Zafari-Shayan, Shirin Moradkhani and Dara Dastan
Medicinal Plants and Natural Products Research Center, Hamadan University of Medical sciences, Hamadan, Iran
Department of Pharmacognosy and Pharmaceutical Biotechnology, School of Pharmacy, Hamadan University of Medical sciences, Hamadan, Iran

Babak Baharvand-Ahmadi
Razi Herbal Medicines Research Center & Madani Heart Hospital, Lorestan University of Medical Sciences, Khorramabad, Iran

Mahmoud Bahmani
Food and Beverages Safety Research Center, Urmia University of Medical Sciences, Urmia, Iran

Zohreh Eftekhari
Production and Research Complex, Pasteur Institute of Iran, Tehran, Iran

Mahyar Jelodari
Faculty of Veterinary, University of Urmia, Urmia, Iran

Mahmoud Mirhoseini
Medical Plants Research Center, Shahrekord University of Medical Sciences, Shahrekord, Iran

Fazeleh Moshfegh and Saeedeh Zafar-Balanezhad
Department of Biology, Mashhad Branch, Islamic Azad University, Mashhad, Iran

Javad Baharara
Research Center for Animal Development Applied Biology, Mashhad Branch, Islamic Azad University, Mashhad, Iran

Farideh Namvar
Department of Medicine, Mashhad Branch, Islamic Azad University, Mashhad, Iran

Lobat Jafarzadeh
Medical Plants Research Center, Shahrekord University of Medical Sciences, Shahrekord, Iran

Amit Gupta
Department of Immunology and Virology, Vidya Pratishthan's School of Biotechnology (VSBT, Research Centre affiliated to Savitribai Phule Pune University), Baramati-413133, Maharashtra, India

Sushama R Chaphalkar
Department of Microbiology, Vidya Pratishthan Arts, Science and Commerce College, Baramati-413133, Maharashtra, India

Index

www.ingramcontent.com/pod-product-compliance
Lightning Source LLC
LaVergne TN
LVHW081038210926
848485LV00004B/1048